STANDARD PRECAUTIONS

FOR INFECTION CONTROL

Wash Hands (Plain soap)
Wash after touching **blood**, **body fluids**, **secretions**, **excretions**, and **contaminated items**.
Wash immediately **after gloves are removed** and **between patient contacts**.
Avoid transfer of microorganisms to other patients or environments.

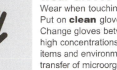

Wear Gloves
Wear when touching **blood**, **body fluids**, **secretions**, **excretions**, and **contaminated items**.
Put on **clean** gloves just **before touching mucous membranes** and nonintact skin.
Change gloves between tasks and procedures on the same patient after contact with material that may contain high concentrations of microorganisms. Remove gloves promptly after use, before touching noncontaminated items and environmental surfaces, and before going to another patient, and wash hands immediately to avoid transfer of microorganisms to other patients or environments.

Wear Mask and Eye Protection or Face Shield
Protect mucous membranes of the eyes, nose and mouth during procedures and patient–care activities that are likely to generate **splashes** or **sprays** of **blood**, **body fluids**, **secretions**, or **excretions**.

Wear Gown
Protect skin and prevent soiling of clothing during procedures that are likely to generate **splashes** or **sprays** of **blood**, **body fluids**, **secretions**, or **excretions**. Remove a soiled gown as promptly as possible and wash hands to avoid transfer of microorganisms to other patients or environments.

Patient-Care Equipment
Handle used patient–care equipment soiled with **blood**, **body fluids**, **secretions**, or **excretions** in a manner that prevents skin and mucous membrane exposures, contamination of clothing, and transfer of microorganisms to other patients and environments. Ensure that reusable equipment is not used for the care of another patient until it has been appropriately cleaned and reprocessed and single use items are properly discarded.

Environmental Control
Follow hospital procedures for routine care, cleaning, and disinfection of environmental surfaces, beds, bedrails, bedside equipment and other frequently touched surfaces.

Linen
Handle, transport, and process used linen soiled with **blood**, **body fluids**, **secretions**, or **excretions** in a manner that prevents exposures and contamination of clothing, and avoids transfer of microorganisms to other patients and environments.

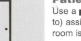

Occupational Health and Bloodborne Pathogens
Prevent injuries when using needles, scalpels, and other sharp instruments or devices; when handling sharp instruments after procedures; when cleaning used instruments; and when disposing of used needles.

Never recap used needles using both hands or any other technique that involves directing the point of a needle toward any part of the body; rather, use either a one-handed "scoop" technique or a mechanical device designed for holding the needle sheath.

Do not remove used needles from disposable syringes by hand, and do not bend, break, or otherwise manipulate used needles by hand. Place used disposable syringes and needles, scalpel blades, and other sharp items in puncture–resistant sharps containers located as close as practical to the area in which the items were used, and place reusable syringes and needles in a puncture–resistant container for transport to the reprocessing area.

Use **resuscitation devices** as an alternative to mouth–to–mouth resuscitation.

Patient Placement
Use a **private room** for a patient who contaminates the environment or who does not (or cannot be expected to) assist in maintaining appropriate hygiene or environmental control. Consult Infection Control if a private room is not available.

The information on this sign is abbreviated from the HICPAC Recommendations for Isolation Precautions in Hospitals.

Form No. **SPR**   BREVIS CORP., 3310 S 2700 E, SLC, UT 84109   © 1996 Brevis Corp.

Fundamentals of Nursing

Standards & Practice

Third Edition

Fundamentals of Nursing

Standards & Practice

Third Edition

Sue C. DeLaune, MN, RN
Assistant Professor
William Carey College
School of Nursing
New Orleans, Louisiana
President and Education Director
SDeLaune Consulting
Mandeville, Louisiana

Patricia K. Ladner, MS, MN, RN
Consultant for Nursing Practice
Louisiana State Board of Nursing
New Orleans, Louisiana

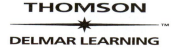

THOMSON

DELMAR LEARNING

Australia   Canada   Mexico   Singapore   Spain   United Kingdom   United States

THOMSON

──────────★──────────

DELMAR LEARNING

Fundamentals of Nursing: Standards and Practice

Third Edition

By Sue C. DeLaune and Patricia K. Ladner

Vice President, Health Care Business Unit:
William Brottmiller

Editorial Director:
Matthew Kane

Acquisitions Editor:
Tamara Caruso

Developmental Editor:
Patricia A. Gaworecki

Editorial Assistant:
Tiffiny Adams

Marketing Director:
Jennifer McAvey

Marketing Coordinator:
Michele McTighe

Technology Director:
Laurie Davis

Technology Project Coordinator:
Carolyn Fox

Production Director:
Carolyn S. Miller

Art and Design Coordinator:
Alexandros Vasilakos

Art and Design Specialist:
Robert Plante

**Assistant to Production and
Technology Directors:**
Kate Kaufman

Production Coordinator:
Mary Ellen Cox

Senior Project Editor:
David Buddle

Library of Congress Cataloging-in-
Publication Data:

DeLaune, Sue C. (Sue Carter)
   Fundamentals of nursing : standards &
practice / Sue C. DeLaune, Patricia K. Ladner.—
3rd ed.
      p. ; cm.
   Rev. ed. of: Fundamentals of nursing / [edited
by] Sue C. DeLaune, Patricia K. Ladner. 2002.
   Includes bibliographical references and index.
   ISBN-13: 978-1-4018-5918-3 (alk. paper)
   ISBN-10: 1-4018-5918-6 (alk. paper)
   1. Nursing. 2. Nursing--Practice.
   [DNLM: 1. Nursing Process. 2. Nursing Care.
WY 100 D342f 2006] I.
Ladner, Patricia K. (Patricia Kelly) II. Title.
   RT41.F8816 2006
   610.73—dc22
                                    2005028584
ISBN-10 1-4018-5918-6
ISBN-13 978-1-4018-5918-3

NOTICE TO THE READER

To Jennifer, Ryan, Katie, and Sarabeth. I especially want to thank my husband and best friend, Jay, for his continued support and belief in me.
SCD

To Wayne, Kelly, Wayne Jr., Gretchen, and Michael.
PKL

We dedicate this book to our grandchildren: Camille Anna Cardinal, Caroline Alexa Cardinal, Leah Marie Ladner, Charles Lee, and Thomas Lee.
"G" and "Mimi"

Contents

Unit II

Nursing Process: The Standard of Care

Unit IV

Promoting Client Health

Unit V

Responding to Basic Psychosocial Needs

Procedures

Contributors

Sheila L. Allen, RN, BSN, CNOR, CRNFA
Consultant, speaker, educator
Meeker, Colorado
*Chapter 40: Nursing Care of the Perioperative
Client*

Carma Andrus, MN, RN, CNS
Dauterive Primary Care Clinic
St. Martinville, Louisiana
Chapter 38: Sensation, Perception, and Cognition

Billie Barringer, RN, CS, APRN
School of Nursing
Northeast Louisiana University
Monroe, Louisiana
Chapter 15: Communication

Barbara Bihm, DNS, RN
Department of Nursing
Loyola University—New Orleans
New Orleans, Louisiana
Chapter 2: Nursing Theory

Barbara Brillhart, PhD, RN, CRRN, FNP-C
College of Nursing
Arizona State University
Tempe, Arizona
Chapter 36: Mobility

Ali Brown, MSN, RN
Assistant Professor
College of Nursing
University of Tennessee
Knoxville, Tennessee
Chapter 7: Nursing Diagnosis

Virginia Burggraf, MSN, RN
Gerontological Nurse Consultant
Kensington, Maryland
Chapter 19: The Older Client

Ann H. Cary, PhD, MPH, RN, A-CCC
Director, Institute for Research, Education,
and Consultation
American Nurses Credentialing Center
Washington, DC
Chapter 3: Research and Evidence-Based Practice

Lissa A. Cash, RN, MSN, CCRN, CEN
Sentara Healthcare eICU
Norfolk, Virginia
Chapter 32: Oxygenation

Beth Christensen, MN, RN, CCRN
Touro Infirmary
New Orleans, Louisiana
Chapter 32: Oxygenation

Jan Corder, DNS, RN
Dean, School of Nursing
Northeast Louisiana University
Monroe, Louisiana
*Chapter 5: Critical Thinking, Decision Making,
and the Nursing Process*

Julie Coy, MS, RN
Pain Consultation Service
The Children's Hospital
Denver, Colorado
Chapter 35: Comfort and Sleep

Mary Ellen Zator Estes, MSN, RN, CCRN
Assistant Professor
School of Nursing
Marymount University
Arlington, Virginia
Chapter 26: Vital Signs and *Chapter 27: Physical
Assessment*

Mary Frost, RN, BSN
Covington, Louisiana
*Chapter 31: Complementary and Alternative
Modalities*

Norma Fujise, MS, RN, C
School of Nursing
University of Hawaii
Honolulu, Hawaii
Chapter 37: Skin Integrity and Wound Healing

Mikel Gray, PhD, CURN, CCCN
Nurse Practitioner/Clinical Investigator
Associate Professor
Department of Urology
University of Virginia Health Sciences Center

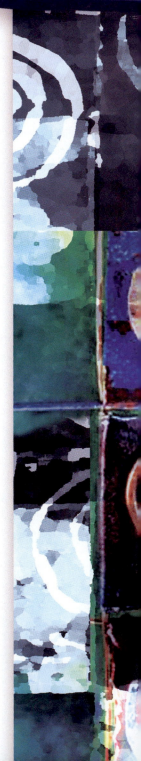

Charlottesville, Virginia *and*
Adjunct Professor
Lancing School of Nursing
Bellarmine College
Louisville, Kentucky
 Chapter 39: Elimination

Janet Kula Harden, RN, MSN
Faculty
Wayne State University
College of Nursing
Detroit, Michigan
 Chapter 30: Medication Administration

T. Heather Herdman, RN, PhD
President-Elect, NANDA-International
Assistant Professor
Bellin College of Nursing
Green Bay, Wisconsin
 Chapter 7: Nursing Diagnosis

Lucille Joel, EdD, RN, FAAN
Professor
College of Nursing
Rutgers—State University of New Jersey
Newark, New Jersey
 Chapter 4: Health Care Delivery, Quality, and the
  Continuum of Care

Georgia Johnson, MS, RN, CNAA, CPHQ
Quality Support Services Coordinator
Southeast Louisiana Hospital
Mandeville, Louisiana
 Chapter 25: Loss and Grief

Claire Lincoln, MN, RN, CS
Psychiatric Mental Health Clinical Nurse Specialist
Touro Infirmary
New Orleans, Louisiana
 Chapter 22: Self-Concept

Tina M. Liske, RN, MSN, CCRN, CNS, NP
SCCM, National AACN, Local AACN
Smithfield, Virginia
 Chapter 32: Oxygenation

JoAnna Magee, MN, RN
School of Nursing
Our Lady of Holy Cross College
New Orleans, Louisiana
 Chapter 2: Nursing Theory

Judy Martin, MS, RN, JD
Nurse Attorney
Louisiana Department of Health and Hospitals
Health Standards Section
Baton Rouge, Louisiana
 Chapter 12: Legal and Ethical Responsibilities

Linda McCuistion, PhD, RN
Assistant Professor
School of Nursing
Our Lady of Holy Cross College
New Orleans, Louisiana
 Chapter 8: Planning and Outcome Identification

Elizabeth "Betty" Hauck Miller, MPH, BSN
Director of Education
Meadowcrest Hospital
Gretna, Louisiana, *and*
JoEllen Smith Regional Medical Center,
New Orleans, Louisianna
 Chapter 25: Loss and Grief

Mary Anne Modrcin-McCarthy, PhD, RN
Associate Professor and Director
 of the Undergraduate Program
College of Nursing
University of Tennessee—Knoxville
Knoxville, Tennessee
 Chapter 7: Nursing Diagnosis

Barbara S. Moffett, PhD, RN
Associate Professor of Nursing
School of Nursing
Southeastern Louisiana University
Hammond, Louisiana
 Chapter 6: Assessment and *Chapter 9: Implementation*

Barbara Morvant, RN, MN
Executive Director
Louisiana State Board of Nursing
Metairie, Louisiana
 Chapter 11: Leadership, Delegation, and Power

Cathy O'Byrne, RN, MN
Tulane University Hospital and Clinic
New Orleans, Louisiana
 Chapter 13: Documentation and Informatics

Brenda Owens, PhD, RN
Associate Professor
School of Nursing
Louisiana State University Medical Center
New Orleans, Louisiana
 Chapter 30: Medication Administration

Roxanne Perucca, MS, CRNI
Infusion Nurse Manager, Clinical Nurse Specialist
University of Kansas Hospital
Kansas City, Kansas
 Chapter 33: Fluids and Electrolytes

Demetrius Porche, DNS, RN, CCRN
Associate Professor and Director
Bachelor of Science in Nursing Program
Nicholas State University
Adjunct Assistant Professor
Tulane University
School of Public Health and Topical Medicine

Chapter 29: Safety, Infection Control, and Hygiene

Suzanne Riche, RN, C, MS
Associate Professor
Charity School of Nursing
New Orleans, Louisiana
  Chapter 6: Assessment

Mary W. Surman, BSN, RN, CWOCN
Wound, Ostomy, Continence Nurses Organization
LSU School of Nursing 1980
Baton Rouge, Louisiana
  Chapter 37: Skin Integrity and Wound Healing

Cheryl Taylor, PhD, RN
Associate Professor of Nursing
North Carolina Agricultural and
  Technical State University
Greensboro, North Carolina

Chapter 20: Cultural Diversity

Lorrie Wong, RN, MS
School of Nursing
University of Hawaii
Honolulu, Hawaii
  Chapter 37: Skin Integrity and Wound Healing

Martha Yager, RN
Assistant Director of Nurses
Bennington Health and Rehabilitation Center
Bennington, Vermont
  Chapter 39: Elimination

Rothlyn Zahourek, MS, RN, CS
Certified Clinical Nurse Specialist
Amherst, Massachusetts
  Chapter 31: Complementary and Alternative Modalities

Reviewers

Marie Ahrens, MS, RN
University of Tulsa
Tulsa, Oklahoma

Kay Baker, MSN, BSN
Pima Community College
Tucson, Arizona

Katie Ball, RN, MSN
Bellin College of Nursing
Green Bay, Wisconsin

Beth A. Beaudet, RW-c, BSN, MS ed., MSN, FNP
Family Nurse Practitioner
Bassett Healthcare
Oneonta, New York

Mary Bliesmer, RN, DNSc, MPH, BS
Mankato State University
Mankato, Minnesota

Billie Bodo
Associate Professor of Nursing
Lakeland Community College
Mentor, Ohio

Lou Ann Boose, RN, BSN, MSN
Assistant Professor
Harrisburg Area Community College
Harrisburg, Pennsylvania

Bonita Cavanaugh, PhD, RN
University of Colorado
Denver, Colorado

Susan K. R. Collins, RN, MSN
Clinical Assistant Professor
Course Chair, Nursing Fundamentals
University of North Carolina at Greensboro
Greensboro, North Carolina

Dauna L. Crooks, RN, DNS
McMaster University
Hamilton, Ontario, Canada
Ernestine Currier
UCLA Center for the Health Sciences
Los Angeles, California

Debbie Dalrymple, RN, MSN, CRNI
Montgomery County Community College
Blue Bell, Pennsylvania

Sharon Decker, RN, CS, MSN, CCRN
Associate Professor of Clinical Nursing
School of Nursing
Texas Tech University Health Sciences Center
Lubbock, Texas

Toni S. Doherty, RN, MSN
Associate Professor
Department Head, Nursing
Dutchess Community College
Poughkeepsie, New York

Colleen Duggan, RN, MSN
Johnson County Community College
Overland Park, Kansas

Mary Lou Elder, RN, MS
Instructor of Nursing
Central Community College
Grand Island, Nebraska

Joanne M. Flanders, MS, RN
Midwestern State University
Wichita Falls, Texas

Kathy Frey, RN, MSN
University of South Alabama
Mobile, Alabama

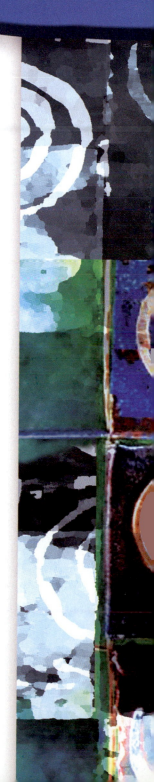

Marcia Gellin, RN, EdD
Erie Community College
Buffalo, New York

Marilyn C. Handley, RN, MSN, PhDc
Instructor
University of Alabama
Capstone College of Nursing
Tuscaloosa, Alabama

Renee Harrison, RN, MS
Tulsa Junior College
Tulsa, Oklahoma

Susan Hauser, RN, MSN, BA
Mansfield General Hospital
Mansfield, Ohio

Judith W. Herrman, PhD, RN
Assistant Chair, Department of Nursing
University of Delaware
Newark, Delaware

Franklin Hicks, RN, MSN, CCRN
Marcella Niehoff School of Nursing
Loyola University
Chicago, Illinois

Kathleen Jarvis, MSN, BSN, RN
School of Nursing
California State University—Sacramento
Sacramento, California

Cecilia Jimenez, RN, MSN, PhD
Marymount University
Arlington, Virginia

Joan Jinks, RN, MSN
Eastern Kentucky University
Richmond, Kentucky

Patricia Jones, RN, MSN
Indiana State University
Terre Haute, Indiana

Jan Kinman, RN
Lane Community College
Eugene, Oregon

Anita G. Kinser, EdD, RN, BC
Assistant Professor
California State University at San Bernardino
San Bernardino, California

Marjorie Knox, RN, MA, MPA
Community College of Rhode Island
Lincoln, Rhode Island

Anne M. Larson, RN, C, PhD
Associate Professor of Nursing
Midland Lutheran College
Fremont, Nebraska

Hope B. Laughlin, BSN, MEd, EdD, MSN
Coordinator of Fundamentals of Nursing Courses
Pensacola Junior College
Pensacola, Florida

Patty Leary, MEd, RN
Mecosta Osceola Career Center
Big Rapids, Michigan

Denise LeBlanc
Humber College
Etobicoke, Ontario, Canada

Patricia M. Lester, RN, MSN
Associate Professor
Cumberland Valley Technical College
Pineville, Kentucky

Sharon Little-Stoetzel, RN, MS
Assistant Professor of Nursing
Graceland University
Independence, Missouri

Patricia Kaiser McCloud, RN, BSN, MS
University of Michigan
Ann Arbor, Michigan

Suzanne McDevitt, RN, MSN, CCRN
University of Michigan
Ann Arbor, Michigan

Chris McGeever
School of Nursing
St. Xavier University
Chicago, Illinois

Myrtle Miller, RN, BSN, MA
Assistant Professor
DeKalb College
Clarkson, Georgia

Maureen P. Mitchell, RN, BScN, MN
Center for Health Studies
Mount Royal College
Calgary, Alberta, Canada

Pertice Moffitt, RN, BSN
Aurora College
Yellowknife, Northwest Territories, Canada

Regina Nicholson, RN
Hospital for Joint Diseases
New York, New York

Katherine Bordelon Pearson, FNP, RN, CS
A. D. N. Department Faculty
Temple College
Temple, Texas

Edith Prichett, RN, MSN
Asheville Buncombe Technical
Community College
Asheville, North Carolina

Carol Rafferty, RN, PhD
Northeast Wisconsin Technical College
Green Bay, Wisconsin

Margaret P. Rancourt, RN, MS
School of Nursing
Quincy College
Quincy, Massachusetts

Anita K. Reed, RN, MSN
Instructor of Nursing
St. Elizabeth School of Nursing
Lafayette, Indiana

Neil Rheiner, RN, MSN, EdD
University of Nebraska
Omaha, Nebraska

Julia Robinson, RN, MS, FNP-C
Associate Professor
California State University
Bakersfield, California

Donna Roddy, RN, BSN, MSN
Chattanooga State Practical Nursing
  and Surgical Technological Programs
Chattanooga, Tennessee

Julie Sanford, DNS, RN
Assistant Professor of Nursing
Spring Hill College
Mobile, Alabama

Ruth Schaffler, RN, MSN, MA, ARNP
Pacific Lutheran University
Tacoma, Washington

Barbara Scheirer, RN, MSN
Assistant Professor of Nursing
Grambling State University
Grambling, Louisiana

Sandy J. Shortridge, RN, MSN
Southwest Virginia Community College
Keenmtu, Virginia

Gail Smith, MSN, RN
Department of Nursing
Miami-Dade Community College
Miami, Florida

Maria A. Smith, DSN, RN, CCRN
School of Nursing
Middle Tennessee State University
Murfreesboro, Tennessee

Sharon Staib, RN, MS
Assistant Professor
Ohio University
Zanesville, Ohio

Paula P. Thompson, BSN, RN
Educator
Carilion Roanoke Memorial Hospital
School of Practical Nursing
Roanoke, Virginia

Anita Thorne, RN, MA
Arizona State University
Tempe, Arizona

Elizabeth K. Whitbeck, MS, RN
Assistant Professor of Nursing
Maria College
Albany, New York

Preface

We are extremely excited to share the third edition of *Fundamentals of Nursing: Standards and Practice* with you! It is hoped that this text will encourage the student to develop an inquiring stance based on the joy of discovery and a love of learning.

As we enter the 21st century, nursing is facing new challenges in delivering quality care to clients in a variety of settings. The settings for delivery of care are rapidly expanding and challenge nurses to "think outside the box" in applying best practices based on current research. This edition presents the most current advances in nursing care and nursing education including research relative to the demands of delivering care across a continuum of settings. At the core, multiple theories of nursing are embraced, and nursing's metaparadigm elements of theory—human beings, environment, health, and nursing—are threaded throughout this text. The organization of units and chapters is sequential; however, every effort has been made to allow for varying needs of diverse curricula and students. Each chapter may be used independently of the others according to the specific curriculum design.

This comprehensive edition addresses fundamental concepts and skills to help prepare novice graduate nurses to apply an understanding of human behavior to those encountered in clinical settings. Physiologic and psychosocial responses of both client and nurse are addressed in a holistic manner. Integrative modalities are presented in an environment that encourages clients to participate in determining their care.

Up-to-date clinical information is based on sound theoretical concepts and provides a rationale for practice. Scientific evidence is applied to the implementation of nursing interventions. Many of the chapter contributors are representatives of specialty nursing organizations that determine standards of professional practice.

Conceptual Approach

A major goal of this edition is to present in-depth material in a clear, concise manner using language that is easy to read, by linking related concepts and encouraging students to integrate principles of health and nursing. Nursing knowledge is formulated on the basic concepts of scientific and discipline-specific theory, health and health promotion, the environment, holism, client teaching, spirituality, research and evidence-based practice, and the continuum of care. Emphasis is placed on cultural diversity, care of the older adult, and ethical and legal principles.

The nursing process provides a consistent approach for presenting nursing care information. Assessment tools specific to topics are presented to assist students with pertinent data collection. Professional nursing practice is emphasized by the incorporation of NANDA nursing diagnoses, the Nursing Interventions Classification (NIC), and the Nursing Outcomes Classification (NOC) into the planning and outcome phase of the process. Therapeutic nursing interventions reflect standards of practice and emphasize safety, communication skills, interdisciplinary collaboration, and effective delegation in delivering nursing care. Critical thinking and reflective reasoning skills are integrated throughout the text. The safe and appropriate use of technology has been incorporated throughout the text to reflect contemporary nursing practice.

The conceptual approach used as an organizational framework for the third edition falls into four categories:

✧ **Individuals.** Viewed as holistic beings with multiple needs and strengths, and the abilities

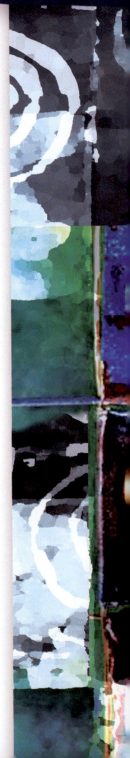

to meet those needs. Holism implies that individuals are treated as whole entities rather than fragmented parts or problems. Each person is a complex entity who is influenced by cultural values, including spiritual beliefs and practices. Every person has the right to be treated with dignity and respect regardless of race, ethnicity, age, religion, socioeconomic status, or health status.

◇ **Environment.** A complex interrelationship of internal and external variables. Internal variables include one's self-concept, self-efficacy, cognitive development, and psychological traits. The external environment affects an individual's health status by facilitating or hindering the person's achievement of needs.

◇ **Health.** Viewed as a dynamic force that occurs on a continuum ranging from wellness to death. An individual's actions and choices effect changes in health status. Individuals who are experiencing illness have strengths that they may use to improve their health status. On the other hand, individuals who are experiencing a high degree of health generally have areas that can be improved.

◇ **Nursing.** An active, interpersonal, professional practice that seeks to improve the health status of individuals. Nursing's focus is person-centered and communicates a caring intent. Caring and compassion are demonstrated through nursing interventions. Nursing is a professional practice based on a scientific knowledge base and delivered in an artful manner.

Other important conceptual threads used to direct the development of this book include:

◇ **Health promotion** encourages individuals to engage in behaviors and lifestyles that facilitate wellness.

◇ **Standards of practice** are discussed, with information from national and specialty organizations incorporated into each chapter as appropriate.

◇ **Critical thinking** is an essential skill for blending science with the art of nursing.

◇ **Evidence-based practice,** which is derived from scientific research, is emphasized across chapters.

◇ **Cultural diversity** is defined as individual differences among people resulting from racial, ethnic, and cultural variables.

◇ **Continuum of care** is viewed as a process for providing health care services in order to ensure consistent care regardless of the setting.

◇ **Community,** as both client and as setting for delivery of care, is evidenced in the new Chapter 17 and

in the "Community Considerations" critical thinking boxes threaded throughout the text.

◇ **Holism** recognizes the bodymind connection and views the client as a whole person rather than fragmented parts.

◇ **Spirituality**—one's relationship with one's self, a sense of connection with others, and a relationship with a higher power or divine source—is discussed in depth in a new chapter.

◇ **Caring,** a universal value that directs nursing practice, is incorporated throughout the text as well as described in depth in a separate chapter.

◇ **Alternative and complementary modalities** are treatment approaches that can be used in conjunction with conventional medical therapies. Chapter 31 is dedicated to this integrative approach, and related information featuring integrative concepts is included throughout the text.

Organization of Text

This textbook provides student nurses with a bridge to connect theory with clinical practice. The intent of the authors is that students be prepared by becoming proficient critical thinkers who are able to use the nursing process with diverse clients in a variety of settings, aided by the linking of important nursing concepts such as safety and infection control and hygiene. Research-based knowledge and clinical skills that reflect contemporary practice are presented in a reader-friendly, practical manner.

Features that challenge students to use critical thinking skills are incorporated into each chapter, and critical thinking questions appear at the end of each. Critical information is highlighted throughout the text in a format that is easily accessed and understood. Similar concepts have been grouped together to encourage students to learn through association; this method of presentation also prevents duplication of content. In addition, several unique chapters were created as a response to user feedback.

Fundamentals of Nursing: Standards and Practice, Third Edition, presents 40 chapters organized in six units:

◇ **Unit I: Nursing's Perspective: Past, Present, and Future** provides a comprehensive discussion of nursing's evolution as a profession and its contributions to health care based on standards of practice. The theoretical frameworks for guiding professional practice and the significance of incorporating research into nursing practice are emphasized. Chapters are reflective of the parallel evolution of nursing and nursing education. Examples showing the incorporation of theory into the nursing process are provided. The concept of evidence-based practice is emphasized along with research utilization. Quality is discussed from the perspective of health care delivery and the continuum of care.

⬥ **Unit II: Nursing Process: The Standard of Care** discusses standards of care established by the American Nurses Association, as well as nursing specialty organizations. Each stage of the nursing process is discussed with an emphasis on critical thinking. New comparative content is reflected in the incorporation of Nursing Outcomes Classification (NOC) and Nursing Interventions Classification (NIC). NOC and NIC information is also threaded throughout the text.

⬥ **Unit III: Professional Accountability** describes the nurse's responsibilities to the client, the community, and the profession. The legal aspects of delegation are discussed in Chapter 11, and "Delegation Tips" have been incorporated into the clinical skills. Chapter 12 combines legal and ethical aspects of nursing practice to reflect the interfacing of these concepts. Informatics has been added to Chapter 13 on documentation.

⬥ **Unit IV: Promoting Client Health** was created to integrate information on health promotion, consumer demand, and client empowerment. Chapter 14 provides nursing theoretical perspectives on caring. Chapter 16 provides information from *Healthy People 2010* as an example of health-promoting activities. Emphasis is placed on the nurse's role in empowering clients to assume more personal accountability for their health-related behaviors. Chapter 17 is a new chapter that addresses the health needs of families and communities.

⬥ **Unit V: Responding to Basic Psychosocial Needs** stresses the importance of the holistic nature of nursing. Spirituality is spotlighted in a new chapter in order to emphasize its impact on individuals' health.

⬥ **Unit VI: Responding to Basic Physiological Needs** discusses areas of nursing care that are common to every area of nursing practice. Concepts such as safety and infection control, mobility, fluid and electrolyte balance, skin integrity, nutrition, and elimination are described within the nursing process framework.

New to This Edition

⬥ Clinical skills have been expanded to include content on delegation and nursing tips from the field.
⬥ Nursing Care plans include comparative diagnoses among NANDA, NOC, and NIC.
⬥ Over 400 new photographs and illustrations have been added.
⬥ Evidence-based practice is highlighted across chapters as appropriate.
⬥ Critical thinking questions have been added at the end of every chapter.

Selected chapter-specific enhancements are also highlighted in this edition:

⬥ Chapter 11, Leadership, Delegation, and Power, addresses the important legal issues surrounding the topic of delegation that so many nurses struggle with today.
⬥ Chapter 12, Legal and Ethical Responsibilities, now combines these two topics in one chapter. In this way, the interface between these two concepts can be purposefully illustrated.
⬥ Chapter 13, Documentation and Informatics, thoroughly discusses the impact of technology on nursing practice.
⬥ Chapter 17, Family and Community Health, is a new chapter to address health needs of the family in a community setting.

Extensive Teaching/ Learning Package

The complete supplements package was developed to achieve two goals:

1. To assist students in learning the essential skills and competencies needed to secure a career in the area of nursing
2. To assist instructors in planning and implementing their programs for the most efficient use of time and other resources

Online Companion

Delmar offers a series of Online Companions™ through the Delmar Web site: **www.delmarlearning.com.** The DeLaune/Ladner Online Companion enables users of *Fundamentals of Nursing: Standards and Practice,* Third Edition, to access a wealth of information designed to enhance the book. Included in the Online Companion are:

⬧ Appendices, including NANDA Nursing Diagnoses, Educational Resources for Caregivers, Recommended Dietary Allowances, and Your Guide to Gloves

⬧ Concept maps

⬧ HIPAA information

To access the site for *Fundamentals of Nursing: Standards and Practice,* Third Edition, simply point your browser to **www.delmarhealthcare.com.** Click on Online Companions, and then select the nursing discipline.

Study Guide

ISBN 1-4018-5919-4

Containing over 500 questions in an easy-to-use format, this study aid builds on and reinforces the content presented in the text. Students have an avenue to learn key concepts at a pace that is comfortable for them. Features include:

⬧ Multiple question types—true/false, matching, sequencing, multiple choice, short answer, and essay

⬧ Various levels of difficulty

⬧ Questions built upon the key concepts on a chapter-by-chapter basis

Skills Checklist

ISBN 1-4018-5920-8

This teaching/learning tool contains key steps for every procedure in *Fundamentals of Nursing: Standards and Practice,* Third Edition, by Sue C. DeLaune and Patricia K. Ladner. These checklists may be used to help students evaluate their comprehension and execution of the procedures. Key features include:

⬧ Three categories to document performance: able to perform, able to perform with assistance, and unable to perform

⬧ Comments section at each step for constructive feedback

⬧ Easy-to-follow format

Electronic Classroom Manager

ISBN 1-4018-5921-6

Free to all instructors who adopt *Fundamentals of Nursing: Standards and Practice,* Third Edition, in their courses, this comprehensive resource includes the following:

Instructor's Guide

✦ **Instructional Strategies**—Centered around the competencies at the beginning of each chapter, critical thinking questions, followed by a student activity (group and/or individual), are provided to enhance student comprehension and critical thinking skills.

✦ **Additional Resource Aids**—Additional audiovisual, computer software, and Web sites are included to increase student awareness of current issues, trends, and skills.

✦ **Evaluation Strategies**—Discussion questions are provided for each chapter to enhance student writing and thinking skills.

Computerized Test Bank with Electronic Gradebook

✦ **Testbank**—Computerized testbank includes over 1,000 questions and has been completely rewritten to reflect an NCLEX style of review.

PowerPoint Presentation

A vital resource for instructors, this PowerPoint presentation parallels the content found in the book, serving as a foundation on which instructors may customize their own unique presentations.

Image Library

The Image Library is a software tool that includes an organized digital library of over 700 illustrations and photographs from the text. With the Image Library you can:

✦ Create additional libraries.

✦ Set up electronic pointers to actual image files or collections.

✦ Sort art by desired categories.

✦ Print selected pieces.

Additional Resources

Delmar's Anatomy and Physiology CD-ROM

ISBN 0-7668-2415-2

Intended for any course where a brief review of anatomy and physiology is desired, *Delmar's Anatomy and Physiology CD-ROM* presents anatomy and physiology in an accessible and engaging manner. Organized by body system, the CD-ROM is perfect for self-guided learning or review.

Delmar's Heart and Lung Sounds for Nurses CD-ROM

ISBN 0-7668-2416-0

Auscultation is one of the most difficult skills for student nurses to master. *Delmar's Heart and Lung Sounds for Nurses CD-ROM* is an excellent learning tool that helps nurses identify and interpret normal and abnormal heart and lung sounds. Features include:

✦ An extensive library of normal and abnormal heart and lung sounds for students to reference

✦ A three-part heart sounds module

✦ A skill review section that includes Overview, Step-by-Step (with actions and rationales), Variations, and Tips and Errors

Delmar's Nursing Skills Video Series

Comprehensive: ISBN 1-4018-1078-0
Basic: ISBN 1-4018-1079-9
Intermediate: ISBN 1-4018-1080-2
Advanced: ISBN 1-4018-1081-0
Over 100 skills in video segments equip student and practitioners alike with the skills they need to survive and thrive in a changing health care world. Each segment carefully shows the step-by-step actions, reinforcing concepts and enhancing the learning experience.

How to Use This Text

The following suggests how you can use the features of this text to gain competence and confidence in your assessment and nursing skills.

Procedure 29-7

Removing Contaminated Items

EQUIPMENT

- Disposable gloves
- Labeled bag for disposal of soiled linens; bag should be hot-water soluble; bag may also be colored (red) for easy identification (*Note:* Some agencies may require linens to be double bagged for removal.)
- Self-supporting stand for linen
- Second linen bag if double-bag technique used

ACTION	RATIONALE
REMOVAL OF SOILED LINEN	
1. Wash hands/hand hygiene when entering the client's room or may use an alcohol-based hand rub.	1. Prevents the spread of microor
2. Wear disposable gloves; wear other protective items (gowns, goggles) as determined by the situation and agency's policies.	2. Protects the nurse from contam from blood and body fluids.
3. Place labeled linen bag in stand (see Figure 29-64).	3. Proper labeling or identification linen bag ensures proper handling by

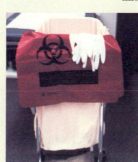

FIGURE 29-64 Biohazard bags and gloves are used to handle and dispose of contaminated items.

(continues)

Procedures

Procedure boxes are step-by-step guides to performing basic clinical nursing skills. This feature will help you gain competence in nursing skills. Use this feature as a study tool to help you understand the rationale behind the nursing interventions, as a guide for mastery of procedures, and as a review aid for future reference.

Evidence-Based Practice and Research Focus boxes

These boxes emphasize the importance of clinical research in nursing by linking theory to practice. As a learning tool, they focus attention on current issues and trends in nursing.

EVIDENCE-BASED PRACTICE

Decreasing Child Abuse and Neglect

Home visits directed at high-risk mothers (identified on the basis of sociodemographic risk factors) have decreased the incidence of child abuse and neglect (Nelson, Nygren, & Qazi, 2004).

▶▶▶▶ RESEARCH FOCUS

Title of Study "Geriatric Rehabiltation: The Influence of Efficacy Beliefs and Motivation."

Author B. Resnick

Purposes (1) To better understand how self-efficacy and outcome expectations are strengthened; (2) to determine how these expectations influence motivation and behavior of older adults in a rehabilitation program.

Methods Interviews were conducted with 77 older adults at an inpatient geriatric rehabilitation program. The 30-minute interviews were conducted privately with the client prior to discharge.

Findings 11 themes were identified as factors that influence efficacy beliefs and motivate people to participate in rehabilitation: (1) personal expectations, (2) personality, (3) role models, (4) verbal encouragement, (5) progress, (6) past experiences, (7) spirituality, (8) physical sensations, (9) individualized care, (10) social supports, and (11) goals.

Implications This study provides a guide to encourage nurses to do a comprehensive evaluation of motivation, and to explore the various factors that influence motivation of older adults.

Source: Resnick, B. (2002). Geriatric rehabilitation: The influence of efficacy beliefs and motivation. Rehabilitation Nursing, 27(4), 152–159.

Nursing Checklist

Reviewing a Chart

✓ Can the assessment data that triggered the nursing diagnosis be identified?
✓ When the defining characteristics of a specific nursing diagnosis are compared to the client's presenting signs and symptoms, is there supporting evidence?
✓ Were critical questions asked during the client interview?
✓ Did the nurse use the data obtained from both the interview and physical assessment in establishing the diagnoses?
✓ Can any assumptions that might have misled the nurse's judgment be identified?
✓ Are the nursing data correlated with the results of the physical examination and findings from diagnostic tests?
✓ Are the expected outcomes realistic?

Nursing Checklist

Nursing Checklist boxes outline important points for you to consider before, during, and after utilizing the nursing process. Checklists are your reference guide to using critical thinking in nursing and to understanding the steps in the nursing process.

Nursing Care Plan

The Client with Ineffective Role Performance

CASE PRESENTATION

Todd Lloyd is a 31-year-old civil engineer who has just left his job of 10 years to care full-time for his newborn daughter, Sarah. He and his wife decided that, after their child was born, she would return to work full-time outside the home, and he would be the primary caregiver for their daughter during the day. Mr. Lloyd presents to you at the clinic stating, "I am very eager and excited about being a full-time dad, but I'm also a little nervous because I really don't know what to expect."

ASSESSMENT

- Lack of knowledge about new parenting role
- Concern over changes in responsibilities

NURSING DIAGNOSIS: *Ineffective role performance* related to change in roles and usual patterns of responsibility, as evidenced by verbalization of concern over lack of knowledge about new role.

NOC: Parenting Performance

NIC: Parent Education: Infant Care

EXPECTED OUTCOMES

The client will:
1. Explain specific concerns about new roles.
2. Demonstrate role competence.
3. Verbalize satisfaction with role performance.

INTERVENTIONS/RATIONALES

1. Encourage the client to express his feelings about his new role. Opens the door to communication and problem solving.
2. Outline with client what aspects of his role(s) will be changing and what will be the same. Helps client identify the ways in which his role is changing, so he can face the changes from a realistic frame of mind. Also highlights similarities, not just differences, between his past and present roles, thus helping client feel less overwhelmed.
3. Assist the client in identifying specific concerns he has regarding the change in roles. Helps the client determine exactly what his concerns are, so they can be addressed.
4. Encourage client to discuss concerns with wife and to seek help together. Support of spouse will be critical to client's success in overcoming concerns about changing roles.
5. Help client gain confidence and competence with new role by demonstrating new role behaviors, offering literature and resources, and providing referral to parenting courses or counselors. Assures client that resources are available to help him meet his needs and helps lessen his anxiety and his feeling of being overwhelmed.
6. Have client return demonstrate new behaviors and offer encouragement and additional teaching. Allows client to try out new behaviors in a "safe" environment and provides

Nursing Care Plan

The Nursing Care Plan walks you through the process of planning care, performing interventions, and evaluating the success of your course of care. These are very helpful in strengthening your understanding of the nursing process in "live" nursing situations, in exercising your critical thinking skills, and for use as a blueprint from which to develop your own complete plans of care.

NURSING ALERT

Consent from Sedated Clients

Sedated clients should never be requested or allowed to sign an informed consent; they may not be capable of understanding the nature of and risks associated with the procedure, so the consent will be invalid, and the nurse and institution will be at legal risk. Wait instead for the client to be competent and free of sedation, or have a legally acceptable family member brought into the decision.

Nursing Alert

As a professional, you will need to be able to react immediately in some situations in order to ensure the health and safety of your patients. Pay careful attention to this feature as it will help you to begin to identify and respond to critical situations on your own, both efficiently and effectively.

REFLECTIVE THINKING

The Media and Health Beliefs

The media are extremely powerful in shaping attitudes and beliefs. Here are some examples of how various media discourage health-promoting behaviors:

Advertising foods with high sugar, salt, and fat content

Promoting alcohol use

Encouraging use of tobacco products

What other examples can you identify? Recently, there seems to be an emerging trend to advertise healthier lifestyles. What examples come to mind?

Reflective Thinking

This feature helps you to develop sensitivity to ethical and moral issues, and guides you to think critically in clinical situations and be active in problem solving. You may choose to read through each one and explore the issues *before* reading the chapter. Then as you read through the chapter, readdress each Reflective Thinking and reevaluate your original thoughts. If you choose to read them as you go through the chapter, perhaps write your thoughts down, then go back and look at them at a later date.

COMMUNITY CONSIDERATIONS

The American Nurses Association and various governing bodies support written medication information for clients that is "scientifically accurate, unbiased in content and tone, sufficiently specific and comprehensive, presented in an understandable and legible format, timely, up to date, and useful." Written medication information should:

◎ Be appropriate to client literacy levels

◎ Reflect print size appropriate to client's visual abilities

◎ Give straightforward instructions

◎ Include brand and trade names

◎ Prominently display drug warnings

◎ Outline indications for use, contraindications, and precautions

◎ List possible adverse reactions and risks, storage, and use

(From American Nurses Association. [1997, March/April]. *The American Nurse, 29* [2], 11)

Community Considerations

Community Considerations spotlight client care in the community environment. Guidelines for care, current trends and issues, and professional protocols are addressed throughout the text.

Client Teaching Checklist

Actions of Parents to Promote Positive Self-Concept in Children

✓ Encourage expression of feelings.

✓ Promote mutual respect and trust by establishing and maintaining open lines of communication; demonstrate a willingness to talk about any subject.

✓ Listen carefully to children, and use words they understand.

✓ Use examples and anecdotes to promote learning.

✓ Teach by example. Role-model problem solving and coping skills.

✓ Encourage children's talents and accept their limitations. Be realistic in your expectations, and avoid comparing one child to another.

✓ Celebrate children's accomplishments.

✓ Demonstrate confidence in their abilities.

✓ Provide children with unconditional love.

Client Teaching Checklist

As a nurse, you will often be a client's main link to health care. The Client Teaching Checklist is a great resource for ensuring success in teaching exercises and procedures, and in relaying critical information to clients.

Acknowledgments

This textbook is the product of many dedicated, knowledgeable, and conscientious individuals. First, we would like to thank Carol Kneisl for initiating our work on this text. We would like to thank all the contributors who persevered to produce an outstanding contribution to the nursing literature. The content for nursing fundamentals has changed greatly over the past 20 years in an effort to incorporate the advances in nursing theory and research and technology. Your clinical expertise is evident in this final product.

Likewise, we need to thank all the reviewers who critically read and commented on the manuscript. Your clinical and academic expertise provided valuable suggestions that strengthened the text.

Our friends and professional colleagues provided encouragement throughout the development of this manuscript. Thank you for sharing so many of your resources and support with us.

We want to thank the nursing department of Ochsner Clinic Foundation Hospital in New Orleans for assisting with the photographs. Also, a special word of thanks goes to these nursing students at the New Orleans campus of William Carey College: Wayne Andras, Katrina Cornin, Tzcanow Cummings, Tanya Johnson, Thuy Nguyen, Karen Patcheco, Kim Richard, Claire Richoux, Brandi Shelley, Jade Simon, Kelly Strahan.

Our families deserve recognition for their daily queries relative to the book, which often stimulated humor, easing a sometimes tedious task. Special thanks to Jay, Jennifer, Katie, and Sarabeth and to Wayne, Kelly, Wayne Jr., Gretchen, and Michael for demonstrating daily understanding and support when the book had to be given priority.

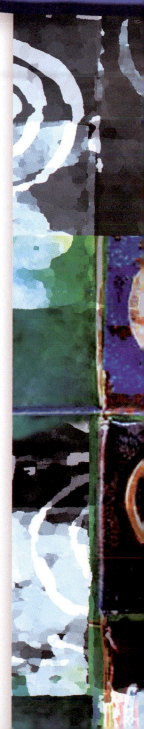

About the Authors

Sue C. DeLaune

Sue Carter DeLaune earned a bachelor of science in nursing from Northwestern State University, Natchitoches, Louisiana, and a master's degree in nursing from Louisiana State University Medical Center, New Orleans. She has taught nursing in diploma, associate degree, and baccalaureate schools of nursing, as well as in RN degree-completion programs. With over 30 years experience as an educator, clinician, and administrator, Sue has taught fundamentals of nursing, psychiatric–mental health nursing, and nursing leadership in a variety of programs. She also presents seminars and workshops across the country that assist nurses to maintain competency in areas of communication, leadership skills, client education, and stress management.

Sue is a member of the American Holistic Nurses Association, Sigma Theta Tau, and the American Nurses Association. She has been recognized as one of the "Great 100 Nurses" by the New Orleans District Nurses Association.

Currently, Sue is an Associate Professor at William Carey College School of Nursing, New Orleans. She also is President of SDeLaune Consulting, an independent education consulting business based in Mandeville, Louisiana.

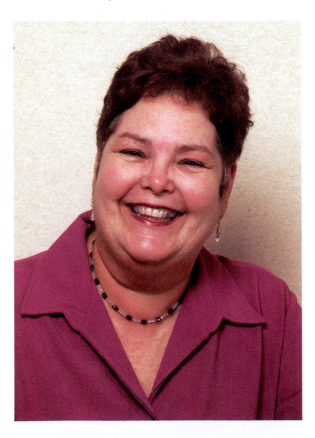

Patricia K. Ladner

Patricia Ann Kelly Ladner obtained an associate degree in science from Mercy Junior College, St. Louis, Missouri, a bachelor of science in nursing from Marillac College, St. Louis, Missouri, a master of science in counseling and guidance from Troy State University, Troy, Alabama, and a master's degree in nursing from Louisiana State Medical Center, New Orleans, Louisiana.

She has taught at George C. Wallace Junior Community College, Dothan, Alabama; Sampson Technical Institute, Clinton, North Carolina; Touro Infirmary School of Nursing and Charity/Delgado School of Nursing in New Orleans, Louisiana. She has also been the Director of Touro Infirmary School of Nursing and a Director of Nursing, Tulane University Medical Center in New Orleans. With 35 years as a clinician and academician, Ms. Ladner has taught fundamentals of nursing, medical-surgical nursing, and nursing seminars while maintaining clinical competency in various critical care and medical-surgical settings. Her professional career has provided her with the necessary knowledge and skills to be an effective lecturer and community leader.

Ms. Ladner received a governor's appointment to serve on an Advisory Committee of the Louisiana State Board of Medical Examiners, and she also served on an Advisory Committee for Loyola University in New Orleans. She maintains membership in Sigma Theta Tau, American Nurses Association, and the Louisiana Organization of Nurse Executives. She served for over 10 years on the Louisiana State Nurses Association's Continuing Education Committee. She is the recipient of the New Orleans District Nurses Association Community Service Award and has been recognized as one of the "Great 100 Nurses" by the New Orleans District Nurses Association.

Ms. Ladner has been listed in *Who's Who in American Nursing.* She is currently the Nursing Practice Consultant for the Louisiana State Board of Nursing.

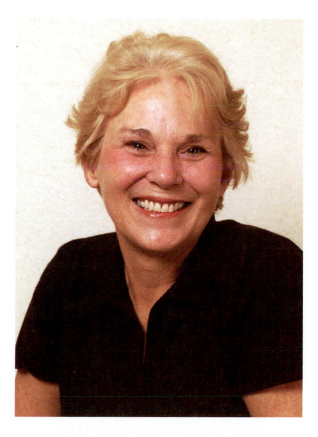

CONTENTS

PREFACE

This text was originally written to fill a long-standing need to treat the topics of stormwater runoff and hydraulics together in one book. It is intended to be used by students of civil engineering, civil engineering technology, and surveying, as well as practitioners in industry and government. The topics presented are relevant to public works, land development, and municipal engineering and planning—in fact, to any designer (both engineer and technician) who must deal with the conveyance of stormwater in any aspect of his/her work.

The book contains features designed to make the learning process more accessible and streamlined, such as:

- Many easy-to-follow examples

- Numerous clear diagrams, charts, and topographic maps to illustrate concepts developed in the text

- Case studies based on real-world projects

- A list of objectives starting each chapter to help focus the readers' attention

- Design charts in the appendices to relate examples and problems to real situations

- A list of current computer software in the appendix

- A comprehensive glossary of important terms

This third edition marks a significant improvement to the text by rearranging material and adding new material. The presentation of open channel hydraulics has been expanded to include an improved treatment of normal depth and critical depth and a new discussion of varied flow. Also, the design of detention facilities has been expanded to more clearly explain the fundamental concepts.

The newly sequenced presentations, as well as the expanded material in the third edition, have resulted in the addition of three new chapters, bringing the total number of chapters to fifteen. In addition, many new figures have been added to help readers gain a clear understanding of the subject matter.

The subjects of hydraulics and hydrology include many more topics than those presented in this text. Hydraulics texts are available that treat engineering hydraulics in a comprehensive manner, and there are hydrology texts that deal only with the engineering aspects of hydrology, but this book pares down the many topics of hydraulics and hydrology to the most basic and common areas dealing with stormwater management encountered by the designer on a day-to-day basis.

Principal topics include the following:

- Background concepts such as historical overview and basic notions of computation and design

- Fluid mechanics

- Fundamental hydrostatics and hydrodynamics

- Flow through hydraulic devices commonly used in stormwater management

- Open channel hydraulics

- Fundamental concepts of rainfall and runoff

- Runoff computation (Rational and NRCS Methods)

- Design of culverts

- Design of storm sewers

- Design of detention basins

One of the outstanding features of the book is the treatment of runoff computations. Thorough analysis and practice of watershed delineation are included to hone this skill, which is so essential to runoff analysis but often lacking in designers' training.

Another outstanding feature of the text is the comprehensive appendix, which includes excerpts from several relevant design manuals in use today. Students and others using the text will continually refer to the design charts located in Appendixes A through D when studying examples and working problems. Mastering the use of the charts is an indispensable benefit in learning the techniques of problem solving in the real world. The student will learn not only the use of the charts but also the theory and rationale used to create them.

For example, when analyzing a culvert problem, the student learns to recognize the correct chart in Appendix B and then uses it to derive key numerical values needed for the problem's solution. References to specific appendix sections are included throughout the text to guide the reader in their proper use.

One of the overarching premises used in framing the text is the belief that students need to learn engineering principles by solving problems by hand without the aid of computer software. When they are practitioners on the job, they can utilize the software, knowing the processes that are being used to compute the answers. And having worked the problems by hand, they will be able to distinguish meaningful answers from erroneous answers.

In addition to the development of hydraulic theory and runoff computation techniques, one of the goals of the text is to introduce some of the rudimentary stormwater management design processes that are used in civil engineering practice. To accomplish this, realistic design problems and case studies are included that rely on actual design charts. However, the text should not be construed as a complete design manual to be used on the job, nor is it intended to be. Good engineering practice requires the use of a variety of comprehensive sources found in professional publications and design manuals prepared by government agencies.

In developing the various topics throughout the text, the author has assumed certain prior knowledge on the part of the reader. This includes the fundamental concepts of land surveying, interpretation of topographic maps, profiles, and cross sections, and the use of the engineer's scale. Also, other engineering concepts such as the formation of free-body diagrams and the resolution of forces and moments are prerequisites to a full understanding of the text.

SUPPLEMENTS

An instructor *e.resource* on CD is available for this text. This is an educational resource that creates a truly electronic classroom. It is a CD-ROM containing tools and instructional material that enrich your classroom and make instructor's preparation time shorter. The elements of the e.resource link directly to the text and tie together to provide a unified instructional system. With the e.resource you can spend your time teaching, not preparing to teach (ISBN 1-4180-3296-4).

Features contained in the e.resource include:

- **Solutions Manual**. Solutions to end of chapter problems.

- **Syllabus**. A summary outline for the study of hydraulics and hydrology using this text.

- **Chapter Hints**. Teaching hints that provide a basis for a lecture outline that helps you present concepts and material.

- **PowerPoint® Presentations**. Slides for each chapter of the text provide the basis for a lecture outline that helps you present concepts and materials as well. Key points and concepts can be graphically highlighted for student retention.

- **Quizzes**. Additional test questions are provided for each chapter.

ACKNOWLEDGMENTS

We would like to thank and acknowledge the professionals who reviewed the text and revision plan to help us publish this new edition:

Dr. Leslie Brunell
Stevens Institute of Technology
Hoboken, NJ

Dr. Shafiqul Islam
Tufts University
Medford, MA

Dr. Roy Gu
Iowa State University
Ames, IA

Dr. Charles Patrick
Morehead State University
Morehead, KY

Dr. Todd Horton
Parkland College
Champaign, IL

Dr. Richard Vogel
Tufts University
Medford, MA

A special thank you goes to Dr. Pete Scarlatos of Florida Atlantic University, Boca Raton, Florida, for performing a technical edit on the new and rewritten chapters.

The author wishes to thank his family for their support—especially his son, Peter, for his tireless typing.

Introduction to Hydraulics and Hydrology with Applications for Stormwater Management

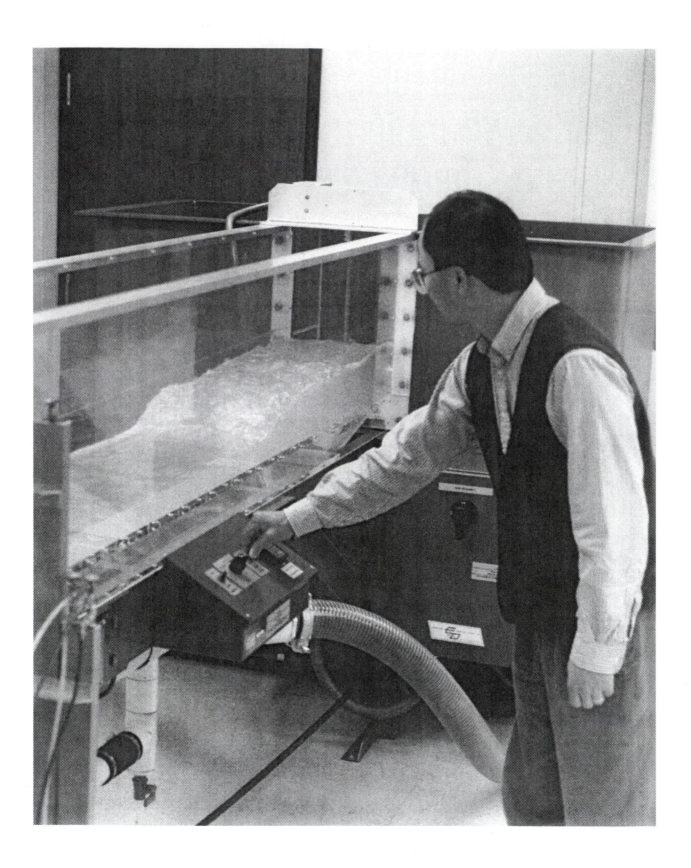

1

Hydraulics and Hydrology in Engineering

Engineers cannot avoid confronting the problems posed by rainfall and its consequent runoff. Some of mankind's earliest endeavors centered on this age-old battle with the forces of nature in the form of water. For most of our history, engineers and their predecessors dealt with water problems by utilizing various rule-of-thumb solutions, that is, whatever seemed to work. Only in recent times have these endeavors taken on a systematic body of laws and quantitative formulas.

In this chapter, we take a brief trip through the world of engineering hydraulics and hydrology of yesterday and today. We will look at the various aspects of modern stormwater management and review some general principles of engineering design.

OBJECTIVES

After completing this chapter, the reader should be able to:

- Place hydraulic/hydrologic engineering in a historical perspective
- Define stormwater management
- Explain the roles of public agencies in stormwater management
- Recognize the factors involved in engineering design
- Perform computations using the appropriate significant figures
- Convert between metric units and English units

1.1 HISTORY OF WATER ENGINEERING

People first started manipulating water on a large scale as a response to the need for irrigation in early agrarian society. The first known large-scale irrigation project was undertaken in Egypt approximately five thousand years ago. In the following millennia, many other water projects sprang up in the Mediterranean and Near

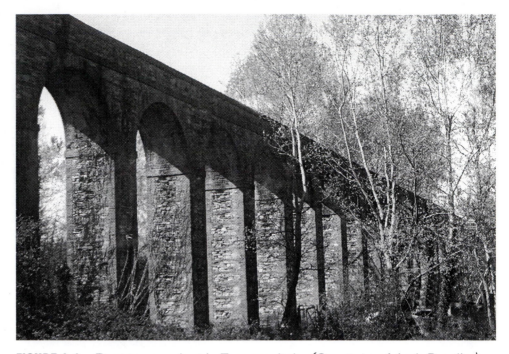

FIGURE 1-1 Roman aqueduct in Tuscany, Italy. *(Courtesy of Jack Breslin.)*

Eastern worlds. These included dams, canals, aqueducts, and sewer systems. The conveyance of water through pipes was also developed in ancient times. In China, bamboo pipes were used as early as 2500 B.C., and the Romans utilized lead and bronze pipes by 200 B.C.

The Romans' prowess as engineers was amply demonstrated in their hydraulic systems. The famous aqueducts were among the wonders of the world and remained in use through two millennia (see Figure 1-1). The Greeks, although not the engineers that the Romans were, nonetheless made significant contributions to the theories of hydraulics. Archimedes is considered the earliest contributor to hydraulics based on truly scientific work. In about 250 B.C., he published a written work on hydrostatics that presented the laws of buoyancy (Archimedes' Principle) and flotation. He is generally considered the Father of Hydrostatics.

During the period from 500 B.C. to the Middle Ages, irrigation and water supply systems were constructed and maintained in such diverse locations as China, the Roman Empire, and North America. Such engineering was designed and constructed by artisans using rules of thumb, artisans who, despite Archimedes' work, lacked the benefits of scientific inquiry. The great Roman engineers, for example, did not understand the concept of velocity, and it was not until A.D. 1500 that the connection between rainfall and streamflow was taken seriously.

As the Roman Empire declined, many of the advances made during the Greco-Roman period were forgotten, only to be rediscovered during the Renaissance. It was during this period that hydraulics began to be developed as a science.

The first effort at organized engineering knowledge was the founding in 1760 of the *Ecole des Ponts et Chaussées* in Paris. In 1738, Daniel Bernoulli published his famous **Bernoulli equation**, formulating the conservation of energy in hydraulics. During the eighteenth and nineteenth centuries, referred to as the classical period of hydraulics, advances in hydraulic engineering laid the groundwork for further developments in the twentieth century.

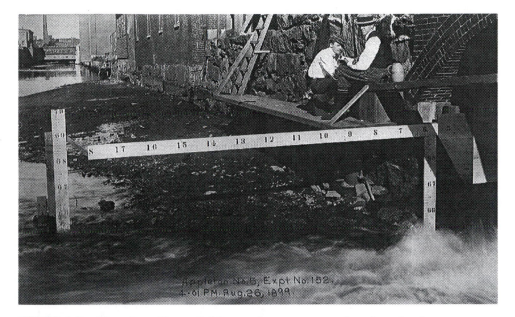

FIGURE 1-2   The city of Lowell, Massachusetts, was the site of a famous series of water power experiments conducted by James Francis and Uriah Boyden. The publication of the results in 1855 contributed greatly to the field of hydraulic engineering. Here, two assistants are shown measuring water levels. *(Courtesy of University of Massachussets Lowell, Locks and Canal Collection.)*

Despite the domination of the French during the classical period, work was conducted in other countries as well. In England, for instance, John Smeaton was very active in many aspects of hydraulic engineering and was the first to call himself a **civil engineer**.

As late as 1850, however, engineering designs were still based mainly on rules of thumb developed through experience and tempered with liberal factors of safety. Since that time, utilization of theory has increased rapidly. Today, a vast amount of careful computation is an integral part of most project designs. Figure 1-2 depicts one of many hydraulic experiments conducted in Lowell, Massachusetts, in the mid-1800s that contributed greatly to the field of hydraulic engineering.

1.2   MODERN PRACTICE OF STORMWATER MANAGEMENT

Civil engineers work with water wherever it affects the structures and infrastructure of civilization. The role of the civil engineer and technician in connection with the many diverse effects of water may be grouped into three broad categories:

1. Flood control—managing the natural flow of stormwater to prevent property damage and loss of life
2. Water resources—exploiting the available water resources for beneficial purposes such as water supply, irrigation, hydroelectric power, and navigation
3. Water quality—managing the use of water to prevent its degradation due to pollutants both natural and man-made

Although the first role listed above, flood control, constitutes the primary focus of this text, the other two are of no less importance. All three areas constitute projects designed and carried out by people working in both the private and public sectors.

As an example of private endeavors in flood control, imagine that an entrepreneur wishes to construct a factory surrounded by a parking area. He or she must engage a civil engineer to design proper grading and a storm sewer system to convey any rainfall occurring on the site. In addition, a detention basin might be required to prevent any adverse effect of runoff from the factory site to adjacent properties.

Although these problems will be solved by an engineering firm contracting directly with the owner, public agencies become involved as well, since all designs affecting the public welfare must be reviewed and approved by the appropriate local, county, and state agencies.

Examples of public endeavors in flood control are many and may be as simple as the design of a pipe culvert under a newly constructed road to allow free passage of a stream or as complex as the extensive levee and pump system surrounding the city of New Orleans, Louisiana. The disastrous flooding that resulted from Hurricane Katrina in 2005 showed how important flood control can be. Each of these public projects may be designed by engineers employed by public agencies or by private engineers contracting directly with the appropriate public agency.

In a typical privately owned land development project, the engineer representing the developer works with the engineer representing the regulating agency to solve any stormwater runoff problems. The relationship between the engineers is at once adversarial and cooperative as they work to protect the respective interests of the private developer and the public. In this way, they create the best possible project.

The term **stormwater management** as used in this text refers to the engineering practices and regulatory policies employed to mitigate the adverse effects of stormwater runoff. These endeavors usually are associated with runoff problems resulting from various types of land development.

1.3 LEGAL AND ENVIRONMENTAL ISSUES

Over the past three decades, legal and environmental issues have dramatically changed the way civil engineers practice their art, and hydraulic/hydrologic engineering is no exception. Stormwater management was once based on the principles of good engineering practice, but now design must also satisfy a myriad of regulations enforced by several levels of public agencies.

When hydraulic and hydrologic design affects the public, there is a legal issue, and when it affects the environment, there is an environmental issue. These two issues usually overlap, since anything that affects the environment most often affects the public. Although legal and environmental issues abound throughout all areas of civil engineering, we will look at only a few that affect stormwater management on a regular basis.

When rain falls from the sky, it strikes the earth and then runs downhill, impelled by gravity across the land to join the streams and rivers that eventually carry it to the sea. Our society considers all such motion of water to be naturally occurring, and if the water does damage along its path, such as erosion or flooding, no legal blame is assigned to any person. But the minute people alter their land in such a way as to change the course of the stormwater, they become liable for any damage done as a result of the alteration. The two ways in which land development generally affects downstream property are by concentrating the flow of stormwater and by increasing the quantity of that flow.

The practice of stormwater management must take these problems into consideration and mitigate them. Mitigation is achieved by a variety of methods, including rerouting the flow, dispersing the flow, lining the ground with erosion protection, and providing a detention basin.

Another problem that occurs in hydraulic and hydrologic design is the pollution of stormwater. Development of the land can and usually does result in several unwanted pollutants mixing into the stormwater as it runs off the developed site. These include salts and oils from paved areas or fertilizer, pesticides, and silt particles from vegetated areas. Stormwater management mitigates these problems by such measures as providing vegetative filters, siltation basins, catch basins, and recharge basins.

Wetlands are an environmental feature that has come into prominence throughout the past two decades. Wetlands are areas of land, usually naturally occurring, that retain water throughout much of the year. They are beneficial to the ecosystem and are particularly sensitive to disruption by the effects of development. Extra care must be taken to identify, delineate, and protect these areas when they are on or adjacent to a land development project.

Design engineers work hand in hand with regulators in addressing and solving the problems raised by legal and environmental issues. In the following section, we will briefly outline the identities of the regulating bodies and the roles they perform.

1.4 PUBLIC AGENCIES

Over the past few decades, life in the United States has become much more regulated than in previous times. Naturally, the field of civil engineering design has acquired its own array of specialized rules. The trend toward increased regulation has generally relied on the concept that the government may regulate anything that affects the health and welfare of the public. In civil engineering, this means that just about everything may be regulated.

Regulating began at the local level with the proliferation of zoning ordinances by municipalities everywhere. Zoning has become more and more complex over the years, especially over the past three decades. Originally the concept was simple: A factory, for instance, cannot be constructed in an area of town reserved for residential development. Today zoning regulates not only the type of development but also details of the infrastructure, such as pavement thicknesses for roads, key parameters in storm sewer design, and detailed methodology for detention design.

Local municipal zoning and land development ordinances are administered by the municipal engineer, a civil engineer employed by or under contract to the municipality, and the zoning officer (also called the building inspector), an employee of the municipality trained in building code enforcement.

One level above municipal is the county in which the project is located. County governments have jurisdiction over certain roads designated as county roads and usually most of the bridges and culverts in the county, except those under state highways. Thus, if the stormwater flowing from a project flows onto a county road or through a county culvert, the county engineering department has limited regulatory power over the project. In addition, the Natural Resources Conservation Service (NRCS), formerly called the Soil Conservation Service, regulates soil erosion aspects of development work through local offices around the country. In many areas, these are called Soil Conservation District (SCD) offices and are semiautonomous regulatory agencies using regulations promulgated by the NRCS, a federal agency.

The next level of regulation consists of a few specially created regional, semi-autonomous agencies that have jurisdiction over certain geographical problem areas. They are usually associated with environmentally sensitive areas, which require more intense scrutiny than the rest of the land to be developed. These include flood control districts, wetland districts, and timberland districts.

The next level of regulation is the state. State laws governing land development are administered by specially created agencies such as the state Department of Environmental Protection, which typically has jurisdiction over any project that affects a state-regulated entity, including, for instance, wetlands, streams, and water fronts or state-owned entities such as highways and culverts.

Finally, the most overreaching level of regulation is the federal government. Federal laws such as the 1972 Clean Water Act are administered by federal agencies including the Environmental Protection Agency (EPA) and the U.S. Army Corps of Engineers. Another federal agency that affects hydraulic and hydrologic design is the Federal Highway Administration, a division of the Department of Transportation. This agency affects local everyday projects principally through the publication of design manuals developed through research.

1.5 ENGINEERING DESIGN

All engineers and technicians, electrical, mechanical or civil, are engaged in design. The civil designer works on projects that can be as daunting in scope as a 500-foot-high dam complete with hydroelectric power station or as mundane as a concrete pipe laid in a trench.

Regardless of the size of the project, the design process requires the complete specification of every aspect of the structure so that it can then be constructed on the basis of the resulting specifications. That is, the engineer or technician must think of every detail of the structure and successfully convey his or her thoughts to the builder.

Design Process

In designing a structure, several important steps are required to transform an initial idea into a clear and fully developed document ready for construction. The example of a storm sewer pipe can be used to illustrate the general steps in performing a typical design:

1. **Concept.** Determine the basic concept of the design. In this case, it is to convey stormwater from one location to another.
2. **Base Map.** Prepare a base map showing the topographic features of the project site together with any pertinent property boundaries. A good base map is essential to the successful design process.
3. **Design Development.** Sketch alternative layouts of the pipe on the base map. Also, research other factors affecting the design, such as soil conditions, structural loading on the pipe, potential interference with other subsurface utilities, drainage area, and meteorological data.
4. **Calculations.** Perform appropriate engineering computations of key design quantities—in this case, the anticipated amount of stormwater to be conveyed by the pipe and the resulting pipe size. The calculations should be in written form and contain any assumptions made. They should be checked by another designer.

5. **Prepare Drawings and Specifications.** Prepare drawings showing the layout in plan and profile including any details and notes needed to describe the structure for use by the builder in constructing the project. Include written specifications if necessary.

Design Outcome

Design is an endeavor that is enriched with experience. As more and more projects are completed, good practitioners start to acquire a deeper appreciation for the larger picture surrounding the design and weave that broader perspective into their work. It is not enough to imagine only the proper functioning of the structure; other factors must also be taken into consideration, such as proper maintenance, cost, safety during construction, and availability of materials. Because the design process is such a complex and ever-growing intellectual endeavor, an exhaustive definition is virtually impossible. However, certain basic elements can be identified.

Design is the process of determining the complete specification of a structure so that it will:

1. Perform its intended function under all foreseeable circumstances without failing
2. Be able to be constructed at a cost within the budget of the owner
3. Be able to be maintained easily and effectively
4. Conform to all applicable local, county, state, and federal laws and regulations
5. Not interfere with other structures or utilities that could be constructed in its vicinity in the future
6. Be able to be constructed in a safe manner
7. Remain intact and functional throughout its intended lifetime
8. Not present a safety hazard to the public throughout its lifetime
9. Not unduly degrade the environment either during construction or throughout its lifetime
10. Be aesthetically pleasing

Each structure must be designed by using all of these factors regardless of its apparent simplicity. In later chapters, we will see how to employ the principles of design listed here in some commonly encountered projects related to hydraulic and hydrologic engineering.

1.6   ENGINEERING COMPUTATIONS

Almost all engineering designs require some computing of numbers. Although the use of calculators and computers makes computing relatively easy, an understanding of certain basic principles of computing is important to a successful design process.

Significant Figures

The concept of significant figures should be familiar to anyone engaged in the various aspects of the design process. The number of significant figures of a quantity is the number of digits used to form the quantity (except for zeros under certain circumstances, as explained below). Thus, the quantities 429, 1.02, and 0.00315 have three significant figures each. The zeros in the third example are not significant because they are only place holders. Zeros can also be used as place holders at the right end of a quantity where the quantity has no decimal point. Thus, the quantities 450, 1500, and 92,000 each have two significant figures. If, however, a decimal point is added to the end of such a quantity, the zeros become significant. Thus, the quantities 450., 1500., and 92,000. have three, four, and five significant figures, respectively.

Numbers subjected to the rules of significant figures generally are quantities that have been measured. For instance, if the length of a pipe is measured as 229 feet, it is said that the length was measured to the nearest foot and the measurement has three significant figures. A pipe measured as 229.0 feet was measured to the nearest tenth of a foot, and the measurement has four significant figures. A pipe measured as 230 feet was measured to the nearest 10 feet, and the measurement has only two significant figures. However, a pipe measured as 230. feet was measured to the nearest 1 foot, and the measurement has three significant figures.

Numbers not subject to the rules for significant figures are pure numbers, which cannot vary to any extent. These numbers include counting numbers and assumed quantities. For example, in the formula $c = 2\pi r$, the number 2 is a counting number and therefore perfectly precise. It is the same as if it was expressed as 2.00000. Also, if the radius, r, is assumed hypothetically to be 4 feet and not measured, then the quantity 4 is also perfectly precise and the same as if it was written 4.00000 feet. (Of course, if r is measured, it should be expressed with the number of significant figures corresponding to the precision of the measurement.)

The rules for computations are as follows:

1. **Multiplication and Division.** The answer to a multiplication or division computation should have no more significant figures than the least number of significant figures in any quantity in the computation.
2. **Addition and Subtraction.** The answer to an addition or subtraction computation should have no more digits to the right of the decimal point than the least number of digits to the right of the decimal point in any quantity in the computation.
3. **Computations in Series.** If a series of computations is to be made where the answer to one is used as a quantity in the next, then only the final answer of the last computation should be rounded to significant figures. In such a case, the number of significant figures would be based on all quantities used in all of the computations.

Example 1-1

Problem

Find the circumference of a pipe having a diameter measured to be 4.00 feet.

Solution

Since the diameter was measured to a precision of three significant figures, it is expressed with three significant figures. The formula for circumference is $c = \pi d$.

$$c = \pi d$$
$$= (\pi)(4.00)$$
$$= 12.6 \text{ ft} \qquad \text{(Answer)}$$

Although the calculator display shows 12.566371, only three significant figures can be used in the answer.

Note: If the measurement had been 4.0 feet, the computed circumference would be 13 feet.

Example 1-2

Problem

Find the circumference of a typical 4-foot diameter pipe.

Solution

In this case, the diameter is a theoretical value and not subject to significant figures.

$$c = \pi d$$
$$= (\pi)(4)$$
$$= 12.566371 \text{ ft} \quad \text{(Answer)}$$

Although all of the figures shown above may be used in the answer, for practical reasons only three or four figures are generally used. If, however, the circumference is to be used in a further computation, as many figures as possible should be used and only the final answer would be subject to rounding to significant figures. See Example 1-3.

Example 1-3

Problem

Find the volume of a cylinder having a diameter measured as 2.3 feet and length measured as 8.25 feet.

Solution

First computation:

$$a = \pi d^2/4$$
$$= \pi(2.3)^2/4$$
$$= 4.1547563 \text{ ft}^2 \quad \text{(shown on calculator)}$$

Second computation:

$$V = aL$$
$$= (4.1547563)(8.25)$$
$$= 34.276739 \text{ ft}^3 \quad \text{(shown on calculator)}$$
$$= 34 \text{ ft}^3 \quad \text{(Answer)}$$

The final answer is rounded to two significant figures because the quantity 2.3 in the first computation has two significant figures.

Note: If the first answer were rounded to two significant figures before performing the second computation, the final answer would have been 35 ft^3.

Accuracy and Precision

One way to appreciate the importance of significant figures is to understand the distinction between accuracy and precision. The term *accuracy* means a value that is close to the actual value. Thus, if the actual length of a pipe is 230.0000 feet, then a length value of 231 feet is accurate within 0.4 percent. On the other hand, a length value of 232.15 feet is less accurate even though it is more precise. The term *precision* refers to the fineness of a measurement. A length of 232.15 feet is precise to within 0.01 feet; that is, it implies a length value somewhere between 232.145 feet and 232.155 feet. Although it is commonly assumed that the true length falls within this range of values, such an assumption is not necessarily correct. Precision does not ensure accuracy.

Sometimes it is tempting to think that increasing the precision of an answer will also increase its accuracy. Thus, it is tempting to express the answer to Example 1-3 as 34.28 ft^3 instead of 34 ft^3. The true answer to Example 1-3 lies in a range between 33.5 ft^3 and 34.5 ft^3. So to state the answer as 34.28 ft^3 is meaningless and misleading.

Engineering calculations must always be accurate. But the accuracy stems from careful measurements and correctly applied scientific principles, not from an overstatement of precision by writing too many significant figures in the answer.

Example 1-4

Problem

Find the cross-sectional area, a, of a circular pipe of diameter not known to you. (True diameter = 2.500 ft.)

Solution

1. Accurate solution: Suppose the diameter is measured as accurately as possible to be 2.4 ft.

   $a = \pi d^2/4$
   $\quad = \pi(2.4)^2/4$
   $\quad = 4.5$ ft^2 (Answer)

   The answer is reported with two significant figures because the value for d had two significant figures.

2. Precise solution: Suppose the diameter is measured sloppily to be 2.7 feet.

   $a = \pi d^2/4$
   $\quad = \pi(2.7)^2/4$
   $\quad = 5.726$ ft^2 (Answer)

   The answer is reported with four significant figures because the calculator displayed at least that many.

Although the *precise* solution looks more accurate, in fact it differs from the theoretical solution of 4.909 ft^2 by a greater percentage than does the *accurate* solution; therefore, it is not acceptable, despite its more precise appearance.

To ensure that computations have the highest degree of accuracy possible, certain techniques should always be employed.

1. Always try to check every computation or measurement by repeating the computation or measurement using an alternate method.

    For instance, if a distance between two stations on a baseline is computed mathematically to be 350 feet, check the answer graphically by measuring the distance on your map with a scale.

    Another example is the measurement of an area on a map. If the area is measured with a planimeter to be 2.35 acres, check the answer by roughly measuring a length and width with a scale and computing the rough area using $a = L \times W$ and comparing with measured area for approximate agreement.

2. Always check the computation by considering whether it seems reasonable.

    For instance, if the volume of a swimming pool is computed to be 150,000 ft^3, a little reflection on the number will reveal that it is far out of the realm of reason. At that point, the calculation should be reviewed for errors.

3. When practical, have another engineer or technician review the entire calculation for agreement with assumptions and computations.

Many computations are performed by using computers. In most cases, these involve relatively inexpensive software loaded on a personal computer. However, before a computer can be used successfully, the principles of design and computation must be understood thoroughly.

Computers

The computer is a tool just as are the calculator and the engineer's scale and all the other design tools utilized by engineers. But it is important to remember that the computer is not a surrogate for sound engineering design judgment. It is essential to good engineering practice to resist the temptation to rely on the answers given by computers as if the software has the ability to make design judgments. All computer computations must be scrutinized and checked as would any other computation performed on a calculator or done longhand.

Design principles presented in the later chapters of this text employ the same methodology utilized by most computer software. Computer applications should be learned elsewhere *after* the governing principles are first acquired. For the reader's convenience, a selected list of computer software relevant to stormwater management problems is included in Appendix E.

Computation and Calculations

In this text, the term *computation* refers to the mathematical manipulation of numbers, while the term *calculations* refers to the overall presentation, including not only the computations but also the statements of explanation that go along with the actual computations.

In addition to being accurate, engineering calculations should be prepared on special forms created for the particular type of calculation used or on engineering calculation paper with each sheet showing the name of the project, the date, and the names of preparer and checker.

Also included in the calculations should be all design assumptions made, identification of the computation methodology and computer software used, and a clear depiction of the results, including diagrams if necessary. In general, the calculations should include all information needed for another engineer who is not familiar with the project to understand the design process and the results.

1.7 METRICATION

Traditionally, hydraulic and hydrologic design calculations have been performed in the United States by using the English system of units. These include feet, pounds, and seconds as base units, with a variety of derived units used as well. However, starting in the 1970s, attempts were made at the federal level to convert the nation to the use of the metric system, also known as the International System of Units (SI). These include meters, kilograms, and seconds as base units. Most of the world is geared to SI units.

Early attempts to "go metric" soon lost momentum, and the conversion was never completed. Another attempt at metrication was mounted in the late 1980s and early 1990s. Federal legislation mandated the use of SI units for projects in certain agencies. An executive order in 1991 required all new federal building construction to be metricized and set the year 2000 as the deadline for highway work conversion.

Although the 2000 deadline was subsequently eliminated, the majority of state highway work became metricized, as reported in January 2000 in *Civil Engineering*, the journal of the American Society of Civil Engineers. In New Jersey, for example, all highway design for the Department of Transportation was required to use SI units.

Despite the progress that has been made, the future of metrication in the United States is in doubt. Opposition to metricized state and federal construction still exists, and some states, including New Jersey, have reverted to English units.

Presentation of design theory and examples in this text is done, to the greatest extent practical, using both systems. Equations that are empirical are presented in both English and SI forms. Rationally derived equations that are valid for any consistent system of units are presented in one form followed by an explanation of appropriate English and SI units. English units are shown first, followed by SI units in parentheses—for example, V = volume, ft^3 (m^3). Unit conversions are presented in Appendix G for the reader's convenience.

Example 1-5

Problem

Find the circumference (in meters) of a pipe having a diameter measured to be 4.00 feet.

Solution

First, convert the diameter to meters.

$$4.00 \text{ feet} \times \frac{1 \text{ m}}{3.28 \text{ ft}} = 1.2195 \text{ m}$$

Next, find the circumference

$$c = \pi d$$
$$= (\pi)(1.2195)$$
$$= 3.83 \text{ m} \qquad \text{(Answer)}$$

Three significant figures are used in the final answer in accordance with the rules for significant figures.

PROBLEMS

1. Find the cross-sectional area of a pipe with diameter measuring 3.04 feet. Express the answer with the proper significant figures.

2. Compute the volume of pavement in a road measured to be 22.0 feet wide and 1.0 mile long. The measured pavement thickness is 0.650 foot. Express the answer in cubic yards using the proper significant figures.

3. If the depth of water in a stream is measured as $6\frac{1}{2}$ inches, find the depth in feet using the proper significant figures.

4. Find the volume of a cylinder with diameter measuring 1.30 feet and length measuring 60. feet. Express the answer in cubic feet using the proper significant figures.

5. Three different lengths of new curb are measured by three different inspectors as follows: 12.25 feet, 151. feet, and 25.0 feet. Find the total length of new curb using proper significant figures.

6. Find the cross-sectional area of a pipe with diameter measuring 36 inches. Express the answer in metric units using the proper significant figures.

7. A rectangular field has dimensions 45.00 feet by 125.00 feet. Find the area using the proper significant figures expressed as (a) square feet, (b) acres, (c) square meters, and (d) hectares.

8. A roadway is to be designed to carry normal vehicular traffic between two existing parallel roadways separated by a distance of approximately 250 feet. Using your imagination, outline as many factors as possible to consider in the design.

9. A pedestrian walkway (sidewalk) is to be installed along one side of an existing paved street. Outline as many factors as possible to consider in the design.

10. A culvert (pipe) is to be designed to convey a small stream through a new road embankment. Outline as many factors as possible to be considered in the design.

FURTHER READING

American Society for Testing and Materials (1993). *Standard Practice for Use of the International System of Units (SI)*. Philadelphia: ASTM.

de Camp, L. (1963). *The Ancient Engineers*. New York: Dorset Press.

Schodek, D. (1987). *Landmarks in American Civil Engineering*. Cambridge, MA: MIT Press.

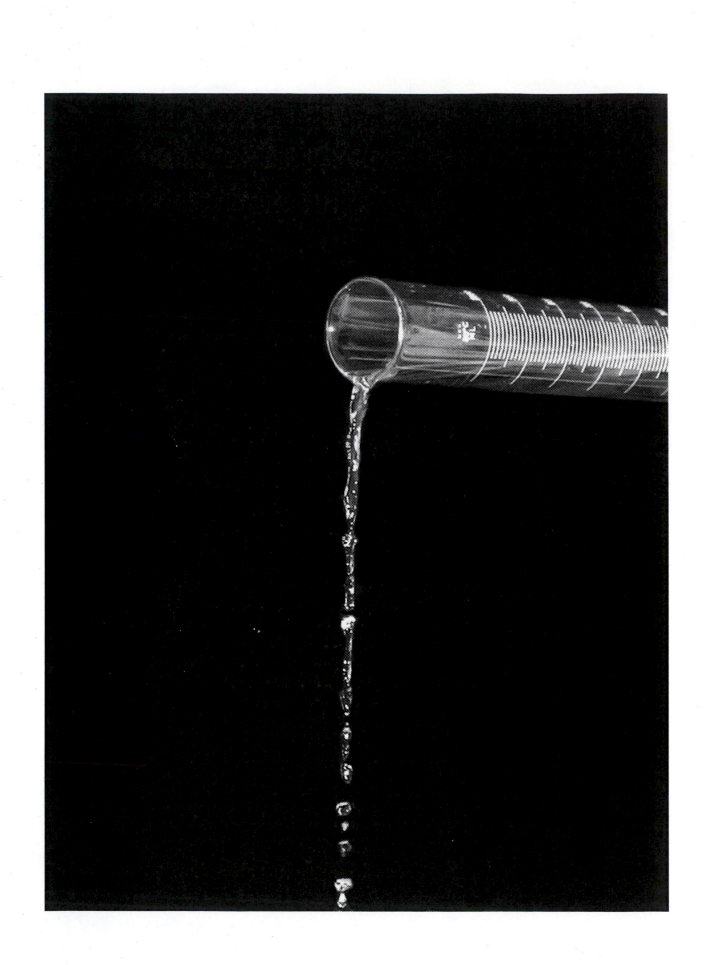

Fluid Mechanics

Fluid is a term that describes both gases and liquids. The forces holding fluid molecules together are much weaker than those of solids, allowing fluids to deform easily under external forces. In the language of mechanics of materials, fluids cannot support shear forces. That is, a fluid will flow under the influence of the slightest stress.

Although most of the principles developed for fluids apply to both gases and liquids, it is liquids, and in particular water, that is of most interest in this text. In this chapter, you will learn some of the fundamental concepts describing the behavior of water as a fluid.

OBJECTIVES

After completing this chapter, the reader should be able to:

- Describe the differences among solid, liquid, and gas
- Describe properties of water such as cohesion, adhesion, and capillarity
- Calculate the specific weight and specific gravity of various liquids
- Calculate the viscosity of a fluid

2.1 FUNDAMENTAL CONCEPTS

All matter encountered on an everyday basis exists in one of three forms: solid, liquid, or gas. Generally, these forms are distinguished by the bonds between adjacent molecules (or atoms) that compose them. Thus, the molecules that make up a solid are relatively close together and are held in place by the electrostatic bonds between the molecules. Therefore, solids tend to keep their shape, even when acted on by an external force.

By contrast, gas molecules are so far apart that the bonds are too weak to keep them in place. A gas is very compressible and always takes the shape of its container. If the container of a gas is removed, the molecules would expand indefinitely.

Between the extremes of solid and gas lies the liquid form of matter. In a liquid, molecules are bonded with enough strength to prevent indefinite expansion but without enough strength to be held in place. Liquids conform to the shape of their container except for the top, which forms a horizontal surface, free of confining pressure except for atmospheric pressure. Liquids tend to be incompressible, and water, despite minute compressibility, is assumed to be incompressible for most hydraulic problems.

In addition to water, various oils and even molten metals are examples of liquids and share in the basic characteristics of liquids.

All liquids have **surface tension**, which is manifested differently in different liquids. Surface tension results from a different molecular bonding condition at the free surface compared to bonds within the liquid. In water, surface tension results in properties called **cohesion** and **adhesion**.

Cohesion enables water to resist a slight tensile stress; adhesion enables it to adhere to another body. Figure 2-1 shows some familiar patterns of water in a container caused by cohesion and adhesion. In Figure 2-1(a), adhesion causes the water in the test tube to wet the side for a short distance above the surface. Figure 2-1(b) shows a meniscus at the top of a test tube caused by surface tension, which results from the cohesion of molecules at the surface of the water.

Capillarity is a property of liquids that results from surface tension in which the liquid rises up or is depressed down a thin tube. If adhesion predominates over cohesion in a liquid, as in water, the liquid will wet the surface of a tube and rise up. If cohesion predominates over adhesion in a liquid, as in mercury, the liquid does not wet the tube and is depressed down. Figure 2-2 shows thin capillary tubes placed in water and mercury. Notice that in the case of water, the meniscus is concave and rises above the surrounding level; the mercury meniscus is convex and is depressed below the surrounding level.

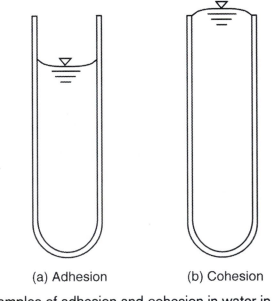

(a) Adhesion   (b) Cohesion

FIGURE 2-1   Examples of adhesion and cohesion in water in a glass test tube.

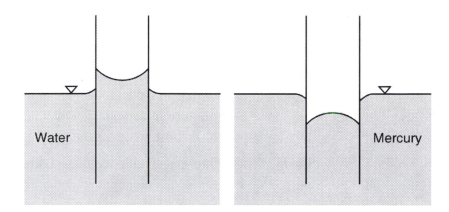

FIGURE 2-2   Capillarity of water versus mercury.

The amount that water rises in a tube depends on the temperature and purity of the water and, especially, the diameter of the tube. A tube with an inside diameter of ¼ inch will cause more capillarity of water than will a tube with a ½-inch inside diameter. Figure 2-3 illustrates this phenomenon.

Certain measuring devices such as manometers and piezometers employ vertical tubes in which water is allowed to rise. It is important, therefore, to use a tube with a large enough diameter to minimize the effect of capillarity, which would cause an error in measurement.

2.2   SPECIFIC WEIGHT AND DENSITY

Any material has a **specific weight**, γ, defined as weight per unit volume. Thus,

$$\gamma = \frac{W}{V} \tag{2-1}$$

where γ = specific weight, lb/ft^3 (N/m^3)
    W = weight, lb (N)
    V = volume, ft^3 (m^3)

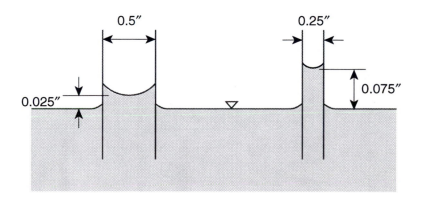

FIGURE 2-3   The effect of tube diameter on the capillarity of tap water.

Specific weight should not be confused with **density**, which is defined as mass per unit volume. Density, ρ, is computed from the expression

$$\rho = \frac{m}{V} \qquad (2\text{-}2)$$

where ρ = density, slugs/ft^3 (kg/m^3)
$\quad m$ = mass, slugs (kg)
$\quad V$ = volume, ft^3 (m^3)

The relationship between specific weight and density is

$$\gamma = \rho g \qquad (2\text{-}3)$$

where g = acceleration due to gravity, 32.2 ft/s^2 (9.81 m/s^2).

Both density and specific weight generally vary with the temperature of a material. This is because thermal expansion results in less mass in a given volume. Water is no exception to this rule.

In Table 2-1, values of specific weight of water at sea level are given for various temperatures. Notice that the specific weight generally decreases by about 4 percent between 32°F and 212°F, which represents the limits of the liquid phase of water. However, within the usual range of temperatures encountered in stormwater management (32°F–80°F), the specific weight of water is quite uniform. The generally accepted value is $\gamma = 62.4$ lb/ft^3 (9.81 kN/m^3).

It is interesting to note in Table 2-1 that a slight rise in specific weight occurs at about 7°F (4°C) above freezing. This is due to a rearranging of the relative positions of molecules that water undergoes when it changes phase from liquid to solid. This phenomenon is unique to water, resulting in a dramatically lower specific weight for ice. Thus, water expands when it freezes, causing ice cubes to float in water.

The expansion of water when it changes to ice can be problematic if it freezes within a container such as a pipe. Expansion can impose excessive stress on the container, sometimes resulting in rupture.

This discussion of specific weight refers to pure water. When impurities are found in water, specific weight is affected. For instance, seawater, containing salt and other impurities, has a specific weight of approximately 64 lb/ft^3, about 3 percent higher than pure water at the same temperature.

The specific gravity of a liquid is the ratio of its specific weight to that of pure water at a standard temperature and should not be confused with the term *specific weight*. Specific gravity is dimensionless. The specific gravity of water under normal conditions encountered in stormwater management is approximately 1.0.

TABLE 2-1 Specific Weight of Water

Temperature			Specific Weight, γ	
°F	(°C)		lb/ft^3	(kN/m^3)
32	(0)	Ice	57.28	(9.003)
32	(0)	Water	62.49	(9.822)
39.16	(3.98)		62.50	(9.823)
50	(10)		62.47	(9.819)
100	(38)		62.00	(9.745)
212	(100)		59.89	(9.413)

2.3   VISCOSITY

When a fluid is subjected to an external stress, its molecules readily yield and slide past one another, resulting in shearing action. However, one fluid will resist shear stress more than another, giving rise to the property of fluids called **viscosity**. Viscosity can be described as a fluid's resistance to shear stress. It can also be thought of as the influence of the motion of one layer of a fluid on another layer a short distance away. Therefore, viscosity has no meaning in a motionless fluid.

Viscosity is sometimes confused with density, but it is very different. Whereas density refers simply to the amount of mass per unit volume, viscosity refers to the ability of fluid molecules to flow past each other. Thus, a very dense fluid could have a low viscosity or vice versa.

The properties of viscosity and density are well illustrated by the example of oil and water. Most oils, as we know, are less dense than water and therefore float on water's surface. Yet despite its lack of density, oil is more viscous than water. This property of viscosity is called **absolute viscosity**. It is designated μ and has units of lb-s/ft^2 (kg-s/m^2). Because it has been found that in many hydraulic problems, density is a factor, another form of viscosity, called **kinematic viscosity**, has been defined as absolute viscosity divided by density. Kinematic viscosity is designated by υ and has units of ft^2/s (m^2/s). Kinematic viscosity of water is taken as 1×10^{-5} ft^2/s (9.29×10^{-7} m^2/s).

The concept of viscosity can be further illustrated by the sliding plate viscometer. This device, shown in Figure 2-4, can be used to measure absolute viscosity. Assume that the lower plate is kept motionless and the upper plate is moved at a certain velocity, v, by applying a force. The portion of fluid in contact with the upper plate moves with velocity v, while the fluid in contact with the lower plate has zero velocity. Therefore, a velocity gradient will be induced throughout the thickness of fluid. If you think of the fluid existing in thin layers parallel to the plates, these layers slide past each other in a shearing action. Different fluids produce different shear stress between layers for a given velocity. Therefore, different fluids have different viscosities.

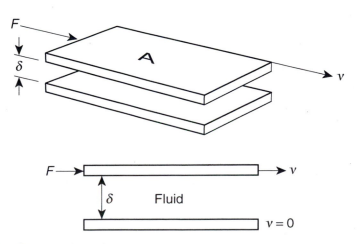

FIGURE 2-4   Sliding plate viscometer.

Referring to Figure 2-4, notice that shear stress, τ, is the force per unit area, or

$$\tau = \frac{F}{A} \tag{2-4}$$

where τ = shear stress, lb/ft^2 (N/m^2)
$\quad\quad F$ = applied force, lb (N)
$\quad\quad A$ = area of plate, ft^2 (m^2)

Also note that the variation of velocity across the plate separation is v/δ. Experimentation shows that the applied force needed to maintain the velocity v is proportional to the velocity and the plate area and inversely proportional to the plate separation, δ. Thus,

$$F \propto \text{(proportional to)} \ \frac{v\,A}{\delta} \tag{2-5}$$

Rearranging Equation 2-5 gives

$$\frac{F}{A} \propto \frac{v}{\delta} \tag{2-6}$$

or

$$\tau \propto \frac{v}{\delta} \tag{2-7}$$

The proportionality constant is called absolute viscosity, μ. Thus,

$$\tau = \mu \frac{v}{\delta} \tag{2-8}$$

Fluids that behave in accordance with Equation 2-8 are called Newtonian fluids. The viscosity of a Newtonian fluid does not vary with the shear stress or the resulting velocity gradient. The viscosity depends only on the condition of the fluid such as temperature. Most fluids encountered in engineering, such as water and oil, are Newtonian fluids.

Example 2-1

Problem

The viscosity of a fluid is to be determined using a sliding plate viscometer. The plate area is 0.16 ft^2, and the separation between plates is 0.070 ft. A force of 0.00020 lb moves the upper plate at a velocity of 6.0 ft/s. What is the absolute viscosity?

Solution

From Equation 2-4, shear stress is

$$\tau = \frac{F}{A}$$
$$= \frac{0.0002}{0.16}$$
$$= 0.00125 \ \text{lb/ft}^2$$

Absolute viscosity is then found by rearranging Equation 2-8. Thus,

$$\mu = \tau \frac{\delta}{v}$$
$$= (0.00125)(0.07)/6.0$$
$$= 0.000015 \ \text{lb-s/ft}^2 \quad \text{(Answer)}$$

The absolute viscosity found in Example 2-1 corresponds to crude oil. To find kinematic viscosity, divide by the density of crude oil, 1.66 slugs/ft^3. Therefore, the kinematic viscosity for Example 2-1 is $0.000015/1.66 = 9 \times 10^{-6}$ ft^2/s.

PROBLEMS

1. What is the weight of 1.0 cubic foot of water?

2. What is the density of water?

3. A can measuring 4.0 inches in diameter and 6.0 inches high is filled with a liquid. If the net weight is 2.0 pounds, what is the specific weight of the liquid?

4. A container measuring 10.0 cm by 20.0 cm is filled with a liquid. If the net weight is 450 N, what is the specific weight of the liquid?

5. What is the specific gravity of SAE 30 oil, which has a specific weight of 57.4 lb/ft^3?

6. What is the specific gravity of kerosene, which has a specific weight of 7.85×10^3 N/m^3?

7. Two capillary tubes are placed vertically in an open container of water. One tube has a diameter of 2.0 mm, and the other a diameter of 1.0 inch. In which tube will the water rise higher?

8. A sliding plate viscometer, as shown below, is used to measure the viscosity of a fluid. The plate area is 0.75 ft^2. A force of 1.5×10^{-4} lb moves the upper plate at a velocity of 10.0 ft/s. What is the absolute viscosity?

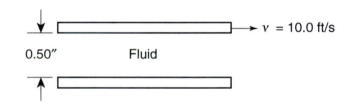

9. A liquid has an absolute viscosity of 2.2×10^{-5} lb-s/ft^2. It weighs 45 lb/ft^3. What is its kinematic viscosity?

10. A liquid has an absolute viscosity of 2.4×10^{-3} N-s/m^2. It weighs 7.85×10^3 N/m^3. What is its kinematic viscosity?

FURTHER READING

Brater, E. F., and King, H. (1996). *Handbook of Hydraulics* (7th ed.). New York: McGraw-Hill.

Douglas, J. F. (2000). *Fluid Mechanics*. Englewood Cliffs, NJ: Prentice Hall.

Franzini, J. B., and Finnemore, E. J. (1997). *Fluid Mechanics with Engineering Applications* (9th ed.). New York: McGraw-Hill.

Lindburg, M. R. (1995). *E.I.T. Review Manual*. Belmont, CA: Professional Publications.

Massey, B. (2005). *Mechanics of Fluids*. Boca Raton, FL: CRC Press.

Mott, R. L. (1994). *Applied Fluid Mechanics* (4th ed.). Englewood Cliffs, NJ: Prentice Hall.

Munson, B. R. (2005). *Fundamentals of Fluid Mechanics*. New York: John Wiley & Sons.

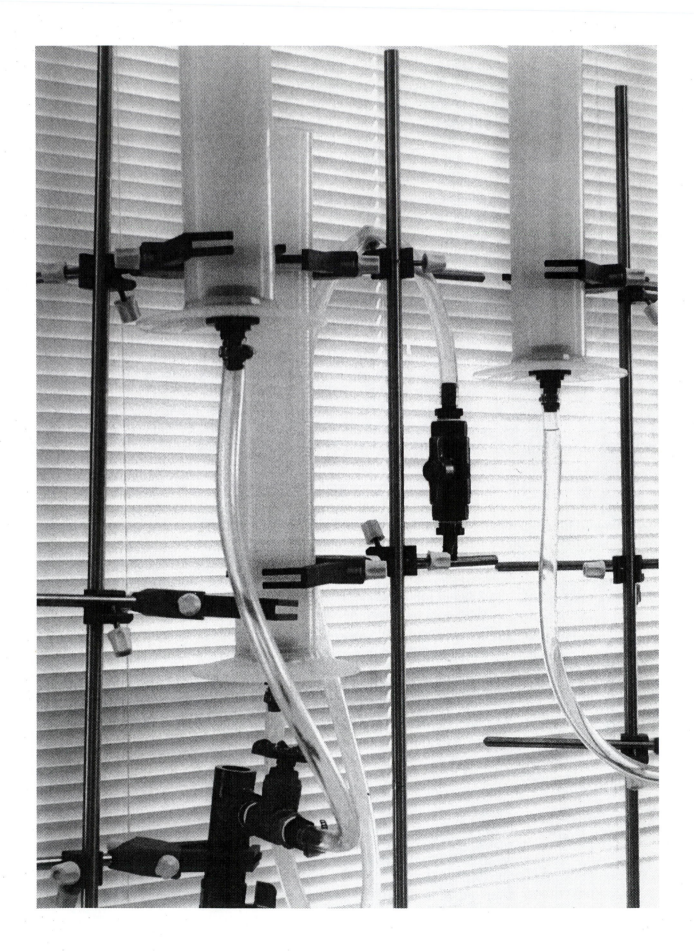

FUNDAMENTAL HYDROSTATICS

The term **hydrostatics** refers to the study of water at rest. Fundamental to the study is the concept of pressure resulting from the weight of water.

In this chapter, you will learn how to quantify the pressure exerted by water on an imaginary submerged surface or on container walls. You will also learn about the pressure exerted by water on a submerged object, giving rise to the concept of buoyancy.

OBJECTIVES

After completing this chapter, the reader should be able to:

- Compute pressure in water at various depths
- Compute the pressure on a submerged vertical surface
- Compute the pressure on a submerged inclined surface
- Compute the pressure on a submerged curved surface
- Compute the buoyant force on a submerged object

3.1 HYDROSTATIC PRESSURE

Pressure is defined as force per unit area. Thus,

$$p = \frac{F}{A}$$

(3-1)

where p = pressure, pounds/ft^2 (N/m^2)
F = force, pounds (newtons)
A = area, ft^2 (m^2)

Water in a container exerts pressure at a right angle, or normal, to the container walls or on any submerged surface. This phenomenon, which is unique to fluids, is due to the inability of water molecules to resist shear stress. Thus, on any submerged surface, only normal force (pressure) and no shear force exists. In a solid, both normal and shear forces exist at any surface due to the nature of the molecules composing the solid.

As a consequence of the absence of shear force in water, the pressure at any point in water at rest is equal in all directions. Figure 3-1 shows infinitesimal elements of water in various shapes. In each case, the pressure acting on the element's surface has the same magnitude.

To compute the pressure at any point in a vessel of water, we can use Equation 3-1, but we must find a way to evaluate F, the force. To determine the force, consider an imaginary horizontal surface or plane located a distance z below the surface, as shown in Figure 3-2.

The weight of a vertical column of water above the surface equals the force exerted there. But the weight, W, of water is expressed as

$$W = \gamma V$$

where γ = specific weight, lb/ft³ (N/m³)   and
V = volume, ft³ (m³).

The specific weight of water is taken as 62.4 lb/ft³ (9.81 kN/m³). The volume, V, is equal to the area of the base times the height, or $V = Az$. Therefore, the pressure can be written as

$$p = \gamma \frac{Az}{A} = \gamma z \qquad (3\text{-}2)$$

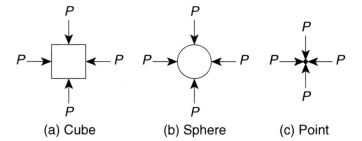

(a) Cube   (b) Sphere   (c) Point

FIGURE 3-1   For each of the infinitesimal elements of water at rest, the pressure acting on each surface in any direction has the same magnitude.

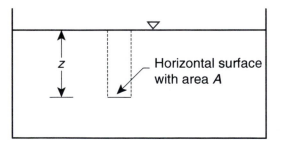

FIGURE 3-2   Pressure at a depth z in a volume of water.

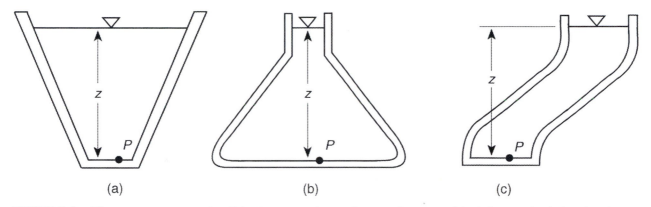

FIGURE 3-3   The pressure at point *P* is the same in each container provided the vertical depth *z* is the same.

Therefore, water pressure at a depth, *z*, below a free surface is computed by Equation 3-2. It is also important to note that the pressure at any given depth depends on only the depth, and not the volume or shape, of the container. Thus, the pressures are equal in the three examples in Figure 3-3.

In Figure 3-3(c), the pressure at point *P* is equal to γz even though there is not an actual vertical column of water from *P* to the surface. The pressure is the same *as though* a vertical column of water with height *z* rested on it.

Example 3-1

Problem

A reservoir of water is connected to a pipe, as shown in the accompanying figure. The pipe valve is closed, preventing any flow. Find the water pressure in the center of the pipe at the valve. The elevation of the reservoir surface is 550.0 feet (NGVD) and that of the center of the valve is 525.0 feet (NGVD).

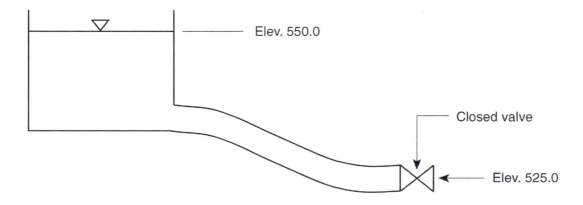

Note: All elevations used in this text are in the National Geodetic Vertical Datum (NGVD), which is given in feet.

Solution

The vertical depth from the surface to the point in question is the difference in elevations:

$$z = 550.0 - 525.0$$
$$= 25.0 \text{ ft}$$

Therefore, using Equation 3-2, we have

$$p = \gamma z$$
$$= (62.4)(25.0)$$
$$= 1560 \text{ lb/ft}^2 \quad \text{(Answer)}$$

The pressure that was discussed above is called **gauge** pressure, meaning pressure in excess of atmospheric pressure. At the surface of water exposed to the atmosphere (called a **free surface**), the actual pressure is equal to that exerted by the atmosphere and increases with depth below the surface. However, by convention, gauge pressure assumes zero magnitude at the surface. All references to pressure in this text will be to gauge pressure as defined above.

3.2 PRESSURE ON PLANE SURFACES

Consider a horizontal plane surface located a depth, z, below the free surface of a container of water. The pressure acts perpendicular to the plane and has a magnitude γz. This can be depicted as a uniformly distributed load, as shown in Figure 3-4.

Keep in mind when interpreting Figure 3-4(a) that both the horizontal plane surface and the pressure distribution extend out of the plane of the paper. Thus, the pressure distribution forms a three-dimensional outline, as depicted in Figure 3-4(b).

The resultant force, F_R, acting on the plane surface is equal to pA where $A = lw$ is the area of the surface. The resultant force acts at the centroid of the pressure

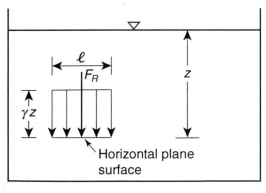

(a) Orthographic View

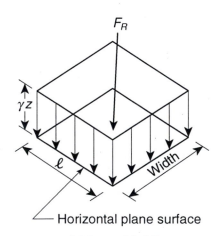

(b) Isometric View

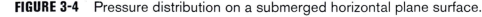

FIGURE 3-4 Pressure distribution on a submerged horizontal plane surface.

distribution. The location of the resultant force is referred to as the **center of pressure**. Thus,

$$F_R = pA$$
$$F_R = \gamma z l w \tag{3-3}$$

where z = depth below surface, ft (m)
l = length of surface, ft (m)
w = width of surface, ft (m)

Notice that Equation 3-3 can be interpreted as follows: The resultant force equals the "area" of the pressure distribution diagram multiplied by the width of the horizontal surface, w. The pressure distribution diagram shown in Figure 3-4(a) has a height γz and a length l and therefore an "area" equal to $\gamma z l$. The "area" described here is only that of the pressure distribution diagram and not a physical entity.

Vertical Surface

If the submerged plane surface is vertical, the pressure distribution takes on one of the shapes shown in Figure 3-5. In this case, the magnitude increases with depth below the free surface. If the vertical plane extends to the free surface, as shown in Figure 3-5(a), the pressure distribution is triangular. If it starts some distance below the free surface, as shown in Figure 3-5(b), the pressure distribution is trapezoidal.

The vertical surfaces shown in Figure 3-5 project out of the plane of the paper just as does the surface in Figure 3-4. Thus, the surface is depicted as a vertical line, and the three-dimensional pressure distribution appears as a two-dimensional shape. For ease of analysis, we will assume that the width is uniform and equal to w.

The centers of pressure and the resultant forces for the surfaces depicted in Figure 3-5 are shown in Figure 3-6. For each case, (a) and (b), the magnitude of the resultant force is equal to the area of the pressure distribution multiplied by w, the width of the surface. Thus, for case (a),

$$F_R = \tfrac{1}{2}(z)(\gamma z)w = \frac{\gamma z^2}{2}w \tag{3-4}$$

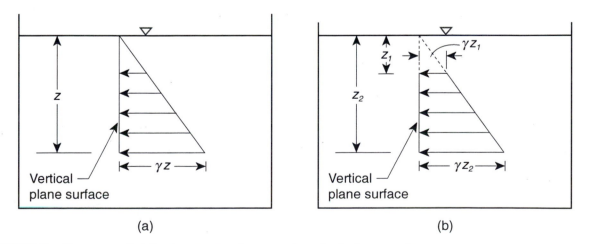

(a)   (b)

FIGURE 3-5   Pressure distribution on a submerged vertical plane surface.

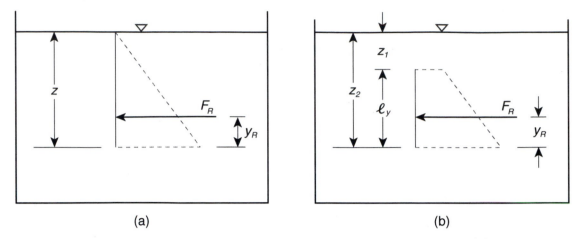

(a)   (b)

FIGURE 3-6 Resultant force and center of pressure for a vertical plane surface, (a) intersecting the surface and (b) completely submerged.

The location of F_R is the center of pressure, which is the centroid of the triangular pressure distribution. Thus,

$$y_R = \frac{1}{3}z \tag{3-5}$$

For case (b),

$$F_R = \left[\frac{\gamma z_1 + \gamma z_2}{2}\right]l_y w = \frac{\gamma l_y}{2}w(z_1 + z_2) \tag{3-6}$$

where $ly = z_2 - z_1$ is the height of the pressure distribution. The location of F_R is determined as the centroid of a trapezoid. Thus,

$$y_R = \frac{l_y}{3}\left[\frac{2z_1 + z_2}{z_1 + z_2}\right] \tag{3-7}$$

Example 3-2

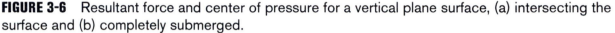

Problem

A vertical surface with height 2.5 feet and width 2.0 feet is submerged 1.0 foot below the water surface. Find the resultant hydrostatic force and the location of the center of pressure.

Solution

Resultant force is computed from Equation 3-6:

$$F_R = \frac{(62.4)(2.5)(2.0)}{2}(1 + 3.5)$$
$$= 702 \text{ lb} \quad \text{(Answer)}$$

The location of the center of pressure is computed from Equation 3-7:

$$y_R = \frac{2.5}{3}\left[\frac{(2)(1)+3.5}{1+3.5}\right]$$
$$= 1.02 \text{ ft} \quad (\text{Answer})$$

Inclined Surface

If the submerged plane surface is inclined, the pressure is perpendicular to the surface, and the pressure distribution is as shown in Figure 3-7.

To derive the resultant force and its location at the center of pressure, we will consider three forces acting on the inclined surface AB, as shown in Figure 3-8:

1. F_H, the resultant force acting on the horizontal projection, BC
2. F_V, the resultant force acting on the vertical projection, AC
3. W, the weight of water occupying the triangular space ABC between the surface and its projections

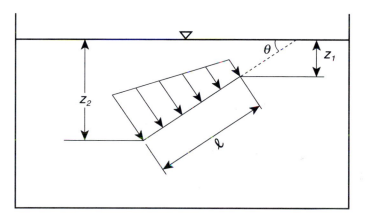

FIGURE 3-7   Pressure distribution on a submerged inclined plane surface.

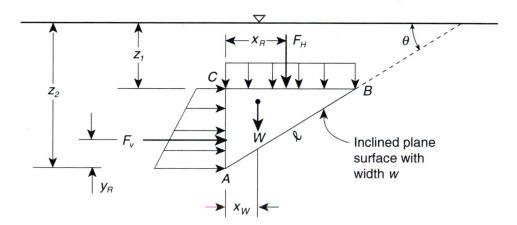

FIGURE 3-8   Free body diagram used to compute pressure on a submerged inclined plane surface.

The value of F_H is computed from Equation 3-3. Thus,

$$F_H = \gamma z_1 wl \cos \theta \tag{3-8}$$

where l is the length of the inclined plane surface. Note that $l_y = l \sin \theta$. Why?

The value of F_V is computed from Equation 3-6. Thus,

$$F_V = \frac{\gamma l_y w}{2}(z_1 + z_2)$$

which can also be written as

$$F_V = \frac{\gamma w}{2}(z_1 + z_2)l \sin \theta \tag{3-9}$$

The value of W is

$$W = \gamma V = \gamma(\tfrac{1}{2}l \sin \theta \, l \cos \theta)w$$
$$= \frac{\gamma w l^2}{2} \sin \theta \cos \theta \tag{3-10}$$

To determine the resultant force F_R, at the center of pressure, find the vector sum of F_H, F_V, and W. Thus, the x-component of F_R is F_V, and the y-component is $F_H + W$. Accordingly, the magnitude of F_R is

$$F_R = \sqrt{F_V^2 + (F_H + W)^2} \tag{3-11}$$

The location of F_R is determined by summing the moments of all forces at A. Thus, using dimensions in Figure 3-8, we have

$$\sum M_A = -F_V(y_R) - W(x_W) - F_H(x_R)$$

But the sum of moments at A can also be expressed in terms of F_R from Figure 3-9 as

$$\sum M_A = -F_R(l_R)$$

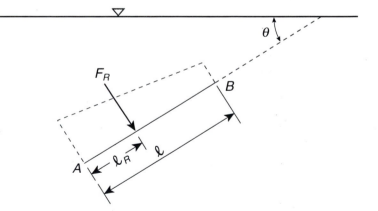

FIGURE 3-9   Resultant force and center of pressure for a submerged inclined plane surface.

where l_R is the location of the center of pressure. Equating the moments yields

$$F_R(l_R) = F_V(y_R) + W(x_W) + F_H(x_R)$$

or

$$l_R = \frac{1}{F_R}\left[F_V(y_R) + W(x_W) + F_H(x_R)\right] \tag{3-12}$$

Example 3-3

Problem

A plane surface with length 4.0 ft and width 3.0 ft is inclined 30 degrees with the horizontal and is submerged 1.0 ft below the free surface of a container of water. Find the resultant hydrostatic force and the location of the center of pressure.

Solution

First, compute the forces F_H, F_V, and W using Equations 3-8, 3-9, and 3-10, respectively:

$$F_H = (62.4)(1.0)(3.0)(4.0)\cos 30° = 648 \text{ lb}$$

$$F_V = \frac{(62.4)(3.0)}{2}(1+3)(4.0)\sin 30° = 749 \text{ lb}$$

$$W = \frac{(62.4)(3.0)(4.0)^2}{2}\sin 30° \cos 30° = 648 \text{ lb}$$

Next, compute z_2:

$$z_2 = z_1 + l\sin 30° = 3.0 \text{ ft}$$

Next, compute the locations of F_H, F_V, and W. The location of F_H is x_R, which is one-half the horizontal projection of the inclined surface. Thus,

$$x_R = \tfrac{1}{2}\, l\cos 30° = 1.73 \text{ ft}$$

The location of F_V is y_R, which is computed by using Equation 3-7. Thus,

$$y_R = \frac{4.0}{3}\left[\frac{2(1)+3}{1+3}\right] = 1.67 \text{ ft}$$

The location of W is x_W, which is one-third the horizontal projection of the inclined surface. Thus,

$$x_W = \frac{1}{3}(4.0)\cos 30° = 1.15 \text{ ft}$$

Next, compute F_R using Equation 3-11. Thus,

$$F_R = \sqrt{749^2 + (648+648)^2}$$
$$= 1497 \text{ lb} \quad \text{(Answer)}$$

Finally, compute l_R, the location of F_R, using Equation 3-12. Thus,

$$l_R = \frac{1}{1497}[749(1.67) + 648(1.15) + 648(1.73)]$$

$$= 2.08 \text{ ft} \quad \text{(Answer)}$$

3.3   PRESSURE ON CURVED SURFACES

Hydrostatic pressure on a submerged curved surface conforms to the general rules developed in the previous section in that pressure is perpendicular to the surface at all points and that the center of pressure is located at the centroid of the pressure distribution. However, computation of these parameters is made more difficult by the geometry that describes the forces. The typical pressure distribution for a circular curved surface is shown in Figure 3-10. Note that as in the previous sections, we are considering a simplified case of submerged curved surfaces: one in which the surface is perpendicular to the paper. The surface may be oriented either convex or concave with respect to the water surface.

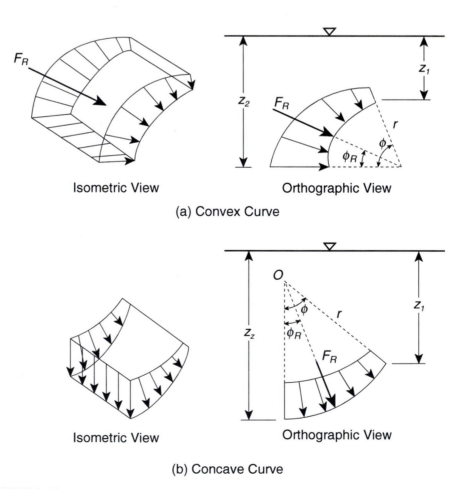

FIGURE 3-10   Pressure distribution on a submerged curved surface.

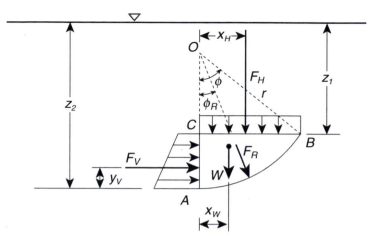

FIGURE 3-11   Resultant force and center of pressure for a submerged curved surface.

To compute the resultant force and location of the center of pressure, refer to Figure 3-11. The curved surface AB shown in Figure 3-11 has a constant radius, r, and constant width, w, projected out of the paper. The line OA is vertical. The three forces acting on the surface F_H, F_V, and W are defined as in the "inclined surface" section in Section 3.2.

The force F_H is the resultant of the pressure acting on the horizontal projection BC of the curved surface. F_H is located at the centroid of the distribution, which is the center of line BC. The force F_V is the resultant of the pressure acting on the vertical projection AC of the curved surface. F_V is located at the centroid of the pressure distribution. The force W is the weight of the wedge of water occupying the volume within ABC. W is located at the centroid of ABC.

The force F_H is the area of the horizontal pressure distribution multiplied by the width, w. Thus,

$$F_H = \gamma z_1 w r \sin \phi \qquad (3\text{-}13)$$

The force F_V is the area of the vertical pressure distribution multiplied by the width, w, which can be computed using Equation 3-9 or by an alternate equation using the geometry of the curved surface. The alternate to Equation 3-9 is

$$F_V = \frac{\gamma w}{2}(z_1 + z_2)(r - r \cos \phi) \qquad (3\text{-}14)$$

The value of W is γV where V is the volume of the wedge of water. Thus,

$$W = \gamma V = \gamma w \left[\frac{\phi}{360} \pi r^2 - \frac{r^2}{2} \sin \phi \cos \phi \right] \qquad (3\text{-}15)$$

where w = width of the surface projecting out of the paper.

To determine the resultant force F_R, find the vector sum of F_H, F_V, and W. The magnitude of F_R is computed from Equation 3-11.

The location of F_R is determined by summing the moments of all forces at A. Thus, using dimensions in Figure 3-11, we have

$$\sum M_A = -F_V(y_V) - W(x_W) - F_H(x_H)$$

But the sum of the moments at A can also be expressed in terms of F_R from Figure 3-10 as

$$\sum M_A = -F_R(r \sin \phi_R)$$

where ϕ_R is the angle made by F_R with the vertical. Equating the moments yields

$$F_R(r \sin \phi_R) = F_V(y_V) + W(x_W) + F_H(x_H)$$

or

$$\phi_R = \sin^{-1}\left\{\frac{1}{rF_R}\left[F_V(y_V) + W(x_w) + F_H(x_H)\right]\right\} \tag{3-16}$$

The dimensions y_V and x_H are the locations of the centroids of the respective force distributions, and x_W is the location of the centroid of the wedge of water ABC over the surface.

Example 3-4

Problem

Find the resultant hydrostatic force and location of center of pressure on the circular portion, AB, of the tank shown here. The tank has a width of 8.0 ft projecting out of the paper.

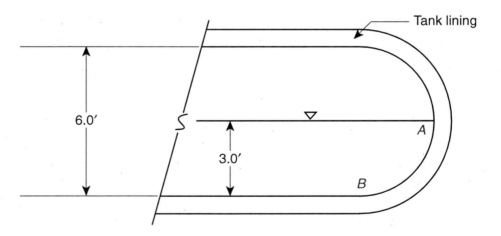

Solution

From the geometry of the problem, the depth to the bottom of the surface, z_2, is 3.0 ft. Also, $z_1 = 0$, $r = 3.0$ ft, and $\phi = 90°$. Forces F_H, F_V, and W are computed by using Equations 3-13, 3-14, and 3-15, respectively:

$$F_H = 0$$

$$F_V = \frac{(62.4)(8.0)}{2}(3.0)(3.0 - 3.0 \cos 90°) = 2246 \text{ lb}$$

$$W = (62.4)(8.0)\left[\frac{90}{360}\pi(3.0)^2 - \frac{(3.0)^2}{2}\sin 90° \cos 90°\right] = 3529 \text{ lb}$$

Next, compute x_H, y_V, and x_W, the locations of the forces:

$$x_H = 0$$

$$y_V = \frac{1}{3}(3.0) = 1.0 \text{ ft}$$

$$x_W = \frac{4(3.0)}{3\pi} = 1.27 \text{ ft}$$

Note: The distance x_W in this case is based on the centroid of a quarter circle, as shown below.

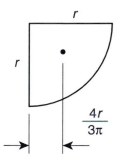

Next, compute F_R from Equation 3-11:

$$F_R = \sqrt{F_V{}^2 + (F_H + W)^2}$$

$$= \sqrt{2246^2 = 3529^2}$$

$$= 4183 \text{ lb}\quad (\text{Answer})$$

Finally, compute ϕ_R using Equation 13-16:

$$\phi_R = \sin^{-1}\left\{\frac{1}{(3.0)(4183)}[(2246)(1.0) + (3529)(1.27) + 0]\right\}$$

$$= 32.4°\quad (\text{Answer})$$

An alternate procedure to locate F_R is to compute the angle of inclination φ_R by simple vector analysis. Since the x-component of F_R is F_V and the y-component is $F_H + W$, the angle between F_R and the vertical axis is

$$\varphi_R = \tan^{-1}\frac{F_V}{F_H + W}$$

$$\varphi_R = \tan^{-1}\frac{2246}{3529}$$

$$\varphi_R = 32.5°\quad (\text{Answer})$$

Note: This procedure is applicable only to curved surfaces because for curved surfaces, the angle φ_R determines the exact position of F_R and for plane surfaces it does not.

3.4. MEASURING PRESSURE

Several devices for the measurement of hydrostatic pressure have been developed over the years. These range from simple devices such as the piezometer and manometer to more complex devices such as the bourdon gauge and the electrical strain gauge. Some of these are described below.

Piezometer

A **piezometer** is a simple tube connected to a body of water with its other end open to the atmosphere, as shown in Figure 3-12. Water enters the piezometer and rises until it reaches a height proportional to the pressure. (A piezometer does not measure pressure directly in lb/in² but rather measures a related quantity called pressure head, a term defined in Chapter 4.) As shown in Figure 3-13, in a static hydraulic system, a piezometer placed at point *B* shows a level equal to the pond level at point *A*. In a dynamic system, a piezometer placed at point *B* with water in motion shows a level less than the pond level at point *A*. This drop in pressure due to the movement of water and the application of piezometers to pressure measurement will be developed in Chapter 4.

To construct a piezometer correctly, its length must be sufficient to accommodate the anticipated rise of water without overflow. Also, the diameter should be sufficiently large to avoid distortion due to adhesion to the tube walls. Usually, a diameter of 0.5 in (12 mm) is sufficient. In addition, if the piezometer will measure water moving in a pipe, the interface between the piezometer tube and the pipe wall should be fashioned carefully to avoid imposing any effect on the water stream. This usually means placing the tube perpendicular to the pipe and making the interface flush.

Manometer

When the water pressure to be measured is relatively high, a piezometer may be inadequate, and a manometer must be used. A high pressure would require a long piezometer tube, but a manometer solves this problem by the use of a heavy liquid such as mercury.

As is shown in Figure 3-14, water pressure in the pipe pushes water up tube *AB*, which in turn forces mercury up tube *CD*. The imbalance of mercury between

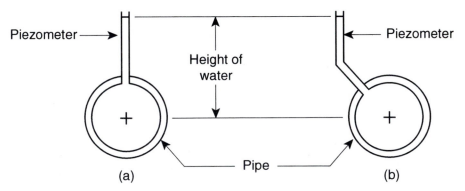

FIGURE 3-12 Piezometer used to measure water pressure in a pipe. In both (a) and (b), if the pressures are equal, the water levels in the piezometers are equal.

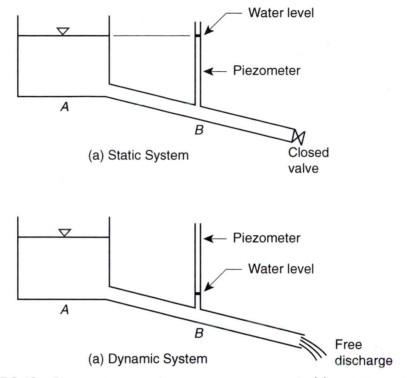

(a) Static System

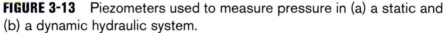

(a) Dynamic System

FIGURE 3-13   Piezometers used to measure pressure in (a) a static and (b) a dynamic hydraulic system.

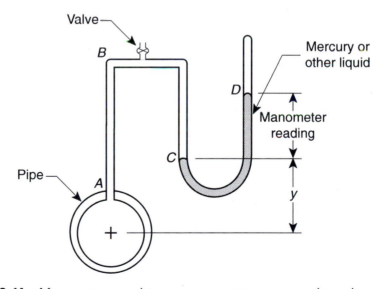

FIGURE 3-14   Manometer used to measure water pressure in a pipe.

points C and D is a measure of the force causing the imbalance. Thus, the vertical distance between C and D is the manometer reading, which together with the distance y is used to find the pipe water pressure.

A valve placed at the high point of the tube assembly is used to relieve any air trapped in the water.

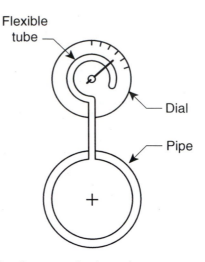

FIGURE 3-15   Schematic diagram of a bourdon gauge.

Manometers can also be used to measure negative pressure (vacuum) in a water pipe. In this case, the mercury level at C would be higher than the level at D. Negative pressure typically is encountered in association with pumping.

Mechanical Gauges

Water pressure is conveniently measured directly in lb/in^2 by use of mechanical gauges such as the bourdon gauge shown schematically in Figure 3-15. In the bourdon gauge, a thin, curved tube connected to the water to be measured deflects under the influence of water pressure and causes a dial to turn. The dial is then calibrated in lb/in^2. Bourdon gauges can also be calibrated to read negative pressure.

An electrical strain gauge is also used to measure water pressure. In this case, the water to be measured is allowed to impinge upon a flexible diaphragm that moves under the influence of changing pressure. The movement is sensed by an electrical strain gauge that is connected to an amplifier and numerical display and/or chart recorder.

3.5. BUOYANCY

Buoyancy is the uplifting force exerted by water on a submerged solid object. Common experience tells us that a heavy rock seems lighter when held under water. This is due to the buoyancy of water.

To understand buoyancy, consider the object shown in Figure 3-16. Essentially, three vertical forces act on the object: pressure downward by the water above the object, pressure upward by the water below the object, and gravity, or the weight of the object. On the upper surface of the object (line BEC), the vertical component of the force is equal to the weight of the volume of water above the object, volume $ABECD$ in Figure 3-16(a). On the lower surface (line BFC), the vertical component of force is equal to the weight of the volume of water above the bottom surface of the object, volume $ABFCD$ in Figure 3-16(b). This is

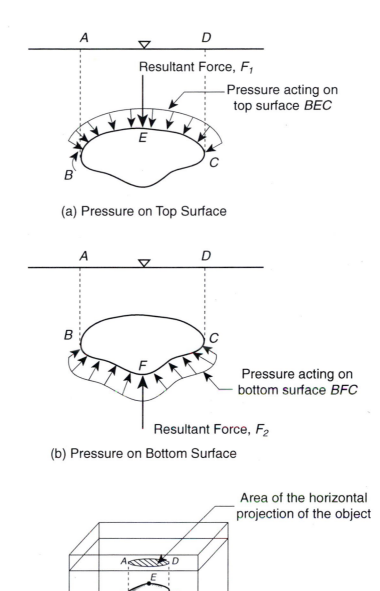

(a) Pressure on Top Surface

(b) Pressure on Bottom Surface

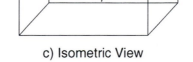

c) Isometric View

FIGURE 3-16   Pressure diagrams for a submerged object.

the imaginary volume of water that would exist if only the bottom surface of the object was present and not the actual object. It follows the rule explained in Section 3.1: Pressure at any point is determined by the depth of the point, whether or not a physical column of water is present directly above, and pressure at any point is equal in all directions.

Since the volume of water above the bottom surface is greater than the volume of water above the top surface, the force pushing up on the object is greater than the force pushing down on the object. The buoyant force, F_B, is the difference between these two forces and is equal to the weight of water that would occupy the space occupied by the object. Thus,

F_1 = weight of water volume $ABECD$
F_2 = weight of water volume $ABFCD$

and

$F_B = F_2 - F_1$
   = weight of water volume $BECF$

If F_B is greater than the weight of the object, the object will rise to the surface of the water. If F_B is less than the weight of the object, the object will sink to the bottom.

Example 3-5

Problem

A 50-pound plastic ball with diameter 2.0 feet is placed in water. What is the buoyant force acting on the ball? Will the ball float or sink?

Solution

The buoyant force is equal to the weight of water displaced by the ball. Thus,

$$F_B = \gamma V$$

where V is the volume of the ball.

$$V = \frac{4}{3}\pi r^3$$
$$= \frac{4}{3}\pi(1)^3$$
$$= 4.19 \text{ ft}^3$$

Therefore,

$$F_B = (62.4)(4.19)$$
$$= 261 \text{ lb} \quad \text{(Answer)}$$

The buoyant force on the ball is 261 pounds. Since the weight of the ball is less than the buoyant force, the ball will float.   (Answer)

PROBLEMS

1. What is the pressure at the bottom of Sunfish Pond, which has a depth of 350 feet?
2. A swimming pool has depths of 4.0 feet and 12.0 feet at the shallow and deep ends, respectively. Find the pressure in lb/ft^2 at each end.
3. A reservoir of water is connected to a 12-inch-diameter pipe 50 feet long and capped at the end. The water surface elevation of the reservoir is 82.5 feet, and

the capped end of the pipe is at elevation 38.0 feet. Find the pressure in psf at the capped end of the pipe.

4. A cylindrical container of water measures 1.75 feet in diameter. The water depth is 8.50 feet. Find the pressure on the bottom surface.

5. In the swimming pool shown below determine the resultant hydrostatic force and locate the center of pressure on surface *AB*. Width = 10.0 ft.

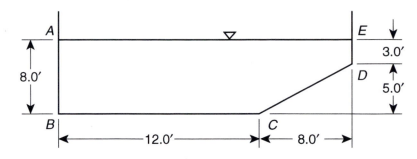

6. In the swimming pool shown in problem 5, determine the resultant hydrostatic force and locate the center of pressure on surface *BC*.

7. In the swimming pool shown in problem 5, determine the resultant hydrostatic force and locate the center of pressure on surface *CD*.

8. Determine the resultant hydrostatic force and locate the center of pressure on the face of the dam shown below.

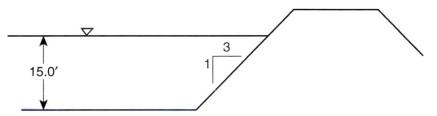

9. For the 2.5-foot by 4.0-foot sluice gate shown below, calculate the resultant hydrostatic force, and locate the center of pressure.

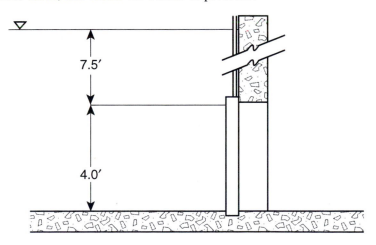

10. Shown below is a portion of a water tank with width 16 feet. Find the resultant hydrostatic force, and locate the center of pressure for surface *AB*.

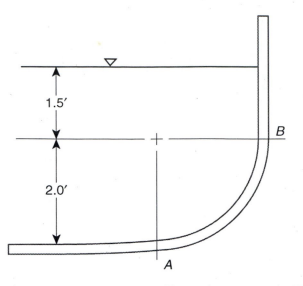

11. Shown below is a concrete ogee-type spillway drawn to scale. The crest length (projecting out of the paper) is 14.0 feet. Using graphical techniques, determine the approximate resultant hydrostatic force on the structure and the location of the center of pressure.

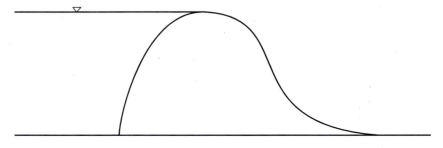

Scale: 1" = 5'

12. Calculate the resultant hydrostatic force and location of the center of pressure on the circular gate shown below.

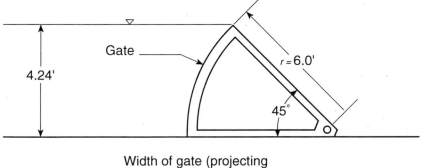

Width of gate (projecting
out of paper) is 8.0 feet.

13. A 0.75-pound can of soda with dimensions 2½ inches by 5 inches is placed in water.

(a) What is the buoyant force acting on the can?

(b) Will the can float or sink?

14. A plastic engineer's scale weighing ¼ pound slips into a reservoir. The scale has a triangular section with each side 1.0 inch and a length of 12.75 inches. Will the scale float or sink?

15. A concrete chamber measuring 8.0 feet by 8.0 feet by 6.0 feet is placed in water. If the chamber weighs 10 tons, will it float or sink?

FURTHER READING

Brater, E. F., and King, H. (1996). *Handbook of Hydraulics* (7th ed.). New York: McGraw-Hill.

Franzini, J. B., and Finnemore, E. J. (1997). *Fluid Mechanics with Engineering Applications* (9th ed.). New York: McGraw-Hill.

Hita, C. E., and Hwang, N. H. C. (1987). *Hydraulic Engineering Systems* (2nd ed.). Englewood Cliffs, NJ: Prentice Hall.

Merritt, F. S. (2004). *Standard Handbook for Civil Engineers* (5th ed.). New York: McGraw-Hill.

Prasuhn, A. L. (1987). *Fundamentals of Hydraulic Engineering*. New York: Holt, Rinehart and Winston.

Simon, A. L., and Korom, S. F. (1997). *Hydraulics* (4th ed.). Englewood Cliffs, NJ: Prentice Hall.

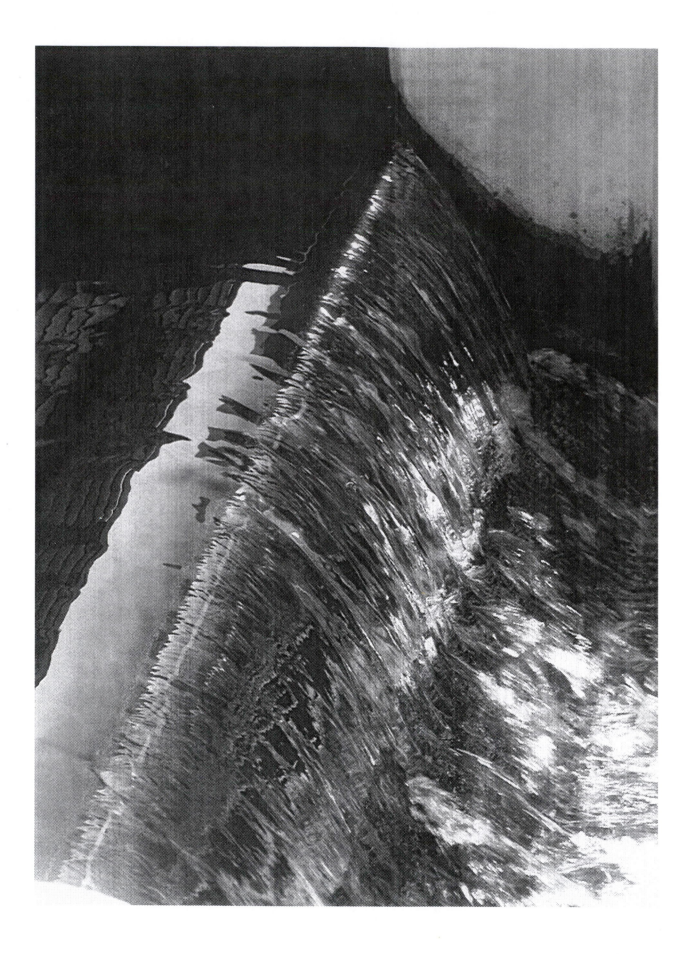

FUNDAMENTAL HYDRODYNAMICS

The term *hydrodynamics* refers to the study of water in motion. The term *hydrokinetics* also is used for this topic. Fundamental to the study are the concepts of conservation of mass and conservation of energy.

In this chapter, you will learn how to describe mathematically the flow of water from a higher location to a lower location using the concepts mentioned above. Included will be an analysis of the Bernoulli equation. You will also learn about methods of measuring the flow of water.

OBJECTIVES

After completing this chapter, the reader should be able to:

- Recognize the types of water flow occurring in different circumstances
- Draw the energy grade line and hydraulic grade line for a simple hydraulic system
- Compute the discharge and velocity of water flowing in a simple hydraulic system
- Measure the discharge and velocity of water flowing in a simple hydraulic system

4.1 MOTION OF WATER

Water can move in all directions (such as when a glass of water is spilled on the floor), or it can be channeled into a prevailing direction such as flow in a pipe. When water flows in a conduit or pipe, all the particles tend to travel together en masse. However, as the particles move uniformly ahead, some move sideways and some move at different speeds. These deviations will be discussed further in Section 4.2. Nevertheless, despite the deviations, all particles of water flowing in a conduit travel generally in the same direction and generally at the same speed.

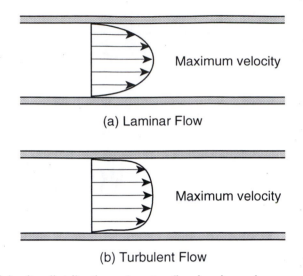

FIGURE 4-1   Velocity distribution of water flowing in a pipe.

Two fundamental parameters are used to describe the motion of water confined to a conduit: velocity, v, and discharge (or rate of flow), Q. Velocity describes the rate of change of position of the water particles as defined in fundamental mechanics. However, since all the particles flowing in a conduit move at slightly different speeds, the velocity of flow is the average speed of all the particles. Figure 4-1 shows a typical velocity distribution of water flowing in a pipe.

Velocity of flow, then, is defined as the average velocity of all water particles crossing an imaginary plane perpendicular to the direction of motion at a particular location along the conduit. Figure 4-2 illustrates the concept. The parameter v is expressed as feet per second (fps) or meters per second (m/s).

Discharge, or rate of flow, Q, describes the amount of water passing through an imaginary plane per unit time at a particular location along the conduit. The parameter Q is measured as volume per unit time, typically cubic feet per second (cfs) or cubic meters per second (m³/s).

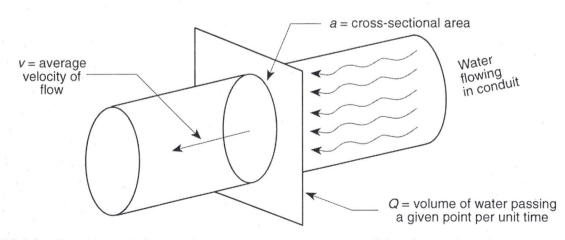

FIGURE 4-2   Definitions of Q, v, and a—parameters used in describing the motion of water.

Flow of water in a conduit may be compared to flow of traffic on a highway. If you sat by the side of the road with a stopwatch and counted the number of cars passing during a particular time, you would have the rate of flow, or the Q-value of the traffic. And if you could measure the speeds of all cars passing you at a given instant and then compute the average, you would have the velocity, or v-value, of the traffic.

4.2   TYPES OF FLOW

Flow of water in a conduit may be classified in various ways to help in the analysis of hydraulic problems. The most basic of these categories are expressed as pairs of opposites, as follows:

- Laminar flow versus turbulent flow
- Steady flow versus unsteady flow
- Uniform flow versus nonuniform flow

Another type of flow, subcritical flow versus supercritical flow, which is applicable to open channels, will be discussed in Chapter 6.

Laminar flow describes smooth flow of water with relatively low velocity. As the water flows in a conduit, it moves in parallel layers with no cross currents. As velocity increases, flow becomes rougher with pulsating crosscurrents within the conduit. This type of flow is called **turbulent flow**. Laminar and turbulent flows are illustrated in Figure 4-3.

The cross currents associated with turbulent flow result in a more uniform velocity distribution across the conduit cross section. Thus, maximum velocity is about 25 percent greater than average velocity, whereas for laminar flow, maximum velocity is twice the average velocity. This is illustrated graphically in Figure 4-1.

Another difference between these types of flow involves energy loss. As water moves along a conduit, energy is lost due to interactions between the water and the

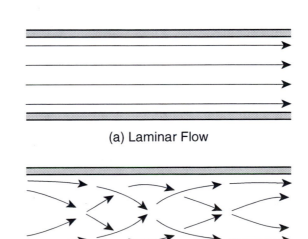

(a) Laminar Flow

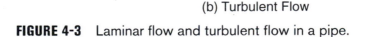

(b) Turbulent Flow

FIGURE 4-3   Laminar flow and turbulent flow in a pipe.

walls of the conduit and between water particles. In turbulent flow, the energy loss is much greater than in laminar flow.

A mathematical method of distinguishing between laminar and turbulent flows was developed by the researcher Osborn Reynolds in 1883. The so-called Reynolds number, N_R, a dimensionless parameter, is defined for circular pipes as

$$N_R = \frac{Dv}{\upsilon} \tag{4-1}$$

where D = inside diameter of pipe, ft (m)

v = average velocity, ft/s (m/s)

υ = viscosity of water, 1×10^{-5} ft^2/s (9.29×10^{-7} m^2/s)

Low values of N_R (up to 2000) describe smooth or laminar water flow, and large values of N_R (above 10,000) indicate turbulent flow. Most flow encountered in hydraulic engineering is turbulent flow.

Steady flow occurs when discharge is unchanged over time. **Unsteady flow** results from a relatively rapid change of discharge, such as the opening of a gate or closing of a valve. Another example of unsteady flow is the emptying of a tank, where the discharge from the tank is a function of the remaining depth.

Even the steadiest flow of water has some fluctuations associated with it. However, for practical purposes, steady flow is that in which the fluctuations are minor and tend to average to zero over time. Also, slowly varying flow, such as that encountered in streams, can usually be analyzed as steady flow. Hydraulic problems addressed in this text are limited to steady flow.

Before leaving the topic of unsteady flow, consider an example of this type of flow called **water hammer**. The phenomenon of water hammer is the extreme variations in water pressure within a pipe caused by an abrupt stoppage of flow. So if, for example, a valve is quickly closed, the pressure against the valve surges due to the collision of the moving water with the closed valve, sending fluctuations of pressure through the pipe due to the conservation of momentum. In this case, water hammer can be recognized by a loud hammering sound in the pipe.

Uniform flow occurs when the cross-sectional area of the conduit remains constant. This type of flow is easily illustrated by flow in pipes or uniformly shaped channels. However, examples of nonuniform flow abound, including a change in pipe size or flow from a reservoir into a channel.

4.3 ENERGY HEAD

In solving hydraulic problems, concepts of energy are used extensively. In Section 4.4, in fact, application of the law of conservation of energy will be presented in some detail. However, when referring to the energy of water, a unique problem is encountered: The fluid nature of water does not allow a given quantity to remain conveniently in place when it moves.

You can easily analyze the energy of a wood block as it slides down an inclined plane because the mass of the block remains intact throughout the slide. But moving water continually exchanges mass throughout its volume as it flows. Therefore, the concept of **head** or **energy head** is used to describe the energy of water in solving hydraulic problems. The term *head* refers to water energy per unit weight of the water and uses units of length, such as feet (meters). This can easily be shown by noting that energy can be expressed as foot-pounds (N-m). Thus,

$$\text{Head} = \frac{\text{Energy}}{\text{Weight}} = \frac{\text{ft-lb}}{\text{lb}} = \text{ft}$$

The concept of head is used to describe mechanical energy, that is, potential and kinetic, as well as energy loss, such as friction and turbulence. Thus, potential energy is described as potential energy head and has length units (not energy units); kinetic energy is described as kinetic energy head, called velocity head, and also has units of length.

It is important to remember that despite the use of head to describe energy, head is not truly energy but is energy per unit weight. As long as you do not lose sight of this distinction, you will find the concept of head a very useful one.

Following are descriptions of the most common forms of energy head:

- **Position head:** describes potential energy per unit weight of a mass of water due to the height of the water above some datum.
- **Pressure head:** describes potential energy per unit weight of a mass of water due to the pressure exerted from above.
- **Velocity head:** describes kinetic energy per unit weight of a mass of water due to kinetic energy resulting from its motion.
- **Head loss:** describes the loss of energy per unit weight of a mass of water due to friction and turbulence.

4.4   CONSERVATION LAWS

When water flows from a higher elevation to a lower elevation, it follows the laws of physics, like any other object. Some of those laws are expressed as conservation laws, such as conservation of energy, momentum, and mass.

We will consider conservation of energy and of mass in our study of hydrodynamics. Conservation of momentum is used to describe hydraulic phenomena beyond the scope of this book and will not be discussed.

Conservation of Energy

Conservation of energy is very important in describing the behavior of water undergoing steady flow. Neglecting friction, potential energy at the higher elevation gives way to kinetic energy at the lower elevation, resulting in the following equation familiar from physics:

$$U_1 + K_1 = U_2 + K_2 \tag{4-2}$$

where U_1 and K_1 represent potential and kinetic energies, respectively, at point 1, and U_2 and K_2 represent potential and kinetic energies respectively at point 2. However, what makes water different from the familiar objects studied in physics is water's inability to maintain a constant shape. Therefore, the energy equation must take on a new form to account for water's fluid nature.

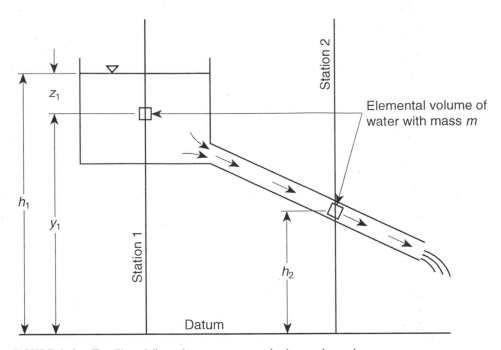

FIGURE 4-4   Profile of flow from a reservoir through a pipe.

To do this, we represent energy as energy head. Thus, Equation 4-2 becomes

$$\frac{U_1}{mg} + \frac{K_1}{mg} = \frac{U_2}{mg} + \frac{K_2}{mg} \tag{4-3}$$

where mg represents the weight of an elemental volume of water as shown in Figure 4-4 as it moves through a hydraulic system. Equations 4-2 and 4-3 are consistent with both English and SI units.

Station 1 and Station 2 are points along the profile of the hydraulic system shown in Figure 4-4. Mathematically, the system is taken as one-dimensional; that is, the energy is considered at any station along the profile as if the system flows in a straight line.

At Station 1, the elemental volume of water is at some depth z_1 below the surface and at some height y_1 above the arbitrary datum. The potential energy head U_1/mg is defined as

$$\frac{U_1}{mg} = \frac{mgy_1}{mg} + \frac{mgz_1}{mg} = y_1 + z_1 \tag{4-4}$$

where the second term, mgz_1/mg, is due to the pressure exerted on the elemental volume by the water above it. This term can be explained as the work in foot-pounds (N-m) required to raise the column of water a distance z_1 for each pound (newton) of the elemental water drop. Equation 4-4 may be expressed in either of the following alternate forms:

$$\frac{U_1}{mg} = y_1 + z_1 = h_1 \tag{4-4a}$$

$$\frac{U_1}{mg} = y_1 + z_1 = y_1 + \frac{p_1}{\gamma} \tag{4-4b}$$

Equation 4-4a follows from Figure 4-4, where you can see that $h_1 = y_1 + z_1$. Equation 4-4b follows from Equation 3-2. Potential energy head for a reservoir with a free surface generally is expressed as Equation 4-4a.

Kinetic energy head (velocity head) at Station 1 is

$$\frac{K_1}{mg} = \frac{\frac{1}{2}mv_1^2}{mg} = \frac{v_1^2}{2g}$$

where v_1 is the velocity of the water element.

At Station 2, the water is contained within a pipe and has no free surface, so for ease of mathematics, we consider the water element to be at the center of the pipe. Potential energy head at Station 2 is expressed in the form of Equation 4-4b,

$$\frac{U_2}{mg} = h_2 + \frac{p_2}{\gamma}$$

where h_2 is the height of the center of the pipe above the datum and p_2 is the pressure exerted by the reservoir above the point. The pressure head term, p_2/γ, can be thought of as the potential energy contained in each pound (newton) of water in the form of pressure. That is, the pressure at Station 2 has the ability to do p_2/γ foot-pounds (N-m) of work on each pound (newton) of water.

Kinetic energy head (velocity head) at Station 2 is

$$\frac{K_2}{mg} = \frac{\frac{1}{2}mv_2^2}{mg} = \frac{v_2^2}{2g}$$

where v_2 is the velocity of the water element at Station 2.

Now Equation 4-3 can be rewritten as

$$h_1 + \frac{v_1^2}{2g} = h_2 + \frac{p_2}{\gamma} + \frac{v_2^2}{2g} \tag{4-5}$$

where h_1 represents the vertical distance from the arbitrary datum to the free surface and $p_1 = 0$. Equation 4-5 is consistent with both English and SI units.

Equation 4-5 is the "energy equation" for an ideal condition in which Station 1 is in a reservoir with a free surface and no friction or other energy losses are present in the pipe.

Example 4-1

Problem

Determine the velocity of water at the outflow end of the pipe shown in Figure 4-4, neglecting friction if the elevation of the center of the pipe is 525 feet (NGVD), and the surface of the reservoir is 550 feet (NGVD).

Solution

Flow in the reservoir has such low velocity that it may be considered to be zero. Therefore, $v_1 = 0$ ft/s. Also, since the outflow has a free surface, the pressure term becomes zero. Substituting into Equation 4-5 then gives

$$550 + 0 = 525 + \frac{v_2^2}{(2)(32.2)}$$

$$v_2^2 = (550 - 525)(2)(32.2)$$

$$= 1610$$

$$v_2 = \sqrt{1610}$$

$$= 40.1 \text{ ft/s} \quad \text{(Answer)}$$

An interesting factor to notice in this example is that the velocity at point 2 does not depend on the size of the reservoir, only on its height. Likewise, the velocity does not depend on the slope of the pipe or the diameter of the pipe. Difference in elevation is the only determining factor.

In general, total energy head at any point along a frictionless pipe can be expressed as the right side of Equation 4-5, or

$$h + \frac{p}{\gamma} + \frac{v^2}{2g}$$

The principle proposed by Daniel Bernoulli in 1738 is that for a frictionless incompressible fluid, total energy head remains constant along the fluid stream. Thus,

$$h + \frac{p}{\gamma} + \frac{v^2}{2g} = \text{constant} \tag{4-6}$$

represents Bernoulli's Principle and is known as the Bernoulli equation. Bernoulli's equation can be expressed in the form of the energy equation (one version of which is Equation 4-5) by equating total energy at one station along a hydraulic system with another.

Because all terms of the energy equation are measured in feet (meters), a graphical representation of energy becomes convenient for hydraulic systems. Thus, the system described in Figure 4-4 can be redrawn as shown in Figure 4-5 to show two important lines used to analyze hydraulic systems.

The **energy grade line** (EGL) depicts total energy (total energy head) at all stations along the system. In this hypothetical case, the energy grade line is horizontal since total energy remains constant (no energy lost to friction). The **hydraulic grade line** (HGL) depicts potential energy (position plus pressure head) at all stations along the system. The vertical separation between the energy and hydraulic grade lines is the velocity head. Wherever there is a free surface, the hydraulic grade line is coincident with it. Why?

A close scrutiny of Figure 4-5 reveals that the hydraulic grade line is coincident with the free water surfaces at both ends. The energy grade line is coincident only with the free surface of the reservoir because, as we have seen, the reservoir velocity is negligible.

To describe the motion of water in the real world better, however, other factors such as friction must be accounted for. Since energy is lost from the system due to

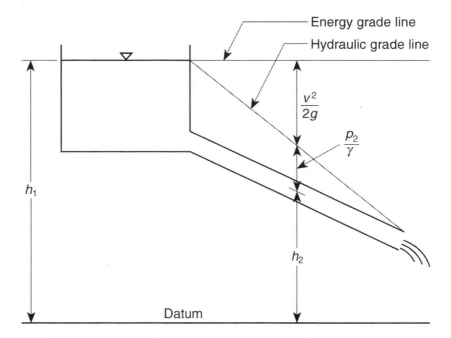

FIGURE 4-5   Energy grade line and hydraulic grade line for a hypothetical hydraulic system with no friction.

friction and other factors, the total energy, or head, at Station 2 will be less than the total energy, or head, at Station 1 by an amount equal to these losses. Thus, Equation 4-5 takes on the form

$$h_1 + \frac{v_1^2}{2g} = h_2 + \frac{p_2}{\gamma} + \frac{v_2^2}{2g} + h_l \tag{4-7}$$

where h_l represents the total amount of head lost to friction and other factors. Equation 4-7 therefore depicts a more realistic form of the energy equation for a hydraulic system with a free surface at Station 1. Figure 4-6 represents the hydraulic system shown in Figure 4-5 except with head losses accounted for.

Close scrutiny of Figure 4-6 reveals that energy losses take place in at least two ways. First, there is a small but sudden drop of the energy grade line at the point where water enters the pipe from the reservoir. This drop, called **entrance loss**, is due to a loss of energy caused by the turbulent motion of the water as it enters from the larger reservoir to the more restrictive pipe. Second, a constant drop in energy takes place along the entire length of the pipe. This drop is due to disruption of the flow caused by turbulence and by contact with the inside surface of the pipe and is called **friction loss**. Total head loss, h_l, is the sum of entrance loss, h_e, and friction loss, h_f. Thus, $h_l = h_e + h_f$.

Further scrutiny of Figure 4-6 indicates that the EGL and the HGL are parallel along the pipe except for a very short distance at the connection with the reservoir. This is because water traveling in a uniform pipe, after a short acceleration, reaches a terminal velocity much the same as an object dropped through the air.

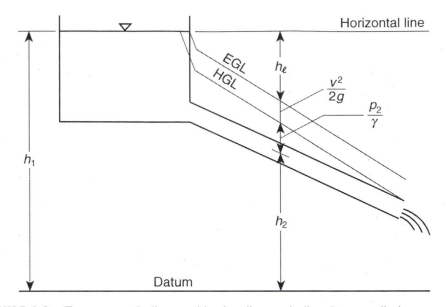

FIGURE 4-6   Energy grade line and hydraulic grade line for a realistic hydraulic system in which friction losses are included.

The amount of friction loss depends on the velocity of flow, as well as the roughness of the pipe. The expression for friction loss for turbulent flow in circular pipes is given by the Darcy-Weisbach formula as follows:

$$h_f = f \frac{Lv^2}{D2g} \tag{4-8}$$

where h_f = friction head loss, ft (m)
 f = friction factor
 L = length of pipe, ft (m)
 D = diameter of pipe, ft (m)
 v = average velocity, ft/s (m/s)
 g = acceleration due to gravity, 32.2 ft/s² (9.81 m/s²)

The dimensionless friction factor f is an empirically derived parameter depending upon a complex set of flow conditions. Figure 4-7 depicts the Moody diagram, which is a graphical solution for f depending on such values as viscosity υ, roughness ε, and Reynolds number N_R. Some selected values of ε are listed in Table 4-1.

Conservation of Mass

In addition to conservation of energy, flow of water is further described by conservation of mass, which asserts that mass is neither created nor destroyed. This means that for an incompressible fluid such as water flowing in a stream or pipe, the quantity of mass passing a cross section at Station 1 per unit time is equal to the quantity of mass passing a cross section at Station 2, or

$$a_1 v_1 = a_2 v_2 \tag{4-9}$$

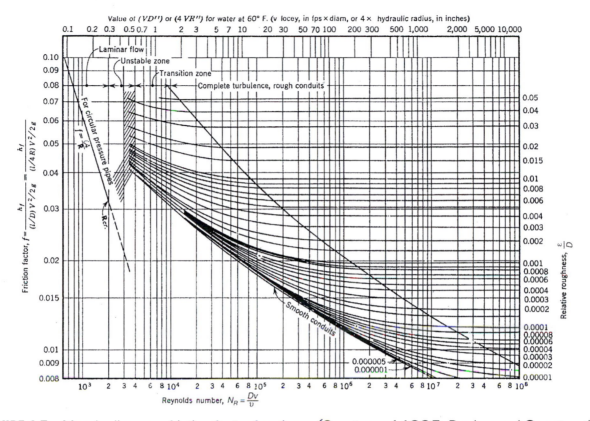

FIGURE 4-7 Moody diagram–friction factor for pipes. *(Courtesy of ASCE, Design and Construction of Sanitary and Storm Sewers.)*

TABLE 4-1 Typical Values of Roughness, ε

Pipe Material	ε (ft)
Riveted steel, few rivets	0.003
Riveted steel, many rivets	0.030
Concrete, finished surface	0.001
Concrete, rough surface	0.010
Wood-stave, smooth surface	0.0006
Wood-stave, rough surface	0.003
Cast iron, new	0.00085
Galvanized iron, new	0.00050
Drawn tubing, new	0.000005

Courtesy of ASCE, Design and Construction of Sanitary and Storm Sewers.

where a_1 = cross-sectional area at Station 1, ft^2 (m^2)
v_1 = average velocity at Station 1, ft/s (m/s)
a_2 = cross-sectional area at Station 2, ft^2 (m^2)
v_2 = average velocity at Station 2, ft/s (m/s).

Equation 4-9 is called the continuity equation and applies to water flowing in any conduit (pipe, channel, stream) as long as no water enters or leaves the conduit between Station 1 and Station 2. The continuity equation also is expressed as

$$Q = va \tag{4-10}$$

where Q = quantity (or rate) of flow in cubic feet per second, cfs (m³/s),
v = average velocity across a given cross section of flow, ft/s (m/s),
a = area of the cross section of flow, ft² (m²).

Figure 4-2 illustrates these parameters.

Example 4-2

Problem

Determine the quantity of flow, Q, at the outflow end of the pipe shown in Figure 4-6 if the elevation of the center of the pipe is 525 feet and the surface of the reservoir is 550 feet. The pipe is composed of smooth concrete and has a diameter of 2.0 feet and a length of 350 feet. Consider friction.

Solution

First, find the velocity, v, by a trial-and-error process using Equation 4-7 and the Moody Diagram.

As in Example 4-1, $v_1 = p_2/\gamma = 0$. Also, assume that $h_e = 0$. Therefore, Equation 4-7 becomes

$$h_1 + 0 = h_2 + 0 + \frac{v_2^2}{2g} + h_f$$

Substituting Equation 4-8 gives

$$h_1 = h_2 + 0 + \frac{v_2^2}{2g} + f\frac{Lv_2^2}{2gD}$$

which can be rearranged to

$$h_1 - h_2 = \left\{1 + f\frac{L}{D}\right\}\frac{v_2^2}{2g} \tag{4-11}$$

Substituting known values gives

$$25 = \left\{1 + f\frac{350}{2}\right\}\frac{v_2^2}{64.4}$$
$$1610 = \{1 + 175f\}v_2^2$$

This equation containing f and v_2 can be solved by using an iteration process as follows:

Assume a value for f, say, $f = 0.02$. Using $f = 0.02$, $v_2 = 18.9$ ft/s from the above equation. From Equation 4-1, the Reynold's number is

$$N_R = \frac{(18.9)(2)}{10^{-5}}$$
$$= 3.78 \times 10^6$$

Now look at the Moody diagram in Figure 4-7 to find the resulting value of f. If the value of f found on the Moody diagram matches the assumed value, then the assumed value was correct and the resulting value of v_2 would be correct as well.

To find f on the Moody diagram, first determine ε/D. From Table 4-1, $\varepsilon = 0.001$. Therefore,

$$\varepsilon/D = 0.0005$$

On the Moody diagram, $N_R = 3.78 \times 10^6$ intersects $\varepsilon/D = 0.0005$ at approximately $f = 0.018$. Since this value of f does not agree with the assumed value of 0.020, choose another f.

Choose $f = 0.018$.

Then, from Equation 4-11, $v_2 = 19.7$ ft/s. The resulting Reynold's number is

$$N_R = \frac{(2)(19.7)}{10^{-5}}$$
$$= 3.9 \times 10^6$$

On the Moody diagram, $N_R = 3.9 \times 10^6$ intersects $\varepsilon/D = 0.0005$ at approximately $f = 0.018$. Therefore, $v_2 = 19.7$ ft/s is correct. Finally, using Equation 4-10, we have

$$Q = v_2 a$$
$$= (19.7)(3.14)$$
$$= 61.9 \text{ cfs} \quad \text{(Answer)}$$

Comparison with Example 4-1 reveals that the velocity at Station 2 was found to be about half the velocity computed assuming no friction. Also, note that even though pipe friction was used in this example, entrance loss was still neglected. In general, entrance loss constitutes a relatively minor portion of the total head loss encountered.

Example 4-3

Problem

Determine the pressure, p, at the center of the pipe shown in Figure 4-6 at a point halfway from the reservoir to the discharge end. Elevations and dimensions are the same as in Example 4-2. The elevation of the bottom of the reservoir is 540 feet. Consider friction.

Solution

First, find the velocity at the discharge end of the pipe, as in Example 4-2. The velocity was found to be 19.7 ft/s. Remembering that velocity is constant throughout the pipe (uniform pipe), the velocity at the halfway point is also 19.7 ft/s.

Use Equation 4-7 with Station 1 in the reservoir and Station 2 at the halfway point of the pipe. Note that the elevation of the center of the pipe at the reservoir is 541 feet. Then $h_1 = 550$ ft and $h_2 = 533$ ft. Also, $v_1 = 0$ and

$$h_f = (0.018)\frac{175}{2}\frac{(19.7)^2}{64.4} = 9.49 \text{ ft}$$

Substituting these values into Equation 4-7 gives

$$550 + 0 = 533 + \frac{p_2}{\gamma} + \frac{(19.7)^2}{64.4} + 9.49$$

Therefore,

$$\frac{p_2}{\gamma} = 1.48 \text{ ft}$$

and

$$P_2 = (1.48)(62.4)$$
$$= 93 \text{ lb/ft}^2 \quad \text{(Answer)}$$

It is interesting to note that if this system were gated at the end and therefore static, the pressure at Station 2 would be (from Equation 3-2) 1061 lb/ft². The dramatic decrease to 93 lb/ft² is due to the loss of potential energy to kinetic energy and to friction.

Example 4-4

Problem

Determine the quantity of flow, Q, in the pipe connecting the two reservoirs in the following diagram. Consider friction.

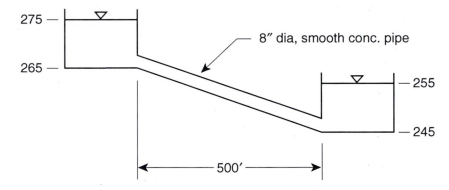

Solution

Use Equation 4-7 with Station 1 in the upper reservoir and Station 2 in the lower reservoir but located at its connection with the pipe. Therefore, v_2 will be the pipe velocity and not zero, as in the case of v_1. However, h_2 will be measured not to the center of the pipe but to the free surface of the lower reservoir. The extra height from the center of the pipe to the free surface accounts for the pressure head at this station.

Now that the station locations are set, the problem can be solved by using trial and error, as in Example 4-2. Assume that $v_1 = 0$ and $p_2/\gamma = 0$. Starting with Equation 4-11 and substituting known values, we have

$$275 - 255 = \left\{ 1 + f \frac{500}{0.67} \right\} \frac{v_2^2}{64.4}$$

or

$$1288 = \left\{ 1 + 750 f \right\} v_2^2$$

This equation containing f and v_2 is solved by using the Moody diagram as follows: Assume a value for f, say, $f = 0.02$. Using $f = 0.02$, $v_2 = 8.97$ ft/s from the above equation. From Equation 4-1, the Reynolds number is

$$N_R = \frac{(8.97)(0.67)}{10^{-5}}$$
$$= 5.98 \times 10^5$$

Now look at the Moody diagram in Figure 4-7 to find the resulting value of f. If the value of f found on the Moody diagram matches the assumed value, then the assumed value was correct, and the resulting value of v_2 would be correct as well.

To find f on the Moody diagram, first determine ε/D. From Table 4-1, $\varepsilon = 0.001$. Therefore, $\varepsilon/D = 0.0015$. On the Moody diagram, $N_R = 5.98 \times 10^5$ intersects $\varepsilon/D = 0.0015$ at approximately $f = 0.022$. Since this value of f does not agree with the assumed value of 0.020, choose another f.

Choose $f = 0.022$.

Then, from Equation 4-11, $v_2 = 8.58$ ft/s. The resulting Reynolds number is

$$N_R = \frac{(8.58)(0.67)}{10^{-5}}$$
$$= 5.72 \times 10^5$$

On the Moody diagram, $N_R = 5.72 \times 10^5$ intersects $\varepsilon/D = 0.0015$ at approximately $f = 0.022$. Therefore, $v_2 = 8.58$ ft/s is correct.

Finally, using Equation 4-10, we have

$$Q = v_2 a$$
$$= (8.58)(0.349)$$
$$= 3.0 \text{ cfs} \quad \text{(Answer)}$$

This value of discharge found for Station 2 is the same throughout the length of the pipe.

Some other examples of hydraulic systems are shown in Figure 4-8. In Figure 4-8(a), water flows from a higher reservoir to a lower reservoir through a pipe. Notice that the energy and hydraulic grade lines are affected slightly by the path taken by the pipe. Where the pipe slope is greater, the EGL and HGL slopes are also greater because they indicate head loss per foot of pipe length. So a sloping pipe has more length per unit length along the profile than does a horizontal pipe.

In Figure 4-8(b), water flowing in a pipe connecting two reservoirs experiences an abrupt increase in pipe diameter. The EGL and HGL provide important information describing the flow expansion phenomenon. First, the vertical separation between EGL and HGL is much greater before the expansion than after, indicating a drop in velocity (predicted by the continuity equation, Equation 4-9). Second, the EGL dips at the transition point, indicating a loss of energy due to turbulence there.

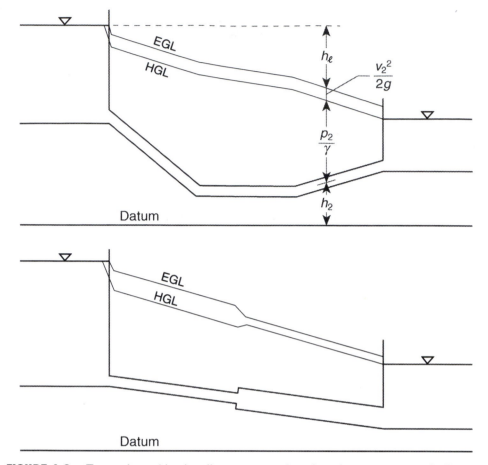

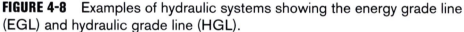

FIGURE 4-8   Examples of hydraulic systems showing the energy grade line (EGL) and hydraulic grade line (HGL).

4.5   MEASURING FLOW

Many methods have been devised over the years to measure the discharge, Q, of water flowing in a conduit. The choice of measuring device depends to a great extent on the type of conduit conveying the flow. For example, in the case of an open channel, various types of weirs are used to measure discharge. As water flows over the weir, a direct correlation is made between the water height and discharge. (These devices are described in Chapter 5.) Also, the Parshall flume, which utilizes the concept of critical depth, is used to measure discharge. Critical depth is discussed in Chapter 6.

One of the most fundamental methods of flow measurement consists of measuring the velocity and then using Equation 4-10 to compute the discharge. The most common methods of velocity measurement are the pitot tube and the current meter.

For pipe flow, the Venturi meter is used. The Venturi meter utilizes Bernoulli's principle to measure discharge directly.

Pitot Tube

In its simplest form, a **pitot tube** consists of an open-ended tube with a 90-degree bend near one end. When the tube is placed in a flow stream with the open end

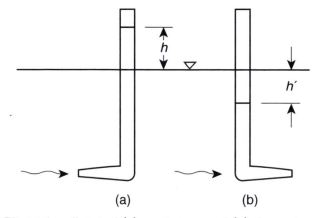

FIGURE 4-9   Pitot tube directed (a) upstream and (b) downstream.

directed upstream, as shown in Figure 4-9(a), water will rise in the tube to a height above the surface equal to $h = v^2/2g$. If the height h can be measured, then velocity v can be computed. In this case, v represents the velocity at the exact position of the tube. To compute Q, the average velocity across the flow cross section must be obtained. This can be accomplished either by taking several measurements and computing an average or by applying a proportionality factor to the measured velocity to compute average velocity directly if such a factor is known. Experimentation indicates that the value of h does not depend on the diameter of the tube or the size of the opening.

A variation of the pitot tube shown in Figure 4-9(b) consists simply of turning the short end of the tube around to point downstream. In this case, a suction is created in the tube, resulting in a water level depressed below the surface by a distance h'. The advantage of this arrangement is that the distance h' may be easier to measure accurately than the distance h. Research has shown an approximate relationship between h' and v as follows:

$$h' \cong 0.43 \frac{v^2}{2g}$$

Many versions of the pitot tube have been developed involving more complex arrangements. These variations provide adaptations to different flow conditions as well as more accurate measurements.

Current Meter

A **current meter** consists simply of a propeller assembly immersed in flowing water together with a mechanism calibrated to convert the turning of the propeller to a velocity. Various designs of the current meter are available for adaptation to different applications from sewer pipes to open channels to large streams.

An example of a current meter used for streams is the Price Type AA shown in Figure 4-10. This meter, which employs rotating cups on one end and fins on the other, is used by the U.S. Geological Survey to measure velocity in streams and rivers. The meter can be lowered from a bridge by cable or in shallow conditions may be attached to a wading rod, as shown in Figure 4-11.

To measure the discharge in a stream using a current meter, the stream is divided by a series of vertical lines, as shown in Example 4-5. At each vertical line, a velocity measurement is taken at 60 percent of the depth, which is the approximate

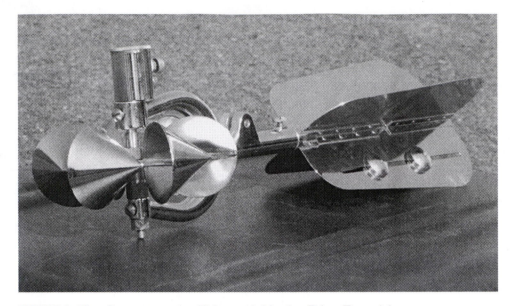

FIGURE 4-10   Current meter. This model is the Price Type AA.

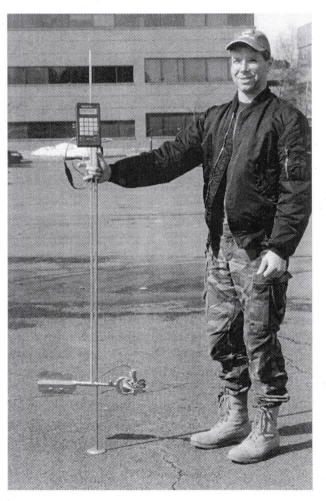

FIGURE 4-11   Price Type AA current meter mounted on a wading rod for use in shallow conditions up to 4 feet deep.

location of the average velocity. Then discharge is computed for each sector of the cross section, and all individual discharge values are summed to give the total discharge.

Example 4-5

Problem

Determine an estimate of the discharge in the stream depicted below using the data in the following tables.

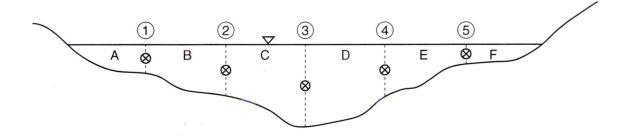

Velocity Measurements

Station	Velocity (ft/s)
1	1.2
2	3.7
3	5.6
4	3.5
5	0.91

Area of Sector

Sector	Area (ft^2)
A	9.8
B	23.2
C	31.0
D	34.8
E	19.6
F	8.5

Solution

The average velocity in Sector A is

$$v_A = \frac{0+1.2}{2} = 0.60 \text{ ft/s}$$

The average velocity in Sector B is

$$v_B = \frac{1.2 + 3.7}{2} = 2.45 \text{ ft/s}$$

Similarly, the remaining average velocities are

$v_C = 4.65$ ft/s
$v_D = 4.55$ ft/s
$v_E = 2.21$ ft/s
$v_F = 0.46$ ft/s

Using Equation 4-10, the discharges in the sectors are

$Q_A = (9.8)(0.60) = 5.88$ cfs
$Q_B = (23.2)(2.45) = 56.84$ cfs
$Q_C = (31.0)(4.65) = 144.15$ cfs
$Q_D = (34.8)(4.55) = 158.34$ cfs
$Q_E = (19.6)(2.21) = 43.32$ cfs
$Q_F = (8.5)(0.46) = 3.91$ cfs

Finally, the total discharge is the sum of the above discharges, or

$$Q = 412.44 \text{ cfs}$$

which is rounded to

$$Q = 410 \text{ cfs}   \text{(Answer)}$$

Venturi Meter

Used to measure discharge in a pipe flowing full, the Venturi meter consists of a carefully designed constriction in the pipe that causes flow velocity to increase in accordance with the continuity equation.

In its simplest form, as shown in Figure 4-12, piezometers are installed at the throat and in the pipe just upstream of the throat. The piezometers measure the drop

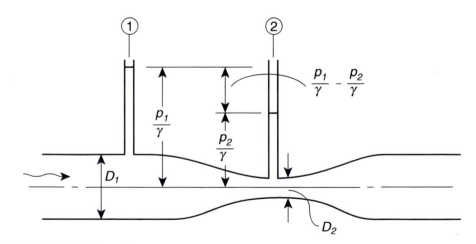

FIGURE 4-12   Venturi meter.

TABLE 4-2   c-Values for Venturi Meters

Throat Diameter (in)	Throat Velocity (ft/s)				
	3	4	5	10	15
1	0.935	0.945	0.949	0.958	0.963
2	0.939	0.948	0.953	0.965	0.970
4	0.943	0.952	0.957	0.970	0.975
8	0.948	0.957	0.962	0.974	0.978
12	0.955	0.962	0.967	0.978	0.981

in pressure head caused by the increase in velocity head. The energy equation, written between the two piezometers, taken at Station 1 and Station 2, respectively, would be

$$\frac{v_1^2}{2g} + \frac{p_1}{\gamma} = \frac{v_2^2}{2g} + \frac{p_2}{\gamma} + h_l \tag{4-12}$$

The datum is taken as the centerline of the pipe. Using the continuity equation and rearranging terms, Equation 4-12 can be written as

$$Q = ca_2 \sqrt{\frac{2g\left(\frac{p_1}{\gamma} - \frac{p_2}{\gamma}\right)}{1 - \left(\frac{D_2}{D_1}\right)^4}} \tag{4-13}$$

where c is a coefficient between zero and one used in place of h_l to account for energy losses. Experimental values of c for various throat diameters are given in Table 4-2.

To yield accurate results, a Venturi meter must be placed in a straight, uniform section of pipe free of turbulence and must have sufficiently rounded corners and gradual diameter transitions.

Example 4-6

Problem

A Venturi meter as shown below is installed in a 6-inch pipe to measure discharge. Piezometer readings from the pipe centerline are as follows:

$p_1/\gamma = 0.95$ ft

$p_2/\gamma = 0.52$ ft

What is the discharge in the pipe?

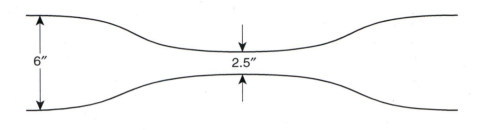

Solution

Substituting known values into Equation 4-13 gives

$$Q = 0.1817c$$

and using Equation 4-10 gives

$$v = 5.343c$$

The value of c can be determined from Table 4-2 using a trial-and-error process. First, choose a value of v and compute the corresponding c-value. From the c-value, compute the resulting value of v. If the computed value of v matches the assumed value, then that value is correct. If not, choose another value of v and repeat the process.

Trial 1: Choose $v = 5$ ft/s. Using Table 4-2 and interpolating, $c = 0.9595$, and the resulting velocity is 5.128 ft/s.

Trial 2: Choose $v = 5.128$ ft/s. Using Table 4-2, $c = 0.95982$, and the resulting velocity is 5.128 ft/s.

Therefore, the velocity is determined to be $v = 5.128$ ft/s and $c = 0.95982$ and

$$Q = (0.1817)(0.95982)$$
$$= 0.174 \text{ cfs} \quad \text{(Answer)}$$

Parshall Flume

Used to measure discharge in an open channel, the Parshall flume consists of a constriction in the channel designed to produce critical depth in the flow stream. The concept of critical depth is explained in Section 6.2. The Parshall flume is one of many flume designs called "critical flow flumes" intended for flow measurement. A Parshall flume is shown in Figure 4-13.

By constricting the flow using a precise configuration, critical flow results, enabling the discharge to be correlated to a single depth, H. As shown in Figure 4-13, a depth monitoring well is placed along the upstream taper section of the flume. The relationship between H and Q is described by different equations for different flow rates and sizes of the flume. The various equations are listed in Table 4-3.

Additional monitoring wells can be placed in the downstream portion to detect high tailwater (high water level at the downstream end of the flume), which could produce a submerged condition. If a Parshall flume operates submerged, the relationship between H and Q must be adjusted.

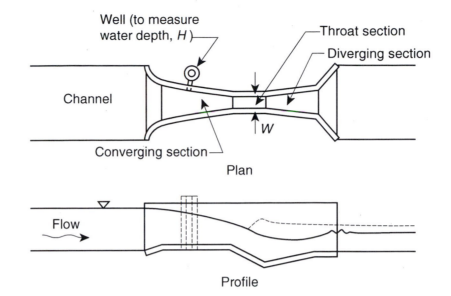

FIGURE 4-13 Parshall flume.

TABLE 4-3 Discharge Equations for a Parshall Flume

Throat Width (W)	Discharge Equation	Free Flow Capacity (cfs)
3 in	$Q = 0.992H^{1.547}$	0.03–1.9
6 in	$Q = 2.06H^{1.58}$	0.05–3.9
9 in	$Q = 3.07H^{1.53}$	0.09–8.9
1 ft–8 ft	$Q = 4WH^{1.522W^{0.026}}$	Up to 140
10 ft–50 ft	$Q = (3.6875W + 2.5)H^{1.6}$	Up to 2000

To yield accurate results, a Parshall flume must be placed in a straight, uniform section of the channel free of downstream obstructions.

PROBLEMS

1. What is the Reynold's number for water flowing in a 24-inch circular pipe at a velocity of 6.21 ft/s? Is the flow laminar or turbulent?

2. Water is flowing in a $2\frac{1}{2}$-inch pipe with a discharge of 0.150 cfs. Find the Reynold's number for this flow. Is the flow laminar or turbulent?

3. Water is flowing in a 300-mm circular pipe with a discharge of 0.250 m³/s. Find the Reynold's number for this flow. Is the flow laminar or turbulent?

4. What is the velocity head of the flow in problem 1?

5. Water in a pipe has a pressure of 22.1 lb/ft². What is the pressure head?

6. Water is flowing in an 8-inch-diameter new cast iron pipe with a velocity of 7.49 ft/s. The friction factor is 0.0215. What is the friction head loss over a length of 115 feet?

7. Water is flowing in a 36-inch concrete pipe (finished surface) with a velocity of 12.5 ft/s. What is the friction head loss over a length of 225 feet?

8. Water is flowing in 2-inch tubing with a velocity of 1.35 ft/s. What is the friction head loss over a length of 25 ft?

9. A reservoir of water is connected to an 8-inch-diameter pipe 50 feet long and discharging freely. The water surface elevation of the reservoir is 410.0, and the elevation of the center of the pipe at its discharge end is 372.5. Neglecting friction, determine the velocity, v, and discharge, Q, at the end of the pipe.

10. Find the velocity, v, and discharge, Q, for the pipe in problem 9 if the pipe is composed of new cast iron and friction is considered.

11. Two reservoirs are connected by a 12-inch concrete pipe (finished surface), as shown below. Determine the velocity and discharge in the pipe. Consider friction, but neglect minor losses.

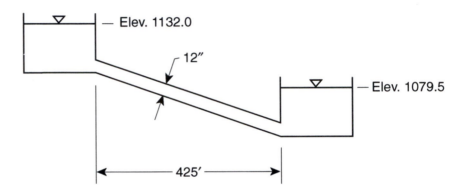

12. A reservoir discharges into a 60-inch concrete pipe (rough surface) that discharges freely, as shown below. What is the pressure in the pipe at point A? Consider friction, but neglect minor losses.

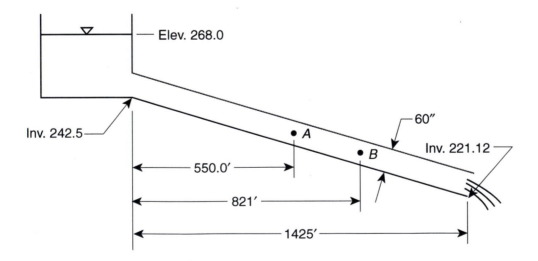

13. In problem 12, if a piezometer is installed on the top of the pipe at point B, what is the elevation of the water level in the piezometer? Consider friction, but neglect minor losses.

14. A reservoir discharges into a 4-inch new cast iron pipe, as shown below. Find the velocity and discharge in the pipe. Consider friction, but neglect minor losses.

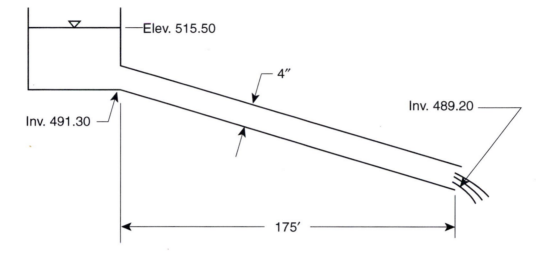

15. Sketch the energy grade line and hydraulic grade line for the hydraulic system shown here:

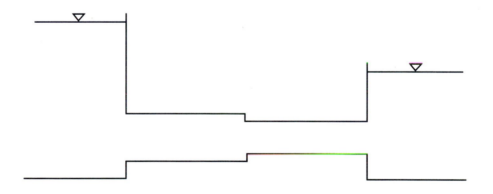

16. Estimate the discharge in the stream cross section shown below using the given data. Determine channel dimensions by scaling.

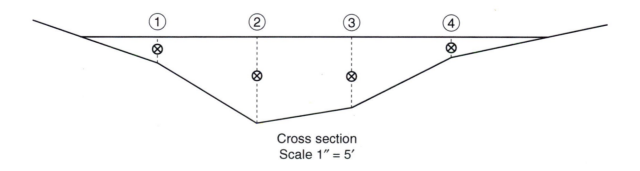

Cross section
Scale 1″ = 5′

Station	Velocity (ft/s)
1	0.86
2	3.15
3	2.59
4	0.46

17. A pitot tube is placed in a flowing channel, as shown below. Estimate the velocity measured by the pitot tube. Speculate on whether the measurement represents average velocity across the cross section. Determine dimensions by scale.

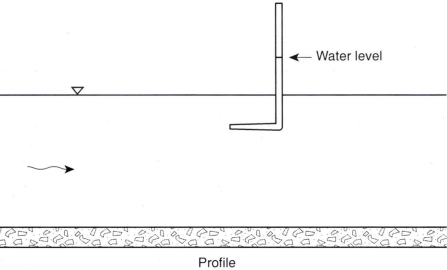

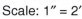

Profile
Scale: 1″ = 2′

18. If the channel flow in problem 17 is reversed so that it moves from right to left and the pitot tube reading is unchanged, what is the new velocity?

19. A Parshall flume is used to measure discharge in a channel. The throat width is 9.0 inches. If the measured depth, H, is 7½ inches, what is the discharge?

20. A Parshall flume with a throat width of 2.50 feet is used to measure discharge. If the measured depth, H, is 1.8 feet, what is the discharge?

21. A Venturi meter with a throat diameter of 4.00 inches is installed in an 8.00-inch-diameter pipe. Piezometer readings from the pipe centerline are as follows: upstream, $p_1/\gamma = 1.64$ ft, and throat, $p_2/\gamma = 0.88$ ft. What is the discharge in the pipe?

22. A Venturi meter with a throat diameter of 10.00 inches is installed in a 24.00-inch pipe. Piezometer readings from the pipe centerline are as follows: upstream, $p_1/\gamma = 2.36$ ft, and throat, $p_2/\gamma = 0.63$ ft. What is the discharge in the pipe?

FURTHER READING

Brater, E. F., and King, H. (1996). *Handbook of Hydraulics* (7th ed.). New York: McGraw-Hill.

Hita, C. E., and Hwang, N. H. C. (1987). *Hydraulic Engineering Systems* (2nd ed.). Englewood Cliffs, NJ: Prentice Hall.

Morris, H. M., and Wiggert, J. M. (1972). *Applied Hydraulics in Engineering* (2nd ed.). New York: Wiley.

Mott, R. L. (1994). *Applied Fluid Mechanics* (4th ed.). Englewood Cliffs, NJ: Prentice Hall.

Prasuhn, A. L. (1987). *Fundamentals of Hydraulic Engineering*. New York: Holt, Rinehart and Winston.

Simon, A. L., and Korom, S. F. (1997). *Hydraulics* (4th ed.). Englewood Cliffs, NJ: Prentice Hall.

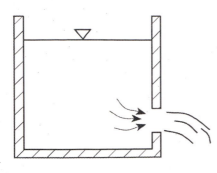

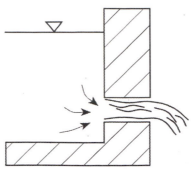

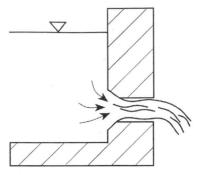

(a) Thin Wall, Square Edge   (b) Thick Wall, Square Edge   (c) Thick Wall, Beveled Edge

FIGURE 5-1   Examples of orifices.

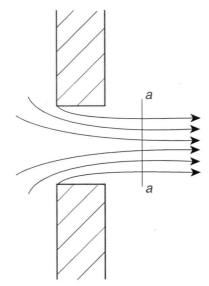

FIGURE 5-2   Jet contraction in a square-edged circular orifice.

Since the velocity is negligible at Station 1, $v_1 = 0$ and since Station 2 is located at a free discharge, $p_2 = 0$, and since the datum runs through the center of the orifice, $h_2 = 0$. Thus, Equation 4-7 becomes

$$h_1 = \frac{v_2^2}{2g} + h_l$$

and

$$v_2 = \sqrt{2g(h_1 - h_l)} \tag{5-1}$$

The term h_1 represents the vertical distance from the center of the orifice to the reservoir free surface and may be simply referred to as h. The energy loss head, h_l, can be accounted for by introducing a coefficient of velocity, c_v. Thus, Equation 5-1 becomes

$$v_2 = c_v \sqrt{2gh} \tag{5-2}$$

Close scrutiny of Figure 5-2 reveals that the cross-sectional area at section a-a (Station 2), a_2, is less than the cross-sectional area of the orifice, a. Thus, $a_2 < a$. These may be related by a coefficient of contraction, c_c. Thus, $c_c = a_2/a$.

The discharge, Q, through the orifice is equal to the discharge at the vena contracta (Station 2). Thus, by utilizing Equation 4-10, Equation 5-2 may be written as

$$\frac{Q}{a_2} = c_v\sqrt{2gh}$$

or

$$Q = a_2 c_v \sqrt{2gh}$$

But replacing a_2 by ac_c gives

$$Q = ac_c c_v \sqrt{2gh}$$

Finally, replacing $c_c c_v$ by a single coefficient, c, called the discharge coefficient, results in

$$Q = ca\sqrt{2gh} \tag{5-3}$$

where Q = discharge, cfs (m³/s)
$\quad\quad\quad c$ = discharge coefficient
$\quad\quad\quad a$ = cross-sectional area of the orifice, ft² (m²)
$\quad\quad\quad h$ = total head, ft (m)

Equation 5-3 is referred to as the *orifice equation*. The discharge coefficient, c, is a dimensionless proportionality constant, which accounts for the reduction of flow due to entrance head loss. The experimental value of c for square-edged orifices varies depending on the size and shape of the orifice and the amount of head. However, for most applications, reliable results can be achieved by using $c = 0.62$.

Example 5-1

Problem

Find the discharge, Q, through a 6-inch-diameter square-edged orifice discharging freely. The water surface elevation of the impoundment is 220.0, and the elevation of the center of the orifice is 200.0.

Solution

First, find the cross-sectional area, converting 6 inches to 0.50 feet:

$$a = \pi r^2$$
$$= \pi(0.25)^2$$
$$= 0.196 \text{ ft}^2$$

Next, find total head as the difference between elevations:

$$h = 220.0 - 200.0$$
$$= 20.0 \text{ ft}$$

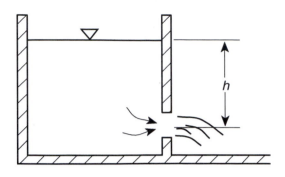

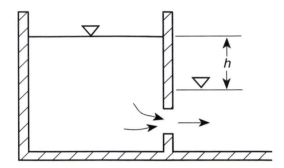

(a) For free discharge, h is measured to the center of the orifice.

(b) For submerged discharge, h is measured to the lower water surface.

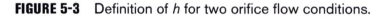

FIGURE 5-3 Definition of h for two orifice flow conditions.

Therefore, using Equation 5-3, we have

$$Q = ca\sqrt{2gh}$$
$$= (0.62)(0.196)\sqrt{(2)(32.2)(20)}$$
$$= 4.4 \text{ cfs} \quad \text{(Answer)}$$

If the water level on the discharge side of the orifice rises above the orifice, it is called a *submerged orifice*. Figure 5-3 illustrates the difference between free-flowing and submerged orifices.

Application of Bernoulli's principle to a submerged orifice results in the same orifice equation used for free-flowing orifices, namely, Equation 5-3. Research has shown that the discharge coefficient, c, varies very little for the submerged case and can be assumed to be the same.

However, in using Equation 5-3 for a submerged orifice, the total head, h, must be computed as the vertical distance from the reservoir surface to the discharge surface, as shown in Figure 5-3(b).

Example 5-2

Problem

Find the discharge Q, through a rectangular orifice 4 inches by 6 inches with square edges discharging submerged. The water surface elevation of the impoundment is 220.0, and the elevation of the water surface of the discharge water is 215.0. The elevation of the center of the orifice is 200.0.

Solution

First, find the cross-sectional area in square feet:

$$a = \left[\frac{4}{12}\right]\left[\frac{6}{12}\right]$$
$$= 0.167 \text{ ft}^2$$

Next, find total head as the difference between elevations:

$$h = 220.0 - 215.0$$
$$= 5.0 \text{ ft}$$

Note that the elevation of the orifice is not relevant. Therefore, using Equation 5-3, we have

$$Q = ca\sqrt{2gh}$$
$$= (0.62)(0.167)\sqrt{(2)(32.2)(5)}$$
$$= 1.9 \text{ cfs}   \text{(Answer)}$$

5.2.   WEIR FLOW

A **weir** is a structure that, like an orifice, regulates the flow of water out of an impoundment or reservoir. Generally, a weir consists of a horizontal surface over which water is allowed to flow. Typical uses include outlet structures for dams and detention basins, as well as other impoundments such as holding tanks in sewage treatment plants. Also, weirs are widely used as measuring devices with such applications as natural streams and treatment works.

Figure 5-4 shows a typical weir discharging freely to a downstream channel. The energy that pushes water over the crest is measured by the head *H* above the crest.

Many different types of weirs have been devised over the years by varying the width and shape of the crest. The most important of these are shown in Figures 5-5 and 5-6.

Close inspection of Figure 5-4(a) reveals that the surface of the impoundment begins to drop as it approaches the weir. This is due to the increase of velocity, which is compensated for by a drop in cross-sectional area in accordance with the continuity equation. Therefore, *H* must be measured at some distance away from the weir crest, where the velocity is virtually zero. Usually, this location is at least a distance 2.5*H* upstream of the crest.

Rectangular Weir

The rate of flow or discharge over a rectangular weir is computed by the weir formula,

$$Q = cLH^{3/2} \tag{5-4}$$

where Q = discharge, cfs
c = discharge coefficient
L = effective crest length, ft
H = head above crest, ft

Equation 5-4 is used for most rectangular weir flow computations using the English system of units. The **discharge coefficient** is an empirically determined

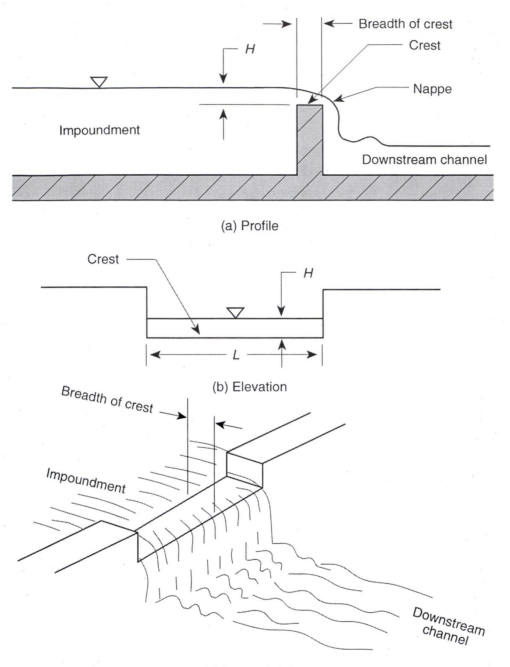

(a) Profile

(b) Elevation

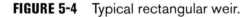

(c) Isometric View

FIGURE 5-4   Typical rectangular weir.

multiplier that accounts for a number of hydraulic factors difficult to describe mathematically. Values of the discharge coefficient depend on the type of weir and the depth of flow. To convert Equation 5-4 for use with the metric system of units, appropriate values of c would be required. Values of c in Appendix A-5 are intended for use with the English system of units.

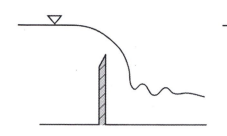
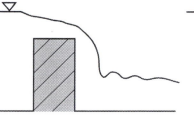

(a) Sharp-Crested Weir   (b) Broad-Crested Weir   (c) Ogee Weir

FIGURE 5-5 Classification of weirs by cross section shape.

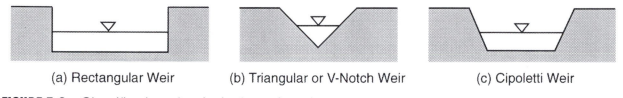

(a) Rectangular Weir   (b) Triangular or V-Notch Weir   (c) Cipoletti Weir

FIGURE 5-6 Classification of weirs by front view shape.

Sharp-Crested Weir

A rectangular, sharp-crested weir is perhaps the most basic type and is used for measuring flow in a channel and also as a simple spillway structure. Computation of the discharge, Q, for this type of weir depends on the dimensions of the weir in relation to the channel and the head, H. Figure 5-7 illustrates the parameters used in determining Q for a sharp-crested weir.

As water flows past the vertical sides of the weir, a loss of energy takes place, which is called **contraction**. This contraction can be accounted for by reducing the actual measured length of the weir to a lesser value called *effective length*. Effective length, L, is computed by

$$L = L' - 0.1nH \qquad (5-5)$$

where L' = actual measured crest length, ft
$\quad n$ = number of contractions
$\quad H$ = head above the crest, ft

If the weir is centered in the channel with L' less than channel width, B, there are two end contractions and $n = 2$. If $L' = B$, there are no end contractions and $n = 0$. If the weir crest is against one side of the channel and not the other, there is one contraction and $n = 1$.

The height of the weir above the channel bottom also has an effect on the discharge, Q. This effect is accounted for by adjusting the discharge coefficient, c, in accordance with the height, P. Thus,

$$c = 3.27 + 0.40\frac{H}{P} \qquad (5-6)$$

where P = height of crest above the channel bottom, ft

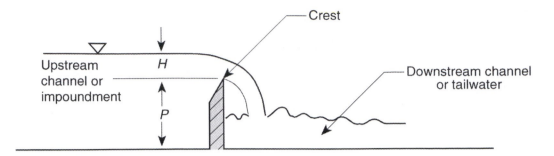

(a) Profile

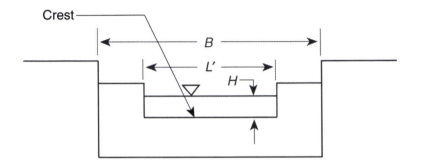

(b) Elevation

FIGURE 5-7   Hydraulic elements of a sharp-crested weir.

Example 5-3

Problem

Find the discharge flowing over a sharp-crested weir, as shown below, if the crest elevation is 282.00 and the impoundment elevation is 283.75.

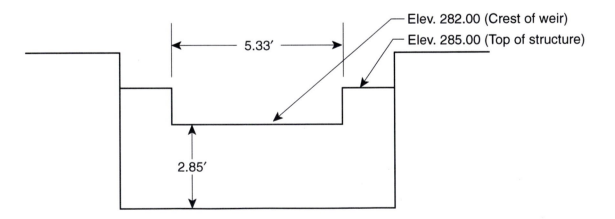

Solution

First, find *H* from the elevations given:

$$H = 283.75 - 282.00$$
$$= 1.75 \text{ ft}$$

Since the weir has two contractions, $n = 2$. Therefore, using Equation 5-5, we have

$$L = L' - 0.1nH$$
$$= 5.33 - (0.1)(2)(1.75)$$
$$= 4.98 \text{ ft}$$

Next, find c using Equation 5-6:

$$c = 3.27 + 0.40\frac{H}{P}$$
$$= 3.27 + (0.40)\frac{1.75}{2.85}$$
$$= 3.516$$

Finally, find Q using Equation 5-4:

$$Q = cLH^{3/2}$$
$$= (3.516)(4.98)(1.75)^{3/2}$$
$$= 40.5 \text{ cfs} \quad \text{(Answer)}$$

V-Notch Weir

A variation of the sharp-crested weir is the triangular, or V-notch weir, which is used to measure flow when very low quantities are expected. Discharge over a V-notch weir is computed by a variation of Equation 5-4:

$$Q = c\left\{\tan\frac{\theta}{2}\right\}H^{5/2} \qquad (5\text{-}7)$$

where θ is the angle (in degrees) made by the notch as shown in Figure 5-8. Although c varies under different conditions, it is taken generally to be 2.5.

Cipoletti Weir

A **Cipoletti weir**, shown in Figure 5-6(c), is a trapezoidal variation of the sharp-crested weir devised to compensate for loss of flow quantity due to contractions at the vertical edges of a rectangular weir. By sloping the edges at approximately 1:4 (horizontal to vertical), the increasing cross-sectional area of flow, as H increases, compensates for loss of flow due to end contraction.

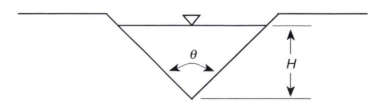

FIGURE 5-8   Hydraulic elements of a V-notch weir.

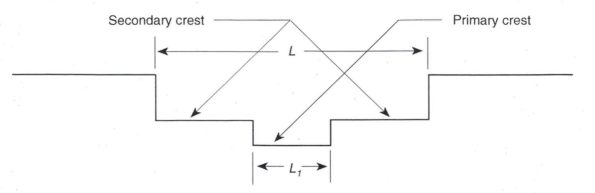

FIGURE 5-9 Front view of a two-stage weir.

Broad-Crested Weir

A **broad-crested weir**, which is rectangular, is commonly employed in outlet structures for dams and detention basins. Discharge is computed using the weir equation, Equation 5-4, with values of c found in Appendix A-5. Correction for side contractions generally is not required for this type of weir. A variation of the broad-crested weir used to regulate discharge more precisely is the multistage weir, as shown in Figure 5-9.

Discharge for the two-stage weir shown in Figure 5-9 is computed by adding the discharge for the primary crest and the discharge for the secondary crest as detailed in Example 5-6.

Example 5-4

Problem

Find the discharge flowing over a 60-degree V-notch weir if $H = 4.0$ inches.

Solution

First, find $\theta/2$:

$$\frac{\theta}{2} = \frac{60}{2} = 30°$$

Next, find H in feet:

$$H = 4.0 \text{ in} = 0.33 \text{ ft}$$

Next, c is assumed to be

$$c = 2.5$$

Finally, find Q from Equation 5-7:

$$Q = c\left\{\tan\frac{\theta}{2}\right\}H^{5/2}$$
$$= (2.5)(\tan 30°)(0.33)^{5/2}$$
$$= 0.090 \text{ cfs} \quad \text{(Answer)}$$

Example 5-5

Problem

Find the discharge flowing over a rectangular broad-crested weir with breadth 9.0 inches, length 4.0 feet, and a head of 1.25 feet.

Solution

First, find c using the chart in Appendix A-5:

$$c = 3.215$$

(The value of c is found by interpolating between values for $H = 1.2$ and $H = 1.4$.) Then compute Q using Equation 5-4:

$$
\begin{aligned}
Q &= cLH^{3/2} \\
&= (3.215)(4.0)(1.25)^{3/2} \\
&= 18 \text{ cfs} \quad \text{(Answer)}
\end{aligned}
$$

Example 5-6

Problem

Find the discharge flowing over a two-stage weir like that shown in Figure 5-9 if the elevation of the impoundment is 235.50. The overall length of the weir is 22.00 feet, and the length of the primary crest is 4.00 feet. The crest breadth is 1.00 foot. The elevation of the primary crest is 233.00, and that of the secondary crest is 233.50.

Solution

Step 1: Find the discharge, Q_1, over the primary crest. Head, H_1, is found from the elevations of the water surface and the crest:

$$
\begin{aligned}
H_1 &= 235.50 - 233.00 \\
&= 2.50 \text{ ft}
\end{aligned}
$$

Then using the chart in Appendix A-5, find c_1:

$$c_1 = 3.31$$

Therefore, discharge Q_1 is

$$
\begin{aligned}
Q_1 &= c_1 L_1 H_1^{3/2} \\
&= (3.31)(4.00)(2.50)^{3/2} \\
&= 52.3 \text{ cfs}
\end{aligned}
$$

Step 2: Find the discharge, Q_2, over the secondary crest. First find head, H_2:

$$
\begin{aligned}
H_2 &= 235.50 - 233.50 \\
&= 2.00 \text{ ft}
\end{aligned}
$$

Then, using the chart in Appendix A-5, find c_2:

$$c_2 = 3.30$$

Therefore, discharge Q_2 is

$$
\begin{aligned}
Q_2 &= c_2 L_2 H_2^{3/2} \\
&= (3.30)(22.0 - 4.00)(2.00)^{3/2} \\
&= 168.0 \text{ cfs}
\end{aligned}
$$

Step 3: Find total discharge, Q:

$$
\begin{aligned}
Q &= Q_1 + Q_2 \\
&= 52.3 + 168.0 \\
&= 220. \text{ cfs} \quad \text{(Answer)}
\end{aligned}
$$

Ogee Weir

A type of rectangular weir that is commonly used as the spillway for a dam is the ogee weir shown in Figure 5-5(c). Its smooth, rounded surface is designed to reduce energy loss by edge contraction as water passes over the crest, thus increasing the discharge Q for a given head H, in comparison to sharp- or broad-crested weirs. Computation of discharge is not included in this text since applications of ogee spillways are not considered.

The geometrical shape of an ogee weir is formed by compound curves with radii dependent on a specific anticipated head. However, the term is commonly applied to weirs that have the general shape shown in Figure 5-5(c).

5.3   FLOW UNDER A GATE

A gate is an opening in an impoundment, usually for the purpose of allowing drawdown or emptying of the impoundment. A gate is also used to provide enhanced discharge quantity to the stream fed by the impoundment. Usually having a rectangular shape, gates are sometimes called head gates, diversion gates, and sluice gates. A sluice gate, shown in Figure 5-10, regulates discharge in a canal. In this case, one of the rectangular gates is completely open. The lifting mechanisms can be seen above the gates.

Flow under a gate is modeled as an orifice provided that the depth of the impoundment is large in comparison to the height of the gate opening. Therefore, calculation of discharge under a gate is performed by using the orifice equation, Equation 5-3. However, because contractions occurring at the edges are different from a square-edged orifice, the value of c is not that used in Section 5-1 but must be determined for each gate individually. Values of c for various actual gates have been determined experimentally and vary generally from 0.70 to 0.85.

Most sluice gates are constructed flush with the bottom of the reservoir, resulting in three edges to cause contractions. If the gate is located above the bottom, as shown in Figure 5-11(b), four contractions would result, and the value of c would be reduced.

When a sluice gate is raised, the resulting flow under the gate may take one of the three forms shown in Figure 5-12. Depending on such factors as the width and slope of the downstream channel and the discharge, the water surface profile

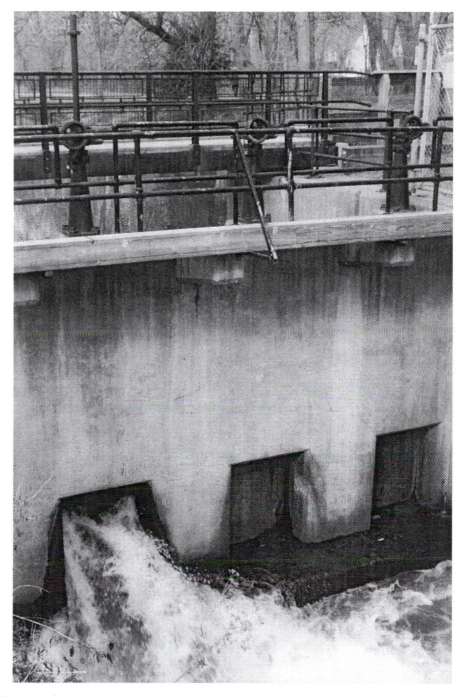

FIGURE 5-10   Sluice gate discharging into a canal.

may form a flat surface similar to that shown in Figure 5-12(a), or a hydraulic jump may occur a short distance downstream, as shown in Figure 5-12(b), or a submerged condition may prevail, as shown in Figure 5-12(c). If a discharging gate is submerged, the value of h in the orifice equation should be measured immediately downstream of the gate and not farther downstream, where the water level is higher.

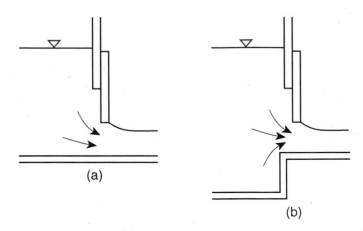

FIGURE 5-11   Vertical gates (a) flush with the bottom of the reservoir and (b) raised above the bottom of the reservoir.

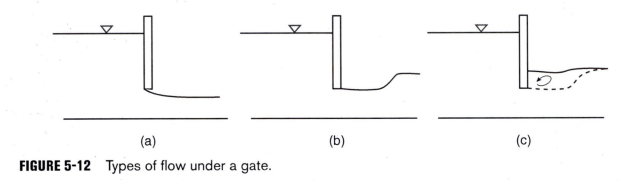

FIGURE 5-12   Types of flow under a gate.

5.4   SIPHON FLOW

A siphon is a pipe used to draw down an impoundment by running up from the impounded water and then down to the downstream channel. For example, if a reservoir impounded by a dam is to be drawn down but no sluice is in place through the dam, a siphon may be used as shown in Figure 5-13.

When the higher portion of the pipe is filled with water, the siphon flows in accordance with Bernoulli's principle. Total energy head driving the flow is the vertical distance from the reservoir surface to the center of the discharge end of the pipe (if the pipe is discharging freely). Flowing over the top of the dam does not hinder discharge because the energy required to push the water from point A to point B in Figure 5-14(a) is balanced by suction in the section from point C to point D.

However, flow in a siphon experiences the same energy losses associated with any full pipe flow. Losses found in the example in Figure 5-14(a) include entrance loss, losses at the four bends of the pipe, and friction loss along the entire length of the pipe.

A siphon is sometimes referred to as a closed conduit that rises above the hydraulic grade line. Figure 5-14 shows the HGL (neglecting entrance loss) for a siphon and a conventional sluice. Notice that a portion of the siphon is located above the HGL, indicating that the water experiences negative pressure there.

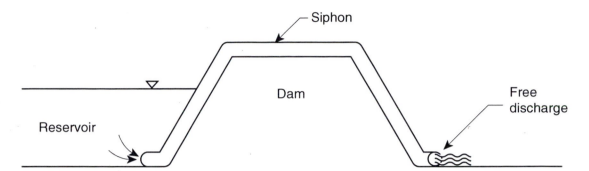

FIGURE 5-13   A siphon used to draw down a reservoir.

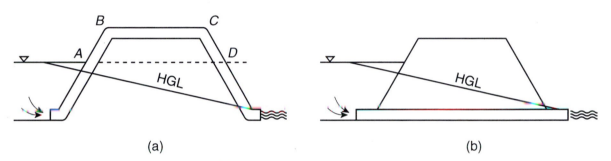

FIGURE 5-14   Comparison between (a) a siphon with flow rising above the HGL and (b) a sluice with flow below the HGL.

Some of the practical problems associated with siphons include starting and stopping flow when the desired drawdown is achieved. Another problem is the accumulation of air in the pipe at the high point. To start a siphon, a pump is used. Water is pumped from the impoundment to the high point to charge the siphon. When the siphon is charged, it will start to run and continue to run on its own. To stop a siphon, a valve could be closed, or air could be introduced at the high point to break the siphon action. If a valve is located at the discharge end of the siphon, closing the valve will stop the siphon and keep it charged, provided that no air leaks compromise the negative pressure.

At the high point of a siphon, air can accumulate as water flows for a period of time. This is the same problem that occurs with pressurized water mains and force mains. To relieve the air and prevent a large buildup, an air release valve should be located at the high point.

Another use of siphons is to provide flow from one reservoir to another if an obstruction is located between them. Figure 5-15 depicts such an arrangement. This siphon, although on a larger scale, would be operated as described above.

Another application of siphons is the siphon spillway for a dam. Shown in Figure 5-16, a siphon spillway consists of an inverted U-shaped conduit with an entrance below normal water level, and the invert of the high point coincides with normal water level. During a rainfall event when the water level rises, water first flows through the conduit without pressure, simulating a weir. When the water level rises high enough to charge the siphon, the conduit flows full, and siphon action takes over.

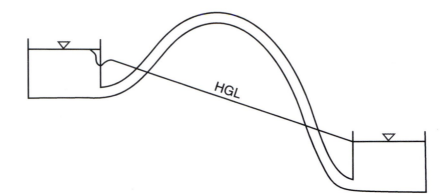

FIGURE 5-15   Siphon connecting two reservoirs.

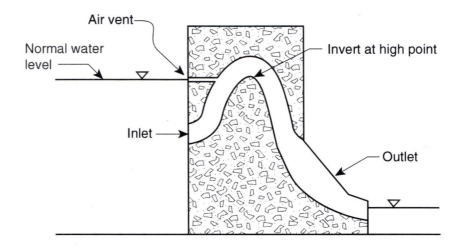

FIGURE 5-16   Siphon spillway.

To prevent the siphon spillway from eventually drawing down the reservoir below normal water level, an air vent is located at normal water level so that as the water level recedes, the air vent is exposed and the siphon action is broken.

PROBLEMS

1. Find the discharge, Q, through a 15-inch-diameter orifice in a vertical wall impounding water at a depth of 6.5 feet above the center of the orifice. The orifice has square edges and discharges freely.

2. An artificial lake is impounded by an earth dam with a square-edged orifice 12 inches by 12 inches for drawdown. The elevation of the surface of the lake is 928.25, and the invert of the orifice is 905.75. When the orifice is opened, what discharge in cfs flows through into the stream below the dam?

3. A reservoir of water is drained by a 10-inch-diameter, square-edged orifice with center at elevation 289.12 that flows directly into a stream with water surface

at elevation 293.49. The elevation of the reservoir surface is 296.85. Find the flow through the orifice.

4. A 150-mm-diameter, square-edged orifice conveys flow from a reservoir with water level at elevation 79.25 m. The center of the orifice is at elevation 66.10 m. Find the discharge for free flow.

5. In problem 4, if the tailwater is at elevation 71.98 m, what is the discharge?

6. A tank measuring 10.0 feet by 10.0 feet by 10.0 feet is completely filled with water. If a 4-inch-diameter, square-edged orifice is located 1.00 foot above the bottom of the tank (to the orifice center), (a) what is the discharge? (b) Estimate the time required to empty the tank halfway.

7. Find the discharge over a 90-degree V-notch weir if the head is 7.5 inches.

8. Find the discharge over the rectangular sharp-crested weir shown below.

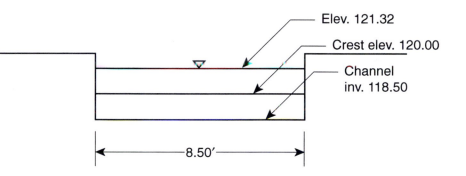

9. Find the discharge over the sharp-crested weir shown below.

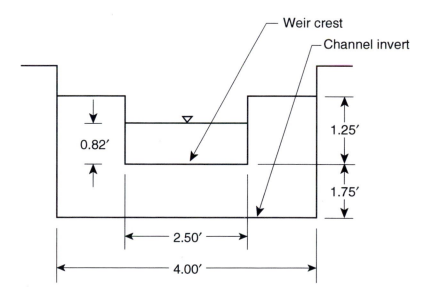

10. Find the discharge over a broad-crested weir with crest breadth of 18 inches and dimensions as shown in problem 8.

11. Find the discharge over the rectangular, two-stage weir shown below if the breadth of each crest is 2.00 feet.

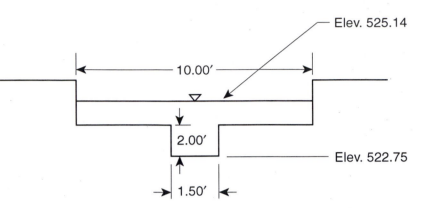

12. A broad-crested weir is formed by cutting a rectangular notch in a 1.0-foot-thick concrete wall. The notch is 2.0 feet deep and 12.0 feet long. If an impoundment rises up to the top of the wall, what is the discharge over the weir?

13. A curved broad-crested weir is shown below. What is the discharge when the reservoir reaches the following levels: (a) 322.10 feet, (b) 324.17 feet, and (c) 325.24 feet? Determine dimensions by scale.

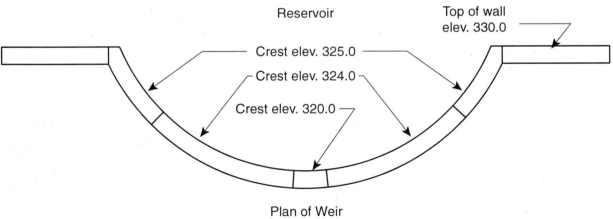

Plan of Weir
Scale: 1″ = 40′

14. A sluice gate in a dam is lifted half its height to allow drawdown of an impoundment. The gate measures 4.00 feet wide by 6.25 feet high. The impoundment water surface is 12.72 feet above the bottom of the gate opening. The discharge coefficient, c, for the gate is 0.77. Find the discharge.

15. A 50-foot, 1-inch diameter hose is used to siphon a swimming pool. The pool measures 8.00 feet by 12.00 feet by 6.0 feet deep. The hose is laid out with its discharge end 10.0 feet below the surface of the pool. Assume that the hose approximates the smoothness of drawn tubing. (a) Find the discharge in the hose. (b) Estimate the time required to draw down the pool to a depth of 2.0 feet.

FURTHER READING

Brater, E. F., and King, H. (1976). *Handbook of Hydraulics*. New York: McGraw-Hill.

Hita, C. E., and Hwang, N. H. C. (1987). *Hydraulic Engineering Systems* (2nd ed.). Englewood Cliffs, NJ: Prentice Hall.

Merritt, F. S. (ed.) (1983). *Standard Handbook for Civil Engineers* (3rd ed.). New York: McGraw-Hill.

Morris, H. M., and Wiggert, J. M. (1972). *Applied Hydraulics in Engineering* (2nd ed.). New York: Wiley.

Mott, R. L. (1994). *Applied Fluid Mechanics* (4th ed.). Englewood Cliffs, NJ: Prentice Hall.

Prasuhn, A. L. (1987). *Fundamentals of Hydraulic Engineering*. New York: Holt, Rinehart and Winston.

Simon, A. L., and Korom, S. F. (1997). *Hydraulics* (4th ed.). Englewood Cliffs, NJ: Prentice Hall.

U.S. Bureau of Reclamation (1977). *Design of Small Dams* (2nd ed.). Denver, CO: U.S. Department of the Interior.

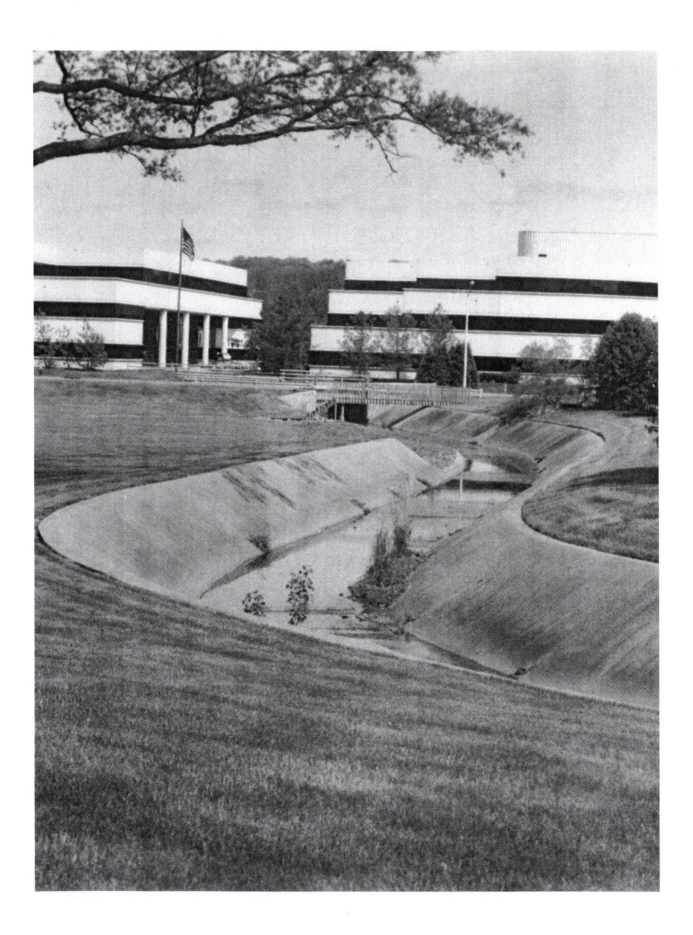

OPEN CHANNEL HYDRAULICS

When water flows downhill in any conduit with the water surface exposed to the atmosphere (free surface), it is said to undergo **open channel flow**. This type of flow is different from pressure flow in a closed conduit but no less complex. Open channel hydraulics is the study of the mechanics of water flowing in open conduits, which generally include channels, streams, and even pipes (not flowing under pressure), as depicted in Figure 6-1. An example of open channel flow is shown in Figure 6-2, which depicts a human-made rectangular channel conveying a stream through a park.

OBJECTIVES

After completing this chapter, the reader should be able to:

- Compute the slope of a channel
- Compute the cross-sectional area, wetted perimeter, and hydraulic radius of a channel
- Identify normal depth in a channel
- Identify and compute critical depth in a channel

6.1 FUNDAMENTAL CONCEPTS

To analyze open channel flow, let us first consider a long, uniform channel such as the concrete trapezoidal channel shown in Figure 6-1(a). A uniform, or **prismatic**, channel is one that maintains a constant shape and slope. The trapezoidal channel is depicted in more detail in Figure 6-3, including a profile and a cross section. The essential elements of the profile are the channel bottom, water surface, and energy grade line (EGL). As we discussed in Section 4.4, the hydraulic grade line (HGL) is coincident with the water surface. Each of these lines has a slope, which may be the same as or different than the others, depending on the type of flow.

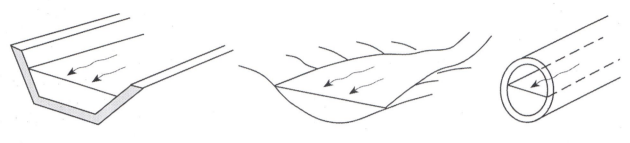

(a) Concrete Channel   (b) Natural Stream   (c) Pipe (not flowing full)

FIGURE 6-1   Examples of open channel flow.

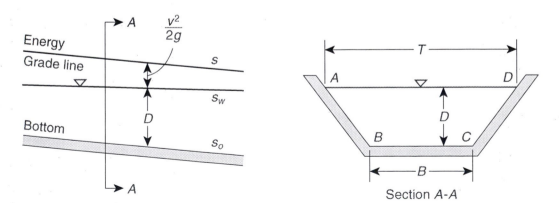

FIGURE 6-2   Open channels are often used to convey stream flow in developed areas. This channel has a rectangular shape with stone sides.

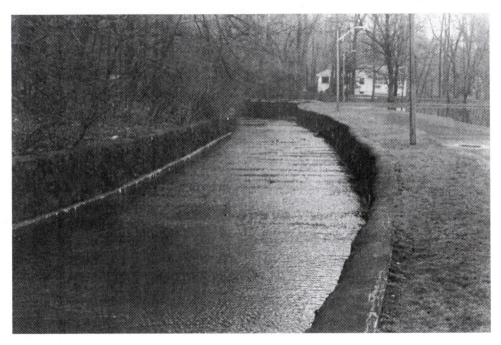

Section *A-A*

FIGURE 6-3   Concrete channel with trapezoidal cross section.

The **slope** of the channel bottom, s_o, is defined as the vertical fall divided by the horizontal run of the bottom. Thus, a channel bottom that drops 1.00 foot (m) in a length of 20.0 feet (m) has a slope of 0.050 ft/ft (m/m). That is,

$$s_o = \frac{\text{drop}}{\text{length}}$$

$$= \frac{1.00}{20.0} = 0.050 \text{ ft/ft (m/m)}$$

Slope can also be expressed as a percentage by multiplying by 100 percent. The slope computed above, expressed as a percent, is 5.0 percent.

Figure 6-3 reveals two other slopes involved with open channel flow, namely, the slope of the water surface, s_w, and the slope of the energy grade line, s. These slopes are defined as drop divided by length, just as with bottom slope.

The **depth** of flow, D, is the vertical distance from the bottom of the channel to the water surface. The **cross-sectional area** of flow, a, is the area of a cross section of the flowing water. In Figure 6-3, the cross-sectional area is the area of the trapezoid, or

$$a = \left(\frac{T + B}{2} \right) D$$

An important concept in open channel hydraulics is **wetted perimeter**. The wetted perimeter, p, is the distance along the channel cross section that is in contact with the flowing water. In Figure 6-3, the wetted perimeter is the sum of the distances AB, BC, and CD. Another important concept is **hydraulic radius**. The hydraulic radius, R, of a channel is defined as the cross-sectional area divided by the wetted perimeter, or

$$R = \frac{a}{p} \tag{6-1}$$

Hydraulic radius is not truly a "radius" in a geometric sense but merely a term defined to give an indication of the hydraulic efficiency of a channel. This concept will be explored further in Chapter 7. Open channel flow may be classified as various types of flow as in any conduit, as defined in Section 4.2. One of these classifications is uniform flow versus varied flow. The distinction between these types is very important, so they will be considered in separate chapters: Chapter 7 for uniform flow and Chapter 8 for varied flow.

Another flow classification is laminar versus turbulent flow. In open channel problems encountered in engineering design, flow is almost always turbulent. However, laminar flow can occur when the depth is very shallow, such as sheet flow, which is encountered in stormwater runoff and discussed in Chapter 10.

Example 6-1

Problem

For the trapezoidal channel shown below, find the slope, s_o; the cross-sectional area, a; the wetted perimeter, p; and the hydraulic radius, R.

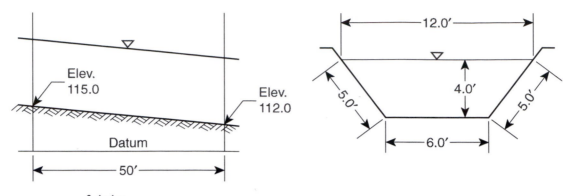

Solution

Slope is computed by using the elevations and the length.

$$s_o = \frac{115.0 - 112.0}{50} = 0.060 \text{ ft/ft} = 6.0\%$$

Cross-sectional area and wetted perimeter are computed by using the dimensions of the cross section. Thus,

$$a = \left(\frac{6.0 + 12.0}{2}\right)4.0 = 36 \text{ s.f.}$$

$$p = 5.0 + 6.0 + 5.0 = 16 \text{ ft}$$

Hydraulic radius is computed by using Equation 6-1. Thus,

$$R = \frac{a}{p} = \frac{36}{16} = 2.25 \text{ ft}$$

Note: When we apply significant figures, the hydraulic radius is 2.3 ft.

6.2   TYPES OF CHANNELS

Channels constructed for the conveyance of water can have many different cross-sectional shapes as well as different slopes and alignments. If a channel changes shape, slope, or alignment, it is nonprismatic, and the flow characteristics are correspondingly affected. Such changes disrupt uniform flow and cause varied flow conditions that require special computational techniques, as discussed in Chapter 8. Typical channel cross sections are shown in Figure 6-4.

Channels are also constructed of many different materials, ranging from grass-lined soil to stone to concrete. The material used to form a channel is referred to as the lining of the channel. The type of material affects the flow because it increases or decreases velocity at the interface between the water and the channel lining. According to the continuity equation (Equation 4-10), if the velocity is affected, the cross-sectional area and consequently the depth are affected.

Maximum velocity occurs just below the free surface in the center of the channel and can reach a magnitude of 2.0 to 2.5 times the average velocity. Figure 6-5 shows typical velocity distributions for rectangular and trapezoidal channels. The lowest velocity is located along the channel lining.

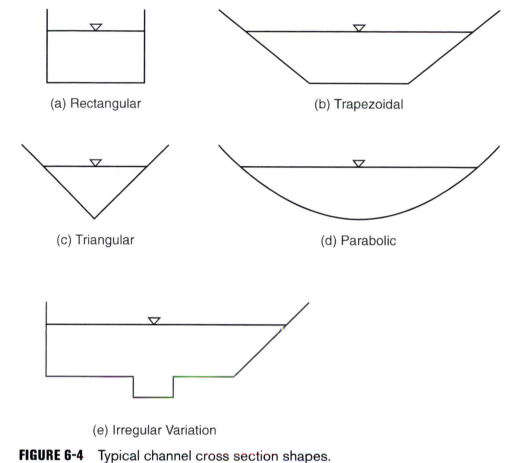

(a) Rectangular

(b) Trapezoidal

(c) Triangular

(d) Parabolic

(e) Irregular Variation

FIGURE 6-4   Typical channel cross section shapes.

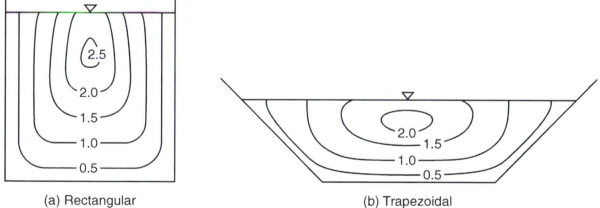

(a) Rectangular

(b) Trapezoidal

FIGURE 6-5   Velocity distributions in rectangular and trapezoidal channels. Values are multiples of average velocity.

6.3   NORMAL DEPTH

When water flows in a uniform channel, after an initial transition, it reaches and maintains a constant velocity and constant depth called **normal depth**, D_n. Flowing water is propelled downstream by its weight, specifically the component of its weight in the direction of the channel. But the friction force produced at the channel lining is equal in magnitude and opposite in direction, thus creating equilibrium that has constant velocity. The energy grade line is parallel to the surface of the water because the velocity, and therefore the velocity head, is constant. That is, all three slopes in Figure 6-3 are equal, or $s_o = s_w = s$ and $D = D_n$.

Another requirement for normal depth is a constant flow rate, Q. For all our work in open channel flow, we will assume constant flow rate.

Normal depth depends on the slope of the channel, the roughness of the channel lining, the dimensions of the channel cross section, and the rate of flow. For greater slopes, D_n is smaller; for lesser slopes, D_n is greater. For rougher channels, D_n is larger; for smoother channels, D_n is smaller. For wider channels, D_n is smaller; for narrower channels, D_n is greater. For smaller values of Q, D_n is smaller; greater values of Q yield greater values of D_n. These characteristics will be quantified in Chapter 7.

6.4 CRITICAL DEPTH

Specific energy, E, is defined as $E = D + v^2/2g$ or total energy head above the channel bed. If we plot values of E against corresponding values of D resulting from variations in depth for the same value of Q, we will obtain a curve like that shown in Figure 6-6.

Close inspection of the specific energy diagram reveals that for very low velocity with very high depth, the specific energy E approaches the value of D. For high velocity, depth approaches zero, meaning that E is composed almost entirely of $v^2/2g$. One particular value of D, called **critical depth**, designated D_c, results in the minimum value of E. Critical depth is a theoretical concept that depends on only the channel shape and the flow quantity Q. It does not depend on the roughness of the channel lining or the slope of the channel. Generally, flow depths greater than critical depth represent more tranquil flow called **subcritical**, and depths below D_c represent more rapid flow called **supercritical**.

The velocity of the water at critical depth is called **critical velocity**. When a channel has a slope that causes normal depth to coincide with critical depth, the

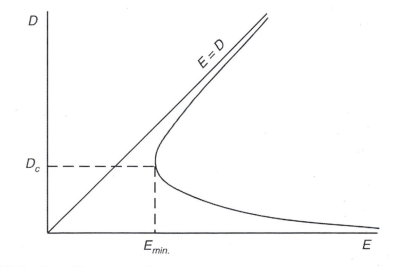

FIGURE 6-6 Specific energy diagram.

slope is called **critical slope**. Critical depth is computed by use of the following relationship, which occurs only at minimum specific energy, E:

$$\frac{a^3}{T} = \frac{Q^2}{g} \qquad (6\text{-}2)$$

where a = cross-sectional area of channel, ft^2 (m^2)
   T = top width of channel, ft (m)
   Q = flow rate, cfs (m^3/s)
   g = acceleration of gravity, 32.2 ft/s^2 (9.81 m/s^2)

Equation 6-2 applies to all channel shapes and must usually be solved by trial and error. However, it is valid only if the flow is gradually varied or parallel to the channel bottom and the channel slope is small (less than 8 percent). For rectangular channels, Equation 6-2 reduces to

$$D_c = \sqrt[3]{\frac{Q^2}{T^2 g}} \qquad (6\text{-}3)$$

For any given channel and flow rate Q, there is a corresponding critical depth. Usually, normal depth in a channel is not equal to critical depth. Only one particular slope results in a normal depth equal to critical depth.

The most common occurrence of critical depth is in gradually varied flow, in which the flow depth varies over a certain distance due to a change in one or more of the channel attributes. The change could be in channel slope or cross-sectional shape. As the depth varies, critical depth can be attained within the transition region. For example, Figure 6-7 shows a profile of a channel transition from subcritical flow to supercritical flow. Depth of flow is at critical depth near the transition point. Notice in Figure 6-7 that theoretical critical depth does not change when the channel slope changes.

A parameter called the **Froude number** may be used to distinguish between subcritical flow and supercritical flow. For a rectangular channel, the Froude number, F, is defined as

$$F = \frac{v}{\sqrt{gD}} \qquad (6\text{-}4)$$

where F = Froude number (dimensionless)
   v = average velocity, ft/s (m/s)
   D = flow depth, ft (m)
   g = acceleration due to gravity, 32.2 ft/s^2 (9.81 m/s^2)

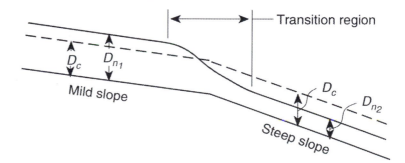
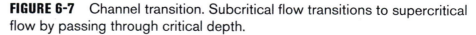

FIGURE 6-7   Channel transition. Subcritical flow transitions to supercritical flow by passing through critical depth.

When $F = 1$, flow is critical. Subcritical flow occurs when $F < 1$ and supercritical when $F > 1$. For nonrectangular channels, the Froude number is defined as

$$F = \frac{v}{\sqrt{gD_h}} \qquad (6\text{-}5)$$

where D_h = hydraulic depth, ft (m).

The hydraulic depth, D_h, is defined as

$$D_h = \frac{a}{T} \qquad (6\text{-}6)$$

where a = cross-sectional area, ft^2 (m^2), and T = top width, ft (m).

The concept of critical depth, although purely theoretical, has many applications in open channel hydraulics. Two major applications of the principle are flow control and flow measurement. In Chapter 8, critical depth is used in the analysis of backwater curves and flow entering a channel. Then in Chapter 9, critical depth is used in analyzing culverts.

Example 6-2

Problem

Find critical depth in a trapezoidal channel having a bottom width of 6.00 feet and 2:1 side slopes and a slope of 1.00 percent. The channel is lined with concrete in good condition and carries a flow of 80.0 cfs.

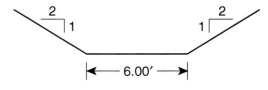

Solution

The condition of the concrete is irrelevant, since D_c does not depend on roughness. Also, the slope is irrelevant, since D_c does not depend on slope. Therefore, first determine the value of Q^2/g, which is the right side of Equation 6-2.

$$\frac{Q^2}{g} = \frac{80^2}{32.2} = 199$$

(This value has meaningless units of ft^5, which we will not bother to write in the computations.)

Trial 1: Let $D_c = 1.00$ foot. Then $a = 8.00$ ft^2 and $a^3 = 512$. Geometry of the channel gives $T = 10.0$ ft.

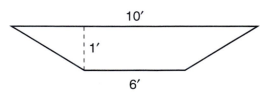

Therefore, $a^3/T = 512/10.0 = 51.2$. This value is then compared to the value of 199 already computed for Q^2/g. Since the value of a^3/T is less than 199, choose a higher value for a^3/T.

Trial 2: Let $D_c = 2.00$ feet. Then $a = 20.0$ ft^2 and $a^3 = 8000$. Geometry of the channel gives $T = 14.0$ feet.

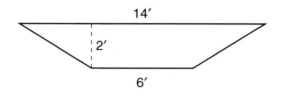

Therefore, $a^3/T = 8000/14 = 571$. Since 571 is greater than 199, the correct value of D_c lies between 1.00 foot and 2.00 feet. An estimate can be made by interpolating between the two sets of numbers computed so far:

D_c	a^3/T
1.00	51.2
x	199
2.00	571

Interpolation:

$$\frac{x-1}{2-1} = \frac{199-51.2}{571-51.2}$$

$$x-1 = \frac{147.8}{519.8}$$

$$= 0.284$$

$$x = 1.28$$

$$D_c = 1.28 \text{ ft}$$

Therefore, an estimate for D_c is 1.28 feet, which must now be checked.

Trial 3: Let $D_c = 1.28$ feet. Then $a = 11.0$ ft^2, $a^3 = 1315$, and $T = 11.12$ ft.

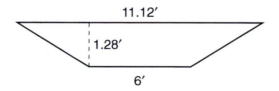

Therefore, $a^3/T = 1315/11.12 = 118$. Since 118 differs from 199 by 41 percent, it is not considered a close enough approximation. Since 118 is less than 199, choose a higher value of D_c, say, $D_c = 1.50$ feet.

Trial 4: Let $D_c = 1.50$ feet. Then $a = 13.5$ ft^2, $a^3 = 2640$, and $T = 12.0$ feet.

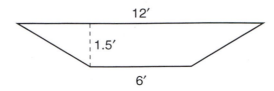

Therefore, $a^3/T = 2460/12 = 205$. Since 205 differs from 199 by 3.0 percent, it is marginal as a close approximation. Therefore, attempt one more trial with $D_c = 1.49$ feet.

Trial 5: Let $D_c = 1.49$ ft. Then $a = 13.38$ ft^2, $a^3 = 2395$, and $T = 11.96$ feet.

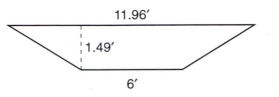

Therefore, $a^3/T = 2395/11.96 = 200$. Since 200 differs from 199 by only 0.5 percent, it is considered a close enough approximation. Therefore, the critical depth has been found to be 1.49 feet.   (Answer)

The above calculation can be performed in a convenient tabular format as follows: First, compute $Q^2/g = 199$. Next, create a table having each parameter to be computed across the top and then proceed to the trials:

Trial	D_c (ft)	a (ft^2)	a^3 —	T (ft)	a^3/T —
1	1.00	8.00	512	10	51.2
2	2.00	20.0	8000	14	571
3	1.28	11.0	1315	11.12	118
4	1.50	13.5	2460	12	205
5	1.49	13.4	2395	11.96	200

This table can be computed by using spreadsheet software.

PROBLEMS

1. A surveyor finds that the bottom of a rectangular channel drops 3.75 feet in a distance of 200.0 feet. What is the slope of the channel?

2. The bottom elevation of a trapezoidal channel is 422.05 at station $1 + 00$ and 423.92 at station $1 + 50$. What is the slope of the channel?

3. A 6.0-foot-wide rectangular channel has a normal depth of 2.45 feet. (a) What is the cross-sectional area of the flow? (b) What is the wetted perimeter? (c) What is the hydraulic radius?

4. A channel conveys a discharge of 210 cfs at a velocity of 5.45 ft/s. Find the cross-sectional area of the channel.

5. Refer to the following channel cross section. Normal depth is 1.50 feet. (a) What is the cross-sectional area of flow? (b) What is the wetted perimeter? (c) What is the hydraulic radius?

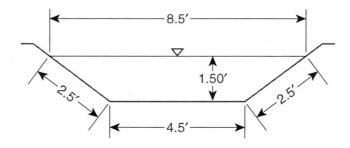

6. Refer to the following channel cross section. Normal depth is 3.0 feet. (a) What is the cross-sectional area of flow? (b) What is the wetted perimeter? (c) What is the hydraulic radius?

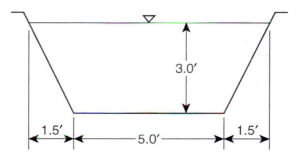

7. Refer to the following channel cross section. (a) What is the normal depth? (b) What is the cross-sectional area of flow? (c) What is the wetted perimeter? (d) What is the hydraulic radius?

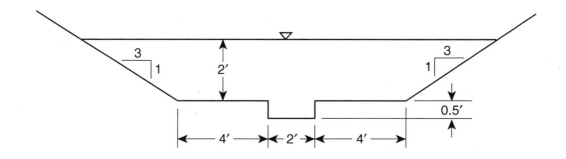

8. A trapezoidal channel with a bottom width of 4.00 feet and side slopes of 2 horizontal to 1 vertical has a normal depth of 5.0 feet. (a) What is the cross-sectional area of flow? (b) What is the wetted perimeter? (c) What is the hydraulic radius?

9. Refer to the following channel cross section. (a) What is the normal depth? (b) What is the cross-sectional area of flow? (c) What is the wetted

perimeter? (d) What is the hydraulic radius? Determine channel dimensions by scaling.

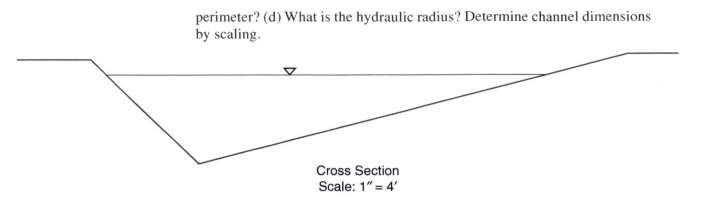

Cross Section
Scale: 1″ = 4′

10. Refer to the following channel cross section. (a) What is the normal depth? (b) What is the cross-sectional area of flow? (c) What is the wetted perimeter? (d) What is the hydraulic radius? Determine channel dimensions by scaling.

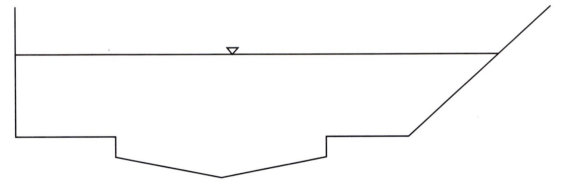

Cross Section
Scale: 1″ = 4′

11. A rectangular channel with a width of 8.0 feet conveys a discharge of 125 cfs. Find the critical depth for the channel.

12. Refer to the channel cross section in problem 6. If the discharge is 100 cfs, what is the critical depth?

13. Refer to the channel cross section in problem 8. If the discharge is 200 cfs, what is the critical depth?

14. Refer to the channel cross section in problem 9. If the discharge is 350 cfs, what is the critical depth?

15. A trapezoidal channel with a bottom width of 10.0 feet and side slopes of 2 horizontal to 1 vertical has a discharge of 650 cfs. What is the critical depth?

16. A trapezoidal channel with a bottom width of 5.0 feet and side slopes of 2 horizontal to 1 vertical has a discharge of 150 cfs. What is the critical depth?

17. A rectangular channel with a width of 6.0 feet conveys a discharge of 115 cfs. If the depth of flow is 3.0 feet, what is the velocity? What is the Froude number? Is the flow subcritical or supercritical?

18. A rectangular channel with a width of 15.0 feet conveys a discharge of 180 cfs. If the depth of flow is 1.2 feet, what is the Froude number? Is the flow subcritical or supercritical?

19. A trapezoidal channel with a bottom width of 4.00 feet and side slopes of 2 horizontal to 1 vertical conveys a discharge of 300 cfs. If the depth of flow is 2.25 feet, what is the Froude number? Is the flow subcritical or supercritical?

20. Water is flowing in a 5.0-foot-wide rectangular channel with a quantity of 100 cfs. Plot a graph of D_n versus E by choosing a variety of flow depths D_n and for each flow depth computing the corresponding value of E using Equation 4-10. Use the graph you plotted to determine critical depth in the channel.

FURTHER READING

Brater, E. F., and King, H. (1996). *Handbook of Hydraulics* (7th ed.). New York: McGraw-Hill.

Chadwick, A. (2004). *Hydraulics in Civil and Environmental Engineering* (4th ed.). London: E and FN Spon.

Chaudhry, M. H. (1993). *Open Channel Flow*. Englewood Cliffs, NJ: Prentice Hall.

Chow, V. T. (1985). *Open Channel Hydraulics*. New York: McGraw-Hill.

Hwang, N. H. C., and Hita, C. E. (1987). *Fundamentals of Hydraulic Engineering Systems* (2nd ed.). Englewood Cliffs, NJ: Prentice Hall.

Merritt, F. S. (2004). *Standard Handbook for Civil Engineers* (5th ed.). New York: McGraw-Hill.

Nalluri, C., and Featherstone, R. E. (2001). *Civil Engineering Hydraulics* (4th ed.). London: Blackwell Science.

Simon, A. L., and Korom, S. F. (1996). *Hydraulics*. Englewood Cliffs, NJ: Prentice Hall.

Strum, T. W. (2001). *Open Channel Hydraulics*. New York: McGraw-Hill.

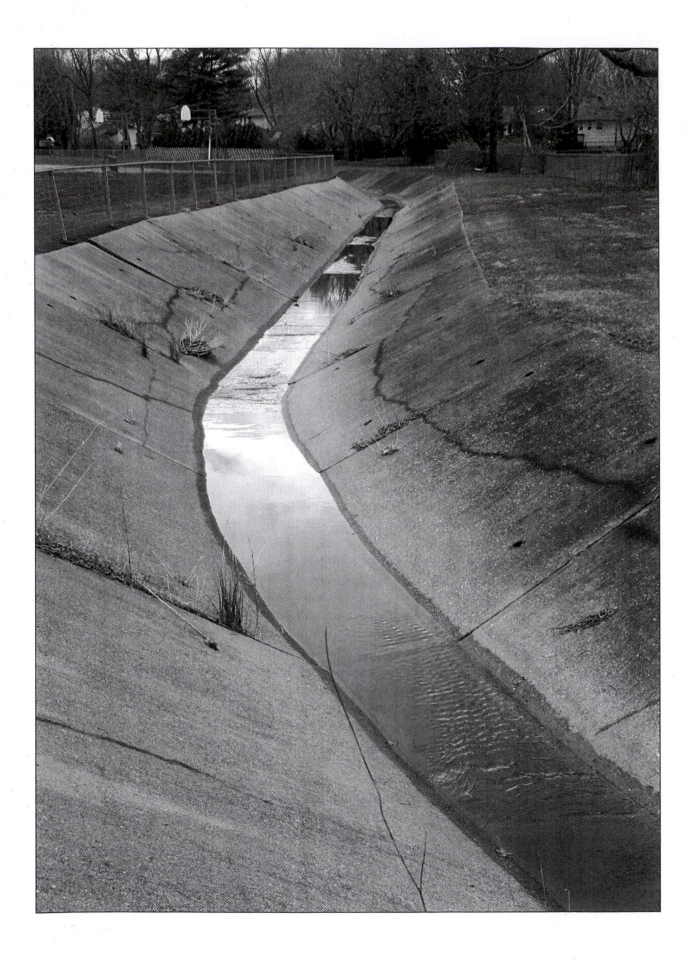

C H A P T E R

7

UNIFORM FLOW IN CHANNELS

In Chapter 6, we saw that in uniform (prismatic) channels, when water flows with a constant rate the resulting water surface profile is parallel to the channel bottom. This type of flow is called **uniform flow** and accounts for most common design conditions, such as long, straight channels and pipes (provided that the pipes are not flowing under pressure). The concept can also be applied to natural streams, even though streams are not strictly prismatic. Also, if a channel undergoes a change of slope or cross section, uniform flow can usually be assumed for the straight sections between transitions.

OBJECTIVES

After completing this chapter, the reader should be able to:

- Compute normal depth in a channel or pipe
- Compute normal depth in a stream including overbanks
- Use the channel and pipe design charts properly

7.1   MANNING'S EQUATION

Various empirical formulas have been devised to compute normal depth in a uniform channel. These formulas bear the names of their creators and include, among others, the Chezy, Darcy, Kutter, and Manning equations. The Chezy formula, developed around 1775 by the French engineer Antoine Chezy, is considered the first uniform flow formula. In 1889, the Irish engineer Robert Manning presented another formula, which has become the most widely used in the United States. The Manning equation for uniform flow is stated as follows:

$$v = \frac{1.49}{n} R^{2/3} s_o^{1/2} \quad \text{(English units)} \tag{7-1}$$

where v = velocity, ft/s
        R = hydraulic radius, ft
        s_o = slope of channel, ft/ft
        n = roughness factor

$$v = \frac{1}{n} R^{2/3} s_o^{1/2} \quad \text{(SI units)} \tag{7-1a}$$

where v = velocity, m/s
        R = hydraulic radius, m
        s_o = slope of channel, m/m
        n = roughness factor

Manning's equation is used to find velocity if normal depth, D_n, is known. Discharge, Q, can then be determined by using the continuity equation $Q = va$. By substituting the continuity equation into Manning's equation, a variation of the equation is created involving discharge, Q, as follows:

$$Q = a \frac{1.49}{n} R^{2/3} s_o^{1/2} \quad \text{(English units)} \tag{7-2}$$

where a = cross-sectional area, ft^2

$$Q = \frac{a}{n} R^{2/3} s_o^{1/2} \quad \text{(SI units)} \tag{7-2a}$$

where a = cross-sectional area, m^2

This variation of Manning's equation can be used to find normal depth if discharge is known. However, a quick look at Equation 7-2 or 7-2a reveals no term for normal depth, even though they are used to calculate normal depth. This seeming contradiction is answered rather easily: Normal depth is calculated indirectly. Manning's equation is used in an iterative (trial-and-error) process to find normal depth. This process will be shown in Example 7-2.

The use of Manning's equation involves various parameters introduced in Section 6.1 plus another term, **roughness factor**, n, an empirical number that describes the roughness of the channel lining. It is similar to f used in Bernoulli's equation but not exactly the same. Values used for f cannot be substituted for n values. Many design manuals contain charts of Manning n values to be used in working with the Manning equation. A selection of such n values is listed in Appendix A-1.

As was mentioned in Section 6.1, hydraulic radius is a measure of the hydraulic efficiency of a channel. The greater the value of R, the more discharge is conveyed by the channel for a given cross-sectional area. Thus, a wide, shallow channel has a relatively large wetted perimeter compared to cross-sectional area and is therefore less efficient than is a square-shaped channel with the same cross-sectional area.

Example 7-1

Problem

Find the hydraulic radius of the two channels shown below having the same cross-sectional area but different wetted perimeters. Which channel will carry more flow?

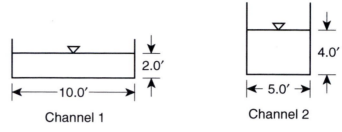

Channel 1   Channel 2

Solution

Channel 1

$$a = (10.0)(2.0) = 20.\ \text{ft}^2$$
$$p = 2.0 + 100. + 2.0 = 14\ \text{ft}$$
$$R = 20./14 = 1.4\ \text{ft} \quad \text{(Answer)}$$

Channel 2

$$a = (5.0)(4.0) = 20.\ \text{ft}^2$$
$$p = 4.0 + 5.0 + 4.0 = 13\ \text{ft}$$
$$R = 20./13 = 1.5\ \text{ft} \quad \text{(Answer)}$$

Channel 2 has greater hydraulic radius than does Channel 1. Therefore, it will carry greater flow, since according to Manning's equation, Q varies directly with $R^{2/3}$.

7.2   CHANNEL FLOW

Typical engineering problems involving uniform flow in channels consist of (1) computing discharge when normal depth is known and (2) computing normal depth when discharge is known. These are illustrated in Examples 7-2 and 7-3, respectively.

Example 7-2

Problem

Find the quantity of flow Q in a concrete rectangular channel having a width of 12.0 feet, a slope of 0.0200 ft/ft, and a normal depth, D_n, of 1.58 feet.

Solution

When D_n is given, Q can be solved directly by using Manning's equation. First, choose the appropriate n value from Appendix A-1. Let $n = 0.013$ for average concrete with trowel finish. Next, find a:

$$a = TD = (12.0)(1.58) = 18.96\ \text{ft}^2$$

Next, find p:

$$p = 1.58 + 12.0 + 1.58 = 15.16\ \text{ft}$$

Next, find R:

$$R = \frac{18.96}{15.16} = 1.25 \text{ ft}$$

Finally, find Q:

$$Q = a\frac{1.49}{n}R^{2/3}s_o^{1/2}$$

$$= (18.96)\frac{1.49}{0.013}(1.25)^{2/3}(0.02)^{1/2}$$

$$= 357 \text{ cfs} \quad \text{(Answer)}$$

The flow velocity can now be easily computed by using Equation 4-10:

$$v = \frac{Q}{a} = \frac{357}{18.96} = 18.8 \text{ ft/s}$$

Example 7-3

Problem

Find normal depth in a 10.0-foot-wide concrete rectangular channel having a slope of 0.0150 ft/ft and carrying a flow of 400. cfs.

Solution

When Q is given, D_n is found by trial and error (iteration). A value for D_n is chosen as a guess (or trial), and the corresponding Q-value is computed. If the computed value of Q is greater than 400. cfs, a second trial using a smaller D_n is made; if Q is less than 400. cfs, a larger D_n is chosen. By trial 3 or 4, D_n can be reasonably approximated.

First, choose the appropriate n value. Let $n = 0.013$.

Trial 1: Let $D_n = 2.00$ feet. Then $a = 20.0$ ft^2, $p = 14.0$ ft, and

$$R = \frac{20}{14} = 1.43 \text{ ft}$$

$$Q = (20)\frac{1.49}{0.013}(1.43)^{2/3}(0.015)^{1/2} = 356 \text{ cfs}$$

Since 356 is less than 400. cfs, choose a larger value of D_n.

Trial 2: Let $D_n = 3.00$ ft. Then $a = 30.0$ ft^2, $p = 16.0$ ft, and

$$R = \frac{30}{16} = 1.88 \text{ ft}$$

$$Q = (30)\frac{1.49}{0.013}(1.88)^{2/3}(0.015)^{1/2} = 640 \text{ cfs}$$

The correct value of D_n lies between 2.00 feet and 3.00 feet. An estimate can be made by interpolating between the two sets of values computed so far. To interpolate, set up a chart of values that have already been determined, where x represents the desired D_n value:

D_n	Q
2.00	356
x	400
3.00	640

Interpolation: $\dfrac{x-2}{3-2} = \dfrac{400-356}{640-356}$

$$\frac{x-2}{1} = \frac{44}{287}$$

$$x - 2 = 0.155$$
$$= 2.15$$

$$D_n = 2.15 \text{ ft}$$

Therefore, an estimate for D_n is 2.15 ft, which must now be checked in trial 3.

Trial 3: Let D_n = 2.15 ft. Then a = 21.5 ft, p = 14.3 ft, and

$$R = \frac{21.5}{14.3} = 1.50 \text{ ft}$$

$$Q = (21.5)\frac{1.49}{0.013}(1.50)^{2/3}(0.015)^{1/2} = 396 \text{ cfs}$$

Since 396 cfs differs from 400. cfs by only 1.0 percent, it is considered a close enough approximation. Therefore, the normal depth has been found to be 2.15 ft.   (Answer)

The above calculations can be performed in a convenient tabular format as follows: First, compute $(1.49/n)s^{1/2}$ because this is the portion of Manning's equation that will not change from one trial to another:

$$\frac{1.49}{n}s_o^{1/2} = 14.04$$

Next, create a table having each parameter to be computed across the top, and then proceed to the trials:

Trial	D_n (ft)	a (ft²)	p (ft)	R (ft)	$R^{2/3}$ —	Q (cfs)
1	2.00	20	14	1.43	1.27	356
2	3.00	30	16	1.88	1.52	640
3	2.15	21.5	14.3	1.50	1.31	396

This tabulation could be easily computed by using standard spreadsheet software such as MS Excel.

Charts for the solution of Manning's equation have been developed for various channel sections. Charts for selected rectangular and trapezoidal channels are found in Appendix A-3. Software packages have also been developed for the solution of Manning's equation. The names of selected hydraulic software are shown in Appendix E.

Hydraulic Design Charts

The design charts presented in Appendix A-3 are accompanied by a one-page explanation of their use. The reader should review the explanation thoroughly before using the charts. To help with the use of the charts, the following description shows how the charts can be used to solve Examples 7-2, 7-3, and 6-2.

For Example 7-2 (finding Q when D_n is known), use Chart 10 in Appendix A-3. First, locate the intersection of the slope and normal depth lines. The line for a slope of 0.0200 ft/ft is shown in the chart, but the normal depth of 1.58 feet is not shown. Normal depth must be interpolated between the lines for 1.5 feet and 2.0 feet. Next, the chosen n-value of 0.013 does not correspond to the calibration of the chart, which is 0.015. Therefore, the Qn scale must be used. From the intersection first located, project a line straight down to the Qn scale, and read the value 4.5. Discharge is found by solving the equation

$$Qn = 4.5$$
$$Q(0.013) = 4.5$$
$$Q = 346 \text{ cfs}$$
$$Q = 350 \text{ cfs} \quad \text{(using significant figures)}$$

This answer is within 2 percent of the computed value of 357 cfs in Example 7-2. Values determined by using the design charts are usually less precise than those obtained by using Manning's equation directly. The lower precision is acceptable if it is precise enough for the application for which it is used.

For Example 7-3 (finding D_n when Q is known), use Chart 9 in Appendix A-3. Start with the Qn scale at the bottom. As in the previous example, the Qn scale is used because $n = 0.013$. For this example,

$$Qn = (400)(0.013)$$
$$Qn = 5.2$$

Locate the value 5.2 on the Qn scale, and project straight up to the 0.015 ft/ft slope line. Using this point, interpolate between adjacent normal depth lines of 2.0 feet and 2.5 feet. The interpolated value is 2.2 feet. This answer is within 2.5 percent of the computed value of 2.15 feet in Example 7-3.

For Example 6-2 (finding D_c when Q is known), use Chart 19 in Appendix A-3. Do not use the Qn scale because critical depth is independent of roughness. Locate the discharge of 80 cfs on the discharge scale, and project straight up to the critical depth line. Using this point, interpolate between adjacent normal depth lines to find critical depth. In this case, the point falls on the 1.5-foot line, so the critical depth is 1.5 feet. This answer is within 1 percent of the computed value of 1.49 feet in Example 6-2.

7.3 PIPE FLOW

When water flows by gravity in a pipe partially full (not under pressure), it conforms to the laws of open channel flow. Normal depth is computed by using the appropriate form of Manning's equation, and critical depth is computed from

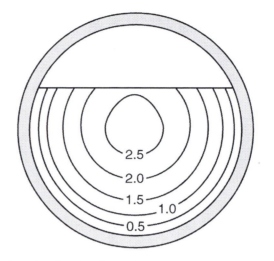

FIGURE 7-1   Velocity distribution in a circular pipe flowing part full. Values are multiples of average velocity.

Equation 6-2. The only difference between pipe flow and rectangular channel flow is the geometry of the cross section.

Velocity distribution in a pipe is similar to that of any open channel, with the distribution influenced by the cross-section shape. Figure 7-1 shows the typical velocity distribution in a pipe flowing part full.

The principal applications of pipe flow are storm sewers, sanitary sewers, and culverts. The following examples illustrate the characteristics of flow in circular pipes.

Example 7-4

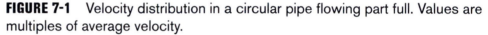

Problem

Find the quantity and velocity of flow in an 18-inch-diameter concrete pipe flowing one-quarter full. The pipe has a slope of 1.00 percent.

Solution

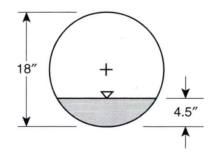

First, choose an n value, say, $n = 0.015$. Next, compute a and p. To find a, the cross-sectional area of flow is recognized as a segment of a circle as described in the geometric analysis following this example. According to the geometric analysis,

$$a = 0.345 \text{ ft}^2$$

To find p, compute the arc length of the circle intersected by the water surface. Again, from geometric analysis, we have

$$p = 1.57 \text{ ft}$$

Next, compute R:

$$R = \frac{a}{p} = \frac{0.345}{1.57} = 0.220 \text{ ft}$$

Finally, compute Q:

$$
\begin{aligned}
Q &= a\frac{1.49}{n}R^{2/3}s_o^{1/2} \\
&= (0.345)\frac{1.49}{0.015}(0.220)^{2/3}(0.01)^{1/2} \\
&= 1.25 \text{ cfs} \quad \text{(Answer)}
\end{aligned}
$$

Also, compute v:

$$v = \frac{Q}{a} = \frac{1.25}{0.345} = 3.62 \text{ ft/s} \quad \text{(Answer)}$$

Geometric Analysis of Circular Pipe Flow

The following analysis illustrates the computation of wetted area, a, and wetted perimeter, p, for use in Manning's equation used for flow in circular pipes. The numbers that are used apply to Example 7-4, but the procedure is applicable to all depths and pipe sizes.

To find a and p, first construct an isosceles triangle using the water surface as the base; then determine the measure of the vertex angle, θ, as shown below. To determine the vertex angle, θ, construct the altitude of the triangle creating the right triangle with angle $\theta/2$, as shown below.

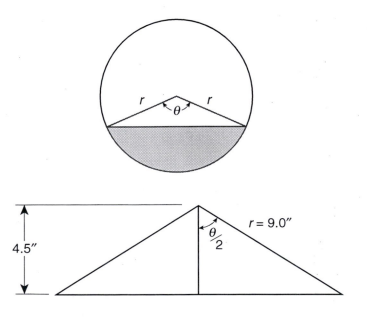

Thus, the angle $\theta/2$ is computed as

$$\cos \frac{\theta}{2} = \frac{4.5}{9.0}$$

$$\frac{\theta}{2} = 60°$$

and the vertex angle, θ, is

$$\theta = 120°$$

Cross-sectional area, a, can now be computed using the formula for a segment of a circle:

$$a = \frac{r^2}{2}\left(\frac{\theta\pi}{180} - \sin\theta\right)$$

or

$$a = \frac{\left(\frac{9.0}{12}\right)^2}{2}\left[\frac{120\pi}{180} - \sin 120°\right]$$
$$= 0.345 \text{ ft}^2$$

Wetted perimeter, p, can be computed by

$$p = \frac{\theta}{360}(2\pi r)$$
$$= \frac{120}{360}(2\pi)\left(\frac{9}{12}\right)$$
$$= 1.57 \text{ ft}$$

Example 7-5

Problem

Find the quantity and velocity of flow in an 18-inch-diameter concrete pipe flowing half full. The pipe has a slope of 1.00 percent.

Solution

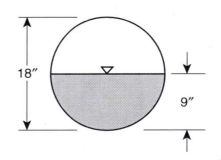

Let $n = 0.015$. Compute a and p:

$$a = \frac{1}{2}\pi\,(0.75)^2$$
$$= 0.884 \text{ ft}^2$$
$$p = \frac{1}{2}\pi\,(1.5)$$
$$= 2.36 \text{ ft}$$

Next, compute R:

$$R = \frac{a}{p} = \frac{0.884}{2.36} = 0.375 \text{ ft}$$

Finally, compute Q:

$$Q = a\frac{1.49}{n}R^{2/3}s_o^{1/2}$$
$$= (0.884)\frac{1.49}{0.015}(0.375)^{2/3}(0.01)^{1/2}$$
$$= 4.56 \text{ cfs} \quad \text{(Answer)}$$

Also, compute v:

$$v = \frac{Q}{a} = \frac{4.56}{0.884} = 5.16 \text{ ft/s} \quad \text{(Answer)}$$

Example 7-6

Problem

Find the quantity and velocity of flow in an 18-inch-diameter concrete pipe flowing 94 percent full. The pipe has a slope of 1.00 percent.

Solution

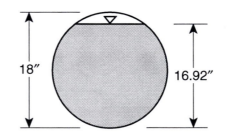

Let $n = 0.015$, and compute a and p. The cross-sectional area, a, is found from geometrical analysis to be

$$a = 1.72 \text{ ft}^2$$

Wetted perimeter, p, also is found from geometrical analysis to be

$$p = 3.97 \text{ ft}$$

Next, compute R:

$$R = \frac{a}{p} = \frac{1.72}{3.97} = 0.433 \text{ ft}$$

Finally, compute Q:

$$Q = a\frac{1.49}{n}R^{2/3}s_o^{1/2}$$

$$= (1.72)\frac{1.49}{0.015}(0.433)^{2/3}(0.01)^{1/2}$$

$$= 9.78 \text{ cfs} \quad \text{(Answer)}$$

Also, compute v:

$$v = \frac{Q}{a} = \frac{9.78}{1.72} = 5.69 \text{ ft/s} \quad \text{(Answer)}$$

Example 7-7

Problem

Find the quantity and velocity of flow in an 18-inch-diameter concrete pipe flowing just full (but not under pressure). The pipe has a slope of 1.00 percent.

Solution

In this case, flowing full means the water surface has just reached the top of the pipe and no pressure results. The pipe may still be considered an open channel for this condition.

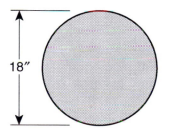

18"

Let $n = 0.015$. Compute a and p:

$$a = \pi r^2 = \pi(0.75)^2 = 1.77 \text{ ft}^2$$
$$p = \pi D = \pi(1.5) = 4.71 \text{ ft}$$

Next, compute R:

$$R = \frac{a}{p} = \frac{1.77}{4.71} = 0.375 \text{ ft}$$

Finally, compute Q:

$$Q = a\frac{1.49}{n}R^{2/3}s_o^{1/2}$$

$$= (1.77)\frac{1.49}{0.015}(0.375)^{2/3}(0.01)^{1/2}$$

$$= 9.14 \text{ cfs} \quad \text{(Answer)}$$

Also, compute v:

$$v = \frac{Q}{a} = \frac{9.14}{1.77} = 5.16 \text{ ft/s} \quad \text{(Answer)}$$

Examples 7-4 through 7-7 illustrate several facts about pipe flow. First, calculating pipe flow is complex and tedious. For this reason, many design charts (including computer software) have been prepared over the years summarizing the solutions to Manning's equation for pipe flow. Appendix A-4 presents one such set of charts to use for problems in this text as well as design projects on the job.

Second, the examples show that the maximum flow in a given circular pipe occurs at a depth of 94 percent of full depth. This odd phenomenon is explained by hydraulic efficiency. As depth approaches the top of the pipe, wetted perimeter (a flow retarder) increases faster than cross-sectional area (a flow increaser). Therefore, the upper 6 percent of a pipe's area contributes nothing to the capacity of the pipe; in fact, it actually decreases the capacity!

Note, however, that when engineers talk about the capacity of a pipe, they generally refer to the Q-value when the pipe is flowing full, not flowing at 94 percent depth, despite the fact that flowing full is a little less than the maximum discharge possible in the pipe. This provides the designer with a modest built-in safety factor.

Another characteristic of pipe flow shown in the examples is that velocity is the same for both half and full flow. Velocity generally increases with depth of flow until it reaches a maximum at 94 percent of full flow. Then it decreases until full flow, where it once again reaches the same value as half-full flow.

Figure 7-2 shows a graph of Q versus depth and v versus depth with values from Examples 7-4 through 7-7 plotted. The pattern that emerges from the plottings illustrates the unique relationships described for discharge and velocity in circular pipes. A graph depicting these relationships for circular pipes in general is shown in Figure 7-3.

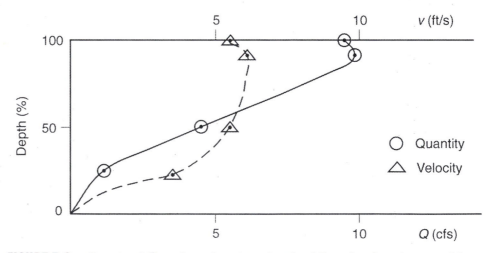

FIGURE 7-2   Graph of Q and v related to depth of flow for the pipe used in Examples 7-4 through 7-7.

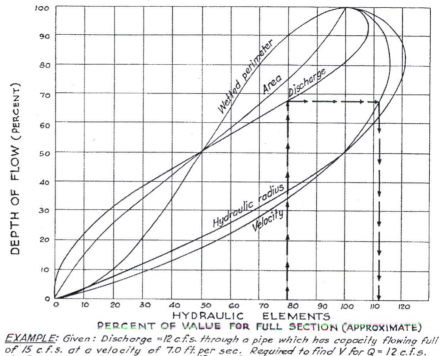

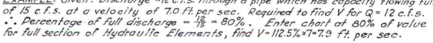

EXAMPLE: Given: Discharge =12 c.f.s. through a pipe which has capacity flowing full of 15 c.f.s. at a velocity of 7.0 ft. per sec. Required to find V for Q = 12 c.f.s.
∴ Percentage of full discharge = 12/15 = 80%. Enter chart at 80% of value for full section of Hydraulic Elements, find V= 112.5%×7=7.9 ft. per sec.

FIGURE 7-3   Hydraulic elements of circular pipe flow. *(Courtesy of E. Seeley, Data Book for Civil Engineers, Vol. 1, John Wiley & Sons, Inc.)*

Critical depth in a pipe flowing as an open channel is computed from Equation 6-2 or taken from the design charts in Appendix A-4. A pipe will have one particular critical depth for each flow quantity Q. The use of Equation 6-2 as an iteration process is quite tedious, and therefore critical depth is normally taken from design charts or computer software.

7.4   STREAM FLOW

Streams are naturally occurring open channels with varying uniformity of cross section and roughness. Figure 7-4 depicts two examples of natural streams. Normal depth can be computed for a stream by using Manning's equation when the stream can be considered uniform and there are no significant obstructions in the stream. Obstructions, such as a bridge crossing, cause a variation in the water surface profile called a **backwater curve**. Backwater curves are plotted by a special computation procedure called a step computation, normally performed by computer. Such computations are described in Chapter 8.

We will limit our analysis of stream flow to uniform flow, in which Manning's equation is used to compute depth and quantity of flow. Natural streams often flow in a flooded condition, that is, with depth above the top of bank elevation. When flooding occurs, we must still be able to compute the depth even though the roughness factors of the overbanks usually differ from that of the channel of the stream. Figure 7-5 shows a typical stream cross section including overbanks. The usual convention for stream cross sections is that they are drawn looking downstream.

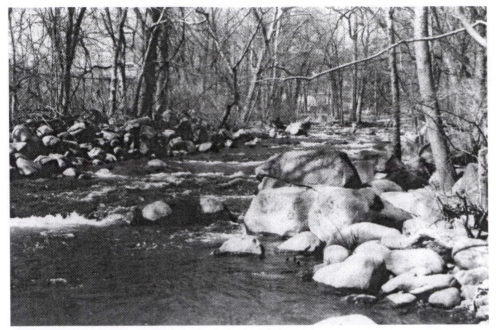

(a) Mountain stream with steep rocky banks.

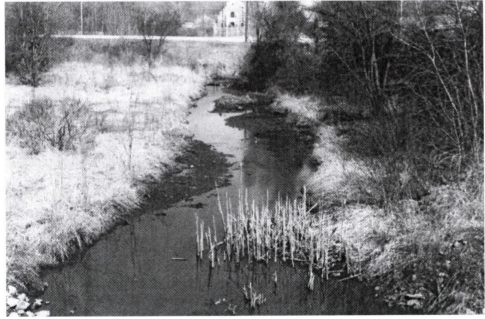

(b) Lowland stream with flat overbanks.

FIGURE 7-4   Examples of natural streams.

Flow Q is computed separately for all three components of the stream: left overbank, channel, and right overbank. Wetted perimeter for the channel is simply the length along the ground in the cross section from top of bank to top of bank. When the water level rises above the top of bank, wetted perimeter does not increase. The following example illustrates the computation of depth in a stream.

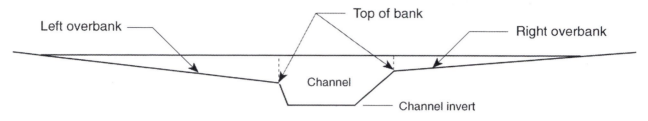

FIGURE 7-5   Typical stream cross section (looking downstream).

Example 7-8

Problem

Find the water surface elevation for the stream depicted below having a flow of 425 cfs and slope of 0.400 percent. Roughness is described as follows:

Left overbank: heavy weeds, scattered brush
Channel: fairly regular section, some weeds, light brush on banks
Right overbank: light brush and trees

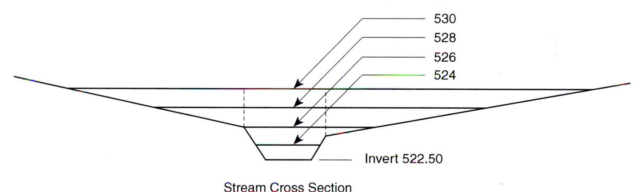

Stream Cross Section
Scale: 1″ = 10′

Solution

First, determine *n* values. Using Appendix A-1, *n* values are estimated as follows:

Left overbank: $n = 0.060$
Channel: $n = 0.042$
Right overbank: $n = 0.070$

Next, compute $\dfrac{149}{n}s_o^{1/2}$ for each stream component:

Left overbank: $\dfrac{1.49}{n}s_o^{1/2} = \dfrac{1.49}{0.06}(0.004)^{1/2} = 1.57$

Channel: $\dfrac{1.49}{n}s_o^{1/2} = \dfrac{1.49}{0.042}(0.004)^{1/2} = 2.24$

Right overbank: $\dfrac{1.49}{n}s_o^{1/2} = \dfrac{1.49}{0.07}(0.004)^{1/2} = 1.35$

Finally, set up a table having each parameter to be computed listed across the top, as shown below, and then proceed to the trials.

Normal Depth Computation for Stream with Overbanks

		Left Overbank					Channel					Right Overbank					Total
Trial	Elev. (ft)	a (ft^2)	p (ft)	R (ft)	$R^{2/3}$ —	Q (cfs)	a (ft^2)	p (ft)	R (ft)	$R^{2/3}$ —	Q (cfs)	a (ft^2)	p (ft)	R (ft)	$R^{2/3}$ —	Q (cfs)	Q (cfs)
1	524	—	—	—	—	—	9	8.3	1.08	1.06	21	—	—	—	—	—	21
2	526	—	—	—	—	—	25.3	12	2.11	1.64	93	3	6	.5	.63	3	96
3	528	10	10.2	0.98	0.99	15	42.9	12	3.58	2.34	225	26.5	17.5	1.51	1.32	47	287
4	530	40	21	1.9	1.54	97	60.5	12	5.04	2.94	399	73	29.5	2.47	1.83	180	676

The elevation corresponding to $Q = 425$ cfs can now be estimated by interpolating between trials 3 and 4. Let x = water surface elevation.

Elev.	Q
528	278
x	425
530	676

$$\frac{x - 528}{530 - 528} = \frac{425 - 287}{676 - 287}$$

$$\frac{x - 528}{2} = \frac{138}{389}$$

$$x - 538 = 0.710$$

$$x = 528.71 \quad \text{(Answer)}$$

Therefore, 528.71 is taken as the water surface elevation corresponding to $Q = 425$ cfs.

Note: In computing the trials, the areas, a, are cumulative; that is, each value for area includes the area for the preceding trial. Also, note that all wetted perimeters for the channel for trial 2 and on are 12 feet. This is because as the water gets above the top of bank, no more contact is made between the water and the ground. For example, in trial 3, a and p are shown as follows:

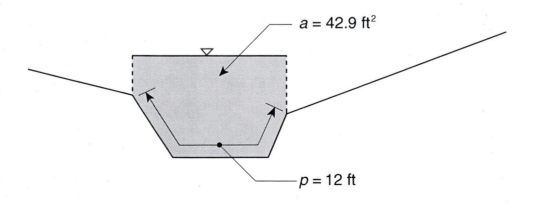

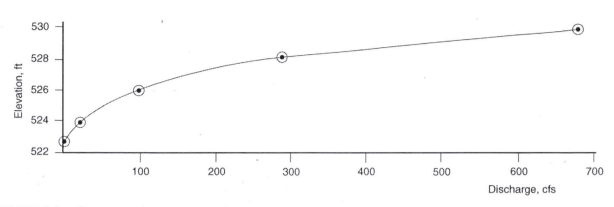

FIGURE 7-6   Stream rating curve for Example 7-8.

Although water does not actually flow with vertical sides (unsupported) as shown above, it is assumed to take on such shape purely for computational purposes. Also, note that the information produced by the trials can be used to plot a graph of discharge, Q, versus water surface elevation. Such a graph is called a **stream rating curve** and is shown in Figure 7-6.

PROBLEMS

1. A rectangular channel lined with concrete ($n = 0.014$) has a bottom width of 5.0 feet and a slope of 2.50 percent. Water is flowing at a depth of 1.25 feet. (a) What is the discharge in cfs? (b) What is the average velocity in ft/s?

2. A rectangular channel lined with brick ($n = 0.016$) has a bottom width of 3.75 feet and a slope of 0.47 percent. Water is flowing at a depth of 2.9 feet. (a) What is the discharge? (b) What is the velocity?

3. A trapezoidal channel lined with grass ($n = 0.027$) has a bottom width of 4.25 feet, side slopes of 2 horizontal to 1 vertical, and a slope of 1.1 percent. Water is flowing at a depth of 2.35 feet. (a) What is the discharge? (b) What is the velocity?

4. A trapezoidal channel lined with stone ($n = 0.024$) has a bottom width of 8.0 feet, side slopes of 2.5 horizontal to 1 vertical, and a slope of 4.2 percent. Water is flowing at a depth of 3.0 feet. (a) What is the discharge? (b) What is the velocity?

5. Refer to the channel cross section shown in problem 7 in Chapter 6. If the channel slope is 1.75 percent and the lining is concrete (trowel finish), what are (a) the discharge and (b) the velocity?

6. Refer to the channel cross section shown in problem 10 in Chapter 6. If the channel slope is 0.62 percent and the lining is concrete (trowel finish), what are (a) the discharge and (b) the velocity?

7. Find the normal depth for a discharge of 350 cfs in a rectangular channel with a bottom width of 20.0 feet. The channel is concrete lined ($n = 0.013$) with a slope of 0.75 percent. Use Manning's equation.

8. Find the normal depth for a discharge of 125 cfs in a trapezoidal channel with a bottom width of 3.00 feet and side slopes of 2 horizontal to 1 vertical. The

channel is lined with riprap (stones) ($n = 0.024$) and has a slope of 1.00 percent. Use Manning's equation.

9. Find the normal depth for a discharge of 225 cfs in a trapezoidal channel with a bottom width of 5.00 feet and side slopes of 2 horizontal to 1 vertical. The channel is lined with concrete ($n = 0.012$) and has a slope of 2.00 percent. Use Manning's equation.

10. Refer to the channel cross section shown in problem 7 in Chapter 6. Disregard the water level shown in the cross section, and find a new normal depth if the channel slope is 1.25 percent and the discharge is 300 cfs. The lining is concrete (trowel finish).

11. Refer to the channel cross section shown in problem 10 in Chapter 6. Disregard the water level shown in the cross section, and find a new normal depth if the channel slope is 2.0 percent and the discharge is 600 cfs. The lining is concrete (trowel finish).

12. A 6.0-foot-wide rectangular channel carries a flow of 56 cfs at a depth of 1.50 feet. What is the average velocity of the flow?

13. A channel conveys a discharge of 210 cfs at a velocity of 5.45 ft/s. Find the cross-sectional area of the channel.

14. A trapezoidal channel with bottom width of 4.00 feet and side slopes of 2 horizontal to 1 vertical carries a flow depth of 2.25 feet at an average velocity of 7.32 ft/s. What is the flow, Q, in the channel?

15. A 36-inch-diameter pipe flowing half full conveys a discharge of 15 cfs. What is the velocity of the flow?

16. Find the capacity of a 15-inch RCP with $n = 0.015$ and $s_o = 1.25$ percent.

17. Find the capacity of a 36-inch RCP with $n = 0.012$ and $s_o = 0.80$ percent.

18. Find normal depth for a discharge of 75 cfs in a 60-inch-diameter concrete pipe ($n = 0.012$). The pipe has a slope of 1.20 percent. Use Manning's equation.

19. Find normal depth for a discharge of 50 cfs in a 48-inch diameter concrete pipe ($n = 0.012$). The pipe has a slope of 1.90 percent. Use Manning's equation.

20. For the stream cross section shown below, find the water surface elevation for a flow of 650 cfs. Determine channel dimensions by scaling. The stream has a slope of 0.110 percent and the following characteristics:

Channel: Fairly regular section, some weeds, light brush on banks.
Overbanks: Heavy weeds, scattered brush.

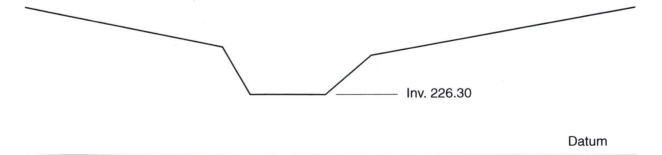

Inv. 226.30

Datum

Stream Cross Section
Scale: 1″ = 10′

FURTHER READING

Brater, E. F., and King, H. (1996). *Handbook of Hydraulics* (7th ed.). New York: McGraw-Hill.

Chadwick, A. (2004). *Hydraulics in Civil and Environmental Engineering* (4th ed.). London: E and FN Spon.

Chaudhry, M. H. (1993). *Open Channel Flow*. Englewood Cliffs, NJ: Prentice Hall.

Chow, V. T. (1985). *Open Channel Hydraulics*. New York: McGraw-Hill.

Hwang, N. H. C., and Hita, C. E. (1987). *Fundamentals of Hydraulic Engineering Systems* (2nd ed.). Englewood Cliffs, NJ: Prentice Hall.

Merritt, F. S. (2004). *Standard Handbook for Civil Engineers* (5th ed.). New York: McGraw-Hill.

Nalluri, C., and Featherstone, R. E. (2001). *Civil Engineering Hydraulics* (4th ed.). London: Blackwell Science.

Simon, A. L., and Korom, S. F. (1996). *Hydraulics*. Englewood Cliffs, NJ: Prentice Hall.

Strum, T. W. (2001). *Open Channel Hydraulics*. New York: McGraw-Hill.

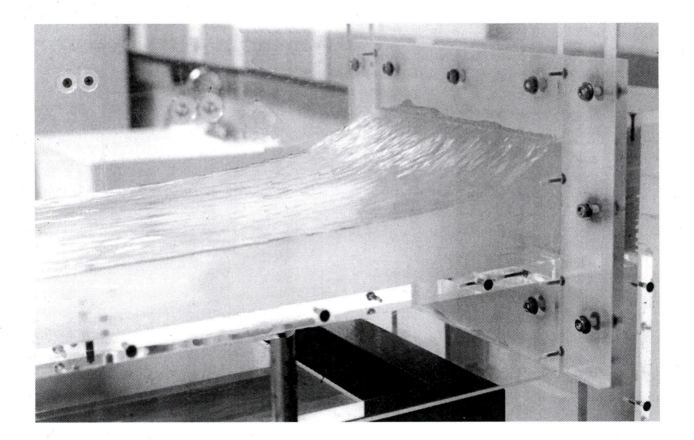

8

VARIED FLOW IN CHANNELS

Water flowing in an open channel sometimes undergoes variations in its depth due to certain conditions in the channel. In Chapter 7, we saw that in uniform channels, when water flows with a constant rate, the resulting water surface profile is parallel to the channel bottom. In this chapter, we will see that obstructions to flow or varying channel conditions result in a water surface profile that is not parallel to the channel bottom. Depending on the type of condition encountered, the flow can be gradually varied or rapidly varied.

OBJECTIVES

After completing this chapter, the reader should be able to:

- Identify water surface profiles for mild- and steep-sloped channels
- Compute a backwater profile using the standard step method
- Compute a water surface profile at an entrance to a channel
- Compute a basic hydraulic jump

8.1 FUNDAMENTAL CONCEPTS

Several conditions can occur in a channel that result in varied flow, either gradual or rapid. Varied flow is considered gradual if it occurs over a relatively long distance. Examples of conditions that cause gradually varied flow include a change in a channel slope, a change in a channel cross section from narrow to wide or from wide to narrow, or an obstruction placed in a channel, such as a culvert or bridge. Examples of rapidly varying flow include a spillway and an energy dissipater. In these cases, high-velocity flow abruptly changes to low-velocity flow over a short distance.

Water surface profiles are categorized according to the slope of the channel bottom and other flow conditions. The slope of the channel bottom can be mild, steep, critical, horizontal, or adverse. These slopes are further described below.

Mild slope (designated M) is a slope resulting in subcritical flow, where normal depth is above critical depth. Steep slope (designated S) is a slope resulting in supercritical flow, where normal depth is below critical depth. Critical slope (designated C) is a slope resulting in critical flow, where normal depth coincides with critical depth. Horizontal slope (designated H) is a perfectly flat slope. Adverse slope (designated A) is a slope pitched in the direction opposite to that of the flow (negative slope). These slopes are illustrated in Figure 8-1.

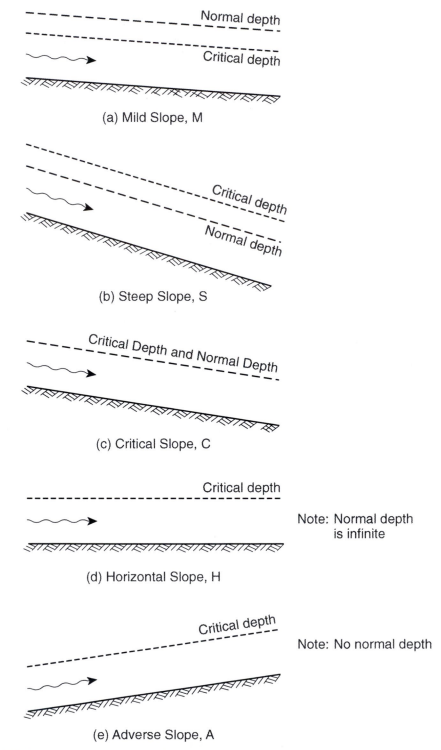

FIGURE 8-1 Classification of channel slopes for varied flow.

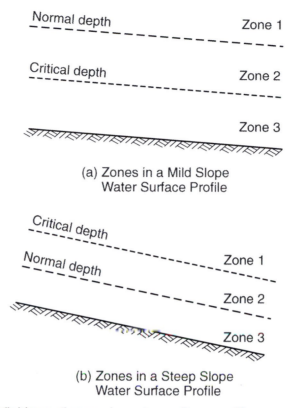

(a) Zones in a Mild Slope
Water Surface Profile

(b) Zones in a Steep Slope
Water Surface Profile

FIGURE 8-2 Definitions of zones in water surface profiles.

A close look at Figure 8-1 reveals that in each case, critical depth is the same. This is because, as was first described in Section 6.4, critical depth depends only on the discharge and channel geometry, not on the channel slope. Normal depth varies with slope conditions. In this text, we are concerned only with the first two conditions shown in Figure 8-1: mild and steep slopes. A more detailed discussion of these conditions follows.

To further analyze water surface profiles in channels with mild and steep slopes, consider three zones within the profile as defined in Figure 8-2.

For mild slopes, Zone 1 comprises the area above the normal depth line, while Zone 2 is the area between the normal depth line and the critical depth line, and Zone 3 consists of the area between the critical depth line and the channel bottom. For steep slopes, the zones are defined similarly except that the normal and critical depth lines are reversed. By using these zone designations, various profiles can be identified for various flow conditions.

Figure 8-3 shows examples of mild slope profiles. The M1 profile shown in part (a) is the typical backwater curve for an obstruction in a channel. This is a common condition in open channel hydraulics and is presented in more detail in Section 8.2.

Figure 8-4 shows examples of steep slope profiles. The obstruction shown in part (a) results in an S1 profile upstream and an S3 profile downstream. If the channel had a mild slope, the resulting profile would resemble that shown in Figure 8-3(a).

A **control section** is a cross section of a channel at which the flow depth can be readily determined. The water surface profile for varied flow is usually sketched by starting at a control section and then proceeding either upstream or downstream,

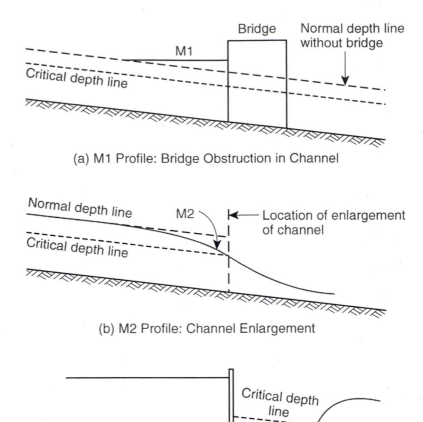

(a) M1 Profile: Bridge Obstruction in Channel

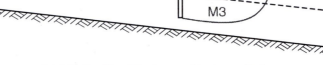

(b) M2 Profile: Channel Enlargement

(c) M3 Profile: Discharge Under a Gate

FIGURE 8-3 Examples of varied flow in mild slope profiles.

depending on flow conditions. For subcritical flow, the control section is always at the downstream end of the channel reach, and the profile is sketched in an upstream direction. For supercritical flow, the opposite is true: The control section is located at the upstream end of the channel reach, and the profile is sketched in a downward direction.

Backwater profiles involving subcritical flow are caused by a downstream condition or obstruction. The obstruction does not allow all the flowing water to pass easily, resulting in a backup or rise of upstream flow similar to traffic backing up when a four-lane road narrows to a two-lane road. However, in the case of supercritical flow, an obstruction does not affect upstream flow because any attempt to back up the water is pushed downstream by the swiftly flowing water. Instead, downstream flow is affected by the obstruction.

8.2 BACKWATER PROFILE

A classic **backwater profile**, or backwater curve, results when an obstruction in a channel causes a pool to form upstream of the obstruction, as shown in Figure 8-3(a).

Computation of a backwater profile can be accomplished either directly by integration of the energy equation or approximately by the so-called step methods.

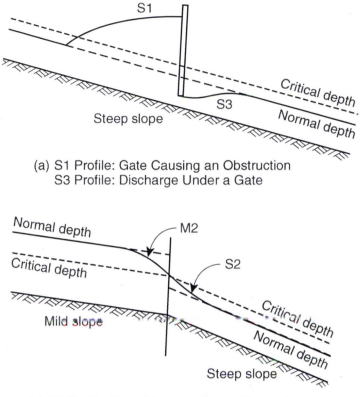

(a) S1 Profile: Gate Causing an Obstruction
S3 Profile: Discharge Under a Gate

(b) S2 Profile: Transition to a Steep Channel

FIGURE 8-4 Examples of varied flow in steep slope profiles.

The step methods involve the calculation of a finite number of points along the profile using the technique of trial and error. In the direct step method, the water surface elevation is known at the control section, and the distance is calculated between that section and another known water surface elevation. The calculation is then repeated along the channel reach. In the **standard step** method, the water surface elevation is known at the control section, and the water surface elevation is calculated at another section of known distance from the control section. The calculation is then repeated along the channel reach. It is the standard step method that is used in the HEC-RAS water surface profile software developed by the U.S. Army Corps of Engineers. Following is a description of this method.

Standard Step Method

The standard step method can be used for both prismatic and nonprismatic channels, including natural streams as well as constructed channels. When used for natural streams, the results are less precise than those for regular channels but precise enough to be useful for design purposes.

Because the flow is varied, there will be locations along the channel causing the varied flow, such as changes in slope, roughness, or cross section. These locations must be determined by inspection of field data, and cross sections must be drawn for each. The distance between cross sections should not exceed that which would result in a change of velocity greater than 20 percent.

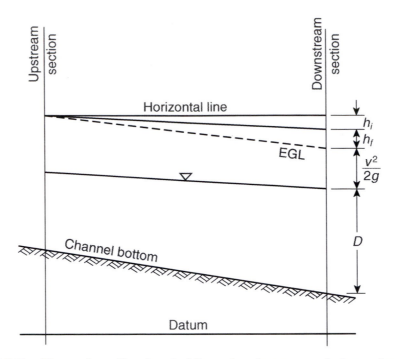

FIGURE 8-5 Channel profile of varied flow showing energy balance for the standard step method.

The water surface profile is computed by balancing total energy from cross section to cross section. Starting at the control section, having known water surface elevation, total energy is computed. Then, by trial and error, the water surface elevation is computed at the next cross section to correspond to the total energy at the control section. The water surface would then be determined in a similar manner for the remaining cross sections. Figure 8-5 shows a schematic diagram of energy balance between sections. Notice that energy head is lost due to friction (designated h_f) and due to eddies (designated h_i). Eddy losses are due to turbulence in the channel caused by uneven surfaces.

The following example illustrates the method.

Example 8-1

Problem

Determine the backwater profile created by an obstruction in a channel causing a backup of 7.00 feet. The channel is rectangular as defined below and conveys a discharge of 500 cfs. Use the standard step method.

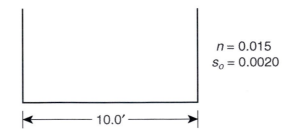

$n = 0.015$
$s_o = 0.0020$

Solution

First, determine whether the flow is subcritical or supercritical by computing normal depth and critical depth. Using Chart 9 in Appendix A-3, we get $D_n = 5.8$ feet and $D_c = 4.3$ feet. Therefore, flow is subcritical, and the control section is the obstruction at the downstream end of the channel reach.

Next, determine the cross section locations and draw the cross sections. Since the channel is uniform (except for the obstruction), cross sections will be placed at regular intervals separated by a distance resulting in a change of velocity less than 20 percent. Use a separation of 200 feet.

To compute the energy balance from section to section, use a table as shown in Table 8-1. Computation results are entered in the table as follows:

Column 1: Station location.

Column 2: Water surface elevation at the station. At the first station (0 + 0), the elevation is equal to the elevation of the channel bottom (102.00 ft) plus the depth of flow (7.00 ft).

Column 3: Depth of flow at the station (equal to the water surface elevation in Column 2 minus the elevation of the channel bottom at the station).

Column 4: Cross-sectional area at the station.

Column 5: Average velocity at the station (equal to the discharge divided by the area in Column 4).

Column 6: Velocity head at the station.

Column 7: Total head at the station (equal to the sum of the values in Columns 2 and 6).

Column 8: Hydraulic radius at the station.

Column 9: Hydraulic radius raised to the four-thirds power.

Column 10: Slope of the energy grade line. Using Manning's equation, we have

$$s = \frac{n^2 v^2}{2.22 R^{4/3}} \tag{8-1}$$

Column 11: Average slope through the reach, that is, between the station and the previous station.

Column 12: Length of the reach (between the station and the previous station).

Column 13: Friction loss in the reach (equal to the product of the values in Columns 11 and 12).

Column 14: Eddy loss in the reach (in this case equal to zero).

Column 15: Total head at the station computed by adding h_f and h_i to the total head value at the lower end of the reach, which is the value in Column 15 in the previous row. If the value thus obtained agrees reasonably with that in Column 7, then the assumed water surface elevation in Column 2 is correct, and the computation proceeds to the next station. (Reasonable agreement is considered to be within 0.01 ft.) If the value obtained does not agree with that in Column 7, however, the water surface elevation in Column 2 is incorrect, and a new value must be assumed and the computations must be repeated.

The resulting backwater profile is drawn by using the values shown in Columns 1 and 2 of Table 8-1. The profile is shown in Figure 8-6. Notice that the profile is

TABLE 8-1   Computation of Backwater Profile for Example 8-1

(1) Station	(2) Elev. (ft)	(3) D (ft)	(4) a (ft²)	(5) v (ft/s)	(6) v²/2g (ft)	(7) H (ft)	(8) R (ft)	(9) R^{4/3}	(10) s	(11) $\bar{s}$	(12) Dist. (ft)	(13) h_f (ft)	(14) h_i (ft)	(15) H (ft)	(16) Checks and exes (x)
0 + 0	107.00	7.00	70.0	7.14	0.79	107.79	2.92	4.17	0.00124	—	—	—	—	107.79	✓
2 + 0	107.30	6.90	69.0	7.25	0.82	108.12	2.90	4.13	0.00129	0.00126	200	0.25	0	108.04	x
2 + 0	107.22	6.82	68.2	7.33	0.83	108.05	2.88	4.11	0.00132	0.00128	200	0.26	0	108.05	✓
4 + 0	107.44	6.64	66.4	7.53	0.88	108.32	2.85	4.01	0.00142	0.00137	200	0.27	0	108.32	✓
6 + 0	107.68	6.48	64.8	7.72	0.92	108.60	2.82	3.99	0.00151	0.00147	200	0.29	0	108.61	✓
8 + 0	107.94	6.34	63.4	7.89	0.97	108.91	2.80	3.94	0.00160	0.00156	200	0.31	0	108.92	✓
10 + 0	108.25	6.25	62.5	8.00	0.99	109.24	2.78	3.90	0.00166	0.00163	200	0.33	0	109.25	✓
12 + 0	108.58	6.18	61.8	8.09	1.02	109.60	2.76	3.88	0.00171	0.00169	200	0.34	0	109.59	✓
14 + 0	108.91	6.11	61.1	8.18	1.04	109.95	2.75	3.85	0.00176	0.00174	200	0.35	0	109.94	✓
16 + 0	109.24	6.04	60.4	8.28	1.06	110.30	2.74	3.82	0.00182	0.00179	200	0.36	0	110.30	✓
18 + 0	109.57	5.97	59.7	8.38	1.09	110.66	2.72	3.80	0.00187	0.00185	200	0.37	0	110.67	✓

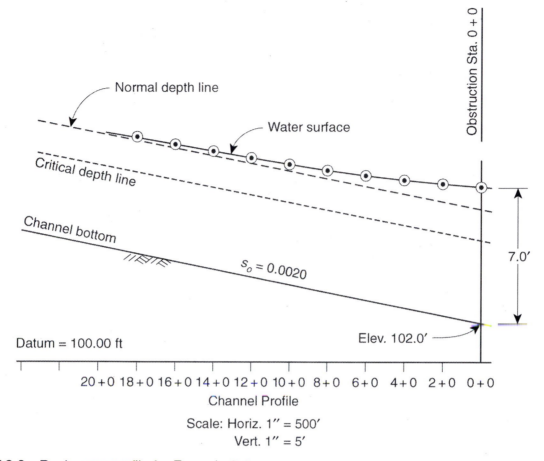

FIGURE 8-6   Backwater profile for Example 8-1.

classified as M1. In Table 8-1, Station 2 + 0 is entered twice because the first entry, with an assumed water surface elevation of 107.40, was incorrect and a second trial was needed. Also, notice that the change of velocity between stations is less than 3 percent, which is well within the allowable 20 percent.

In computing a backwater profile in a natural stream, HEC-RAS software normally is used. However, field data are the same as those needed for a hand calculation. The designer should be extra careful when choosing cross section locations, extent of the overbank included in each cross section, roughness coefficients, and other key parameters. The use of HEC-RAS, as with other application software, can easily lull the user into a false sense of security because the output looks valid whether it is or not.

8.3   ENTRANCE TO A CHANNEL

Another example of varied flow occurs when water flows from a large body such as a reservoir into a channel. This situation is encountered frequently in the design of an emergency spillway for a reservoir or detention basin.

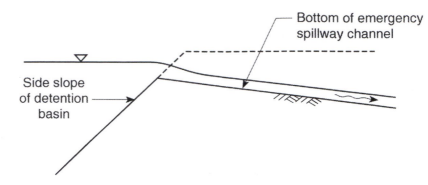

FIGURE 8-7   Profile of an entrance to a channel.

As an example, consider the detention basin depicted in Figure 14-7. Notice that the emergency spillway consists of a channel with its entrance cut into the side of the detention basin. Figure 8-7 shows a profile of a typical entrance to an emergency spillway channel such as the one depicted in Figure 14-7.

To calculate the drop in water surface as it enters the channel, use Bernoulli's equation (see Section 4.4) as applied to the reservoir and the channel. For water depth parameters, refer to Figure 8-8. By using the bottom of the channel at the entrance as a datum, Bernoulli's equation can be written as

$$D_r + \frac{v_r^2}{2g} = D_e + \frac{v_e^2}{2g} + h_e \tag{8-2}$$

where D_r = depth of the reservoir, ft
  v_r = velocity in the reservoir, ft/s
  D_e = depth at the channel entrance, ft
  v_e = velocity at the channel entrance, ft/s
  h_e = entrance head loss, ft

If the velocity in the reservoir is assumed to be zero and the minor entrance losses are considered negligible, Equation 8-2 becomes

$$D_r = D_e + \frac{v_e^2}{2g} \tag{8-3}$$

Substituting the continuity equation, $Q = va$, into Equation 8-3 gives

$$D_r = D_e + \frac{Q^2}{2ga^2} \tag{8-4}$$

where Q = discharge into the channel, cfs
  a = cross sectional area at the entrance, ft^2

If flow in the channel is subcritical ($s_o < s_c$), water enters the channel at normal depth, D_n. Therefore, depth at the entrance is equal to depth throughout the remainder of the channel, and Equation 8-4 can be written as

$$D_r = D_n + \frac{Q^2}{2ga^2} \quad \text{(Subcritical)} \tag{8-5}$$

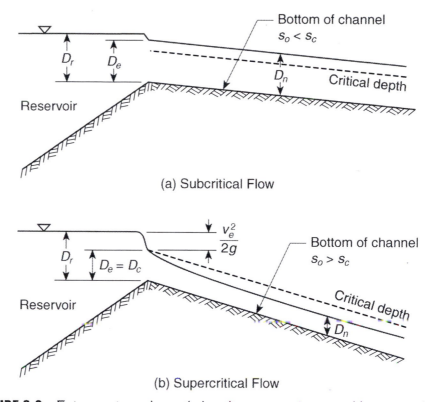

FIGURE 8-8   Entrance to a channel showing parameters used in computing depths of flow.

Values of D_n can be chosen and corresponding values of Q found by using Manning's equation. Then the D_n- and Q-values can be substituted into Equation 8-5 to find corresponding values of D_r.

If flow in the channel is supercritical ($s_o > s_c$), water enters the channel at critical depth, D_c. Therefore, Equation 8-4 can be written as

$$D_r = D_c + \frac{Q^2}{2ga^2} \quad \text{(Supercritical)} \tag{8-6}$$

Values of D_c can be chosen and corresponding values of Q found by using Equation 6-2 or Equation 6-3 (for rectangular channels). Then the D_c- and Q-values can be substituted into Equation 8-6 to find corresponding values of D_r.

Example 8-2

Problem

An emergency spillway for a detention basin is constructed as a rectangular channel with bottom width 12.0 feet and lined with riprap ($n = 0.025$). The slope of the channel is 0.0050 ft/ft. Compute a chart that shows the relationship between reservoir elevation and discharge into the channel.

Solution

First, determine whether the emergency spillway flow will be subcritical or supercritical. Because Q is not yet known, test for a few anticipated values of Q. In this case, values of Q up to 150 cfs indicate $D_n > D_c$, or subcritical flow.

Next, choose a list of D_n-values and find their corresponding Q-values using Manning's equation. Then, using the D_n- and Q-values, calculate corresponding D_r-values using Equation 8-5. Following is a table of the values and the answer to the problem. The table can be used as an outflow rating for the emergency spillway in computing a reservoir routing as presented in Chapter 14.

D_n (ft)	Q (cfs)	D_r (ft)
0.5	15.1	0.60
1.0	45.6	1.22
1.5	85.7	1.85
2.0	133	2.48

Example 8-3

Problem

An emergency spillway for a detention basin is constructed as a rectangular channel with bottom width 12.0 feet and lined with riprap ($n = 0.025$). The slope of the channel is 0.020 ft/ft. Compute a chart that shows the relationship between reservoir elevation and discharge into the channel.

Solution

First, determine whether the emergency spillway flow will be subcritical or supercritical. Because Q is not yet known, test for a few anticipated values of Q. In this case, values of Q up to 150 cfs indicate $D_n < D_c$, or supercritical flow.

Next, choose a list of D_c-values and find their corresponding Q-values using Equation 6-3. Then, using the D_c- and Q-values, calculate corresponding D_r-values using Equation 8-6. Following is a table of the values and the answer to the problem. The table can be used as an outflow rating for the emergency spillway when computing a reservoir routing as presented in Chapter 14.

D_c (ft)	Q (cfs)	D_r (ft)
0.5	24.1	0.75
1.0	68.1	1.50
1.5	125	2.25
2.0	193	3.00

Notice that Examples 8-2 and 8-3 present the same emergency spillway except for the slope of the channel. In Example 8-2, the slope is 0.50 percent (subcritical), and in Example 8-3, the slope is 2.0 percent (supercritical). In which example is the reservoir level higher for a given discharge?

The answer is not readily discernible by looking at the results of the examples. However, if values of D_r versus Q are plotted on a graph, the answer becomes more obvious. Notice in Figure 8-9 that Q-values are slightly higher (by 10 percent) for supercritical flow or D_r-values are lower for given Q-values. This means that if the

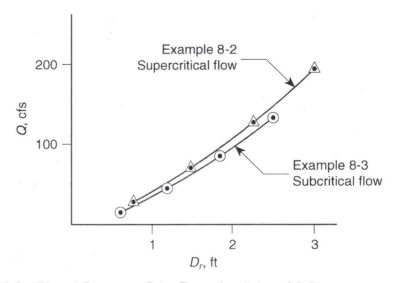

FIGURE 8-9   Plot of D_r versus Q for Examples 8-2 and 8-3.

emergency spillway is constructed with a 2.0 percent slope, the water level in the reservoir will tend to rise less than if the channel slope is flatter (0.5 percent). This could be a design consideration for the detention basin.

8.4   HYDRAULIC JUMP

When water flows down a steep surface such as a spillway and enters a relatively flat channel, the result is a transition from rapid shallow flow to slower, deeper flow. Any abrupt transition from a lower-stage supercritical flow to a higher-stage subcritical flow is referred to as a **hydraulic jump**. Figure 8-10 shows a hydraulic jump.

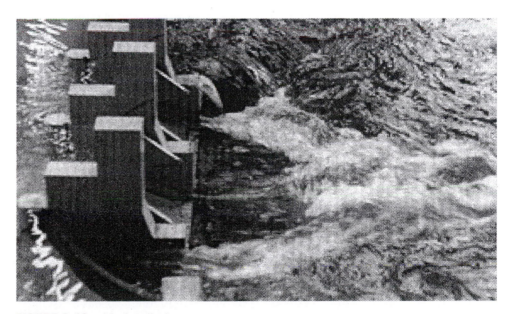

FIGURE 8-10   Hydraulic jump.

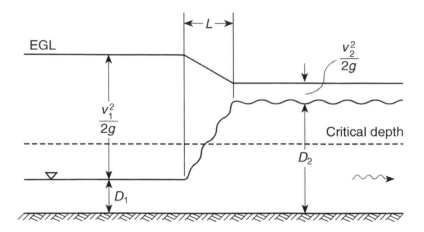

FIGURE 8-11   Typical hydraulic jump showing key parameters.

Hydraulic jumps can occur wherever flow in a channel is very rapid, such as a steep channel transitioning to a flat channel or flow discharging under a sluice gate into a channel. Hydraulic jumps can also be induced at a point of rapid flow to reduce the high velocity and thus control erosion downstream. Typical jump-inducing structures include stilling basins and energy dissipaters consisting of concrete blocks acting as obstructions to the flow.

Hydraulic jumps can be weak or very pronounced depending on flow conditions. A classification of different types of jumps has been developed by the U.S. Bureau of Reclamation according to the Froude number, F, of the incoming flow. The Froude number is discussed in Section 6.4. The value of F must be greater than 1.0 for a hydraulic jump to form. This is because hydraulic jumps always occur when flow transitions from supercritical flow to subcritical flow. According to the classification, the greater the value of F, the stronger is the hydraulic jump. The strongest jumps occur when $F > 9.0$. For values of F between 1.0 and 9.0, the hydraulic jumps that form have various characteristics, including weak, oscillating, and steady.

Typical features of a hydraulic jump are shown in Figure 8-11. Flow depth before the jump, D_1, is called *initial* depth and the depth after the jump, D_2, is called *sequent* depth. The length, L, of the jump cannot be computed mathematically because of the complex motion of the water within the jump. However, values of L have been determined experimentally and can be found in many hydraulic texts. Generally, sequent depth is determined by normal depth in the channel downstream of the hydraulic jump. The location of the jump is determined by the initial velocity and the initial depth relative to the sequent depth. A hydraulic jump will form in a rectangular channel when the following equation is satisfied:

$$D_2 = \frac{1}{2} D_1 \left[\sqrt{1 + 2F_1^2} - 1 \right] \tag{8-7}$$

To illustrate the use of Equation 8-7, consider the following example.

Example 8-4

Problem

Flow in the spillway shown in Figure 8-12 has a discharge of 250 cfs. The spillway is 12.0 feet wide and discharges into a rectangular channel of the same width.

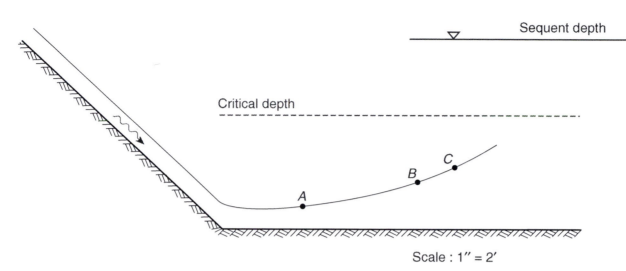

Scale : 1″ = 2′

FIGURE 8-12   Profile of the hydraulic jump in Example 8-4.

Normal depth in the channel is 4.0 feet. The profile of the flow from the spillway is shown in Figure 8-12 to scale. Find the location and height of the hydraulic jump.

Solution

The profile in Figure 8-12, which includes points A, B and C, is an M3 profile computed by a method such as the standard step method. Each of the points represents a possible initial depth, D_1, for the hydraulic jump. By using Equation 8-7 together with Equation 6-4, the sequent depth, D_2, can be computed. The point resulting in a sequent depth matching the normal depth (4.0 feet) corresponds to the location of the hydraulic jump. The following table shows the computations.

Point	D_1 (ft)	a_1 (ft²)	v_1 (ft/s)	F_1	D_2 (ft)	
A	0.5	6	41.7	10.4	7.1	
B	1.0	12	20.8	3.67	4.7	
C	1.28	15.36	16.3	2.54	4.0	OK

Point C, having a depth of 1.28 feet, was found by trial and error. It is the correct location of the hydraulic jump because it is the only point that results in a sequent depth of 4.0 feet, which matches normal depth in the channel.

The height of the jump is the difference between the initial and sequent depths, or

Height = $D_2 - D_1$ = 4.0 – 1.28 = 2.72 feet.   (Answer)

The location of a hydraulic jump can be very important in the design of hydraulic structures. In the case of a spillway such as the one in Example 8-4, the apron would be extended downstream of the hydraulic jump to protect against scour.

Generally, if the sequent depth is increased, the jump occurs more upstream, and if the sequent depth is decreased, the jump occurs more downstream. Usually, an upstream jump location is desirable. However, control of the sequent depth is difficult because varying discharge values result in varying sequent depths and therefore varying locations of the hydraulic jump. Methods of mitigating this problem include constructing a stilling basin or a sloping apron.

PROBLEMS

1. A concrete rectangular channel with a bottom width of 6.0 feet and a slope of 0.5 percent conveys a discharge of 225 cfs ($n = 0.015$). Determine whether the flow is subcritical or supercritical.

2. If the channel in problem 1 has a slope of 1.0 percent, is the flow subcritical or supercritical?

3. A trapezoidal channel with bottom width of 4.0 feet and side slopes of 2 horizontal to 1 vertical and slope of 1.0 percent conveys a discharge of 50 cfs ($n = 0.025$). Determine whether the flow is subcritical or supercritical.

4. Determine the backwater profile created by an obstruction in a channel causing a backup of 8.0 feet. The channel is rectangular as defined below and conveys a discharge of 800 cfs. Use the standard step method.

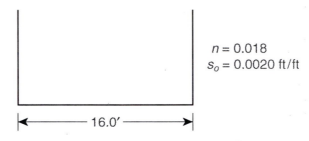

$n = 0.018$
$s_o = 0.0020$ ft/ft

16.0′

5. Determine the backwater profile created by an obstruction in a channel causing a backup of 5.0 feet. The channel is trapezoidal as defined below and conveys a discharge of 200 cfs. Use the standard step method.

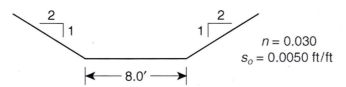

$n = 0.030$
$s_o = 0.0050$ ft/ft

8.0′

6. An emergency spillway for a detention basin is constructed as a rectangular channel with bottom width of 16.0 feet and lined with concrete ($n = 0.015$). The elevation of the crest of the emergency spillway is 1125.00 feet. The slope of the channel is 0.0020 ft/ft. Compute a chart showing the relationship between reservoir elevation and discharge into the channel.

7. Compute a chart for elevation versus discharge for the channel in problem 6 if the channel slope is 0.020 ft/ft.

8. An emergency spillway for a detention basin is constructed as a trapezoidal channel with bottom width of 10.0 feet and side slopes of 2 horizontal to 1 vertical and lined with grass ($n = 0.040$). The elevation of the crest of the emergency spillway is 480.00 feet. The slope of the channel is 0.0080 ft/ft. Compute a chart showing the relationship between reservoir elevation and discharge into the channel.

9. Compute a chart for elevation versus discharge for the channel in problem 6 if the channel slope is 0.050 ft/ft.

10. Flow in a spillway has a discharge of 525.0 cfs. The spillway is 20.0 feet wide and discharges into a rectangular channel of the same width. Normal depth in the channel is 3.20 feet. The profile of the flow from the spillway is shown in the following scale drawing. Find the location and height of the hydraulic jump.

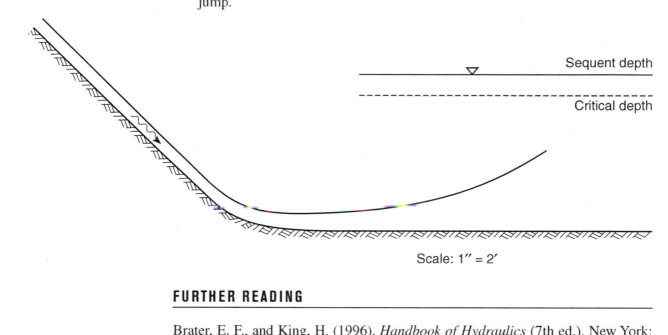

Sequent depth

Critical depth

Scale: 1″ = 2′

FURTHER READING

Brater, E. F., and King, H. (1996). *Handbook of Hydraulics* (7th ed.). New York: McGraw-Hill.

Chaudhry, M. H. (1993). *Open Channel Flow*. Englewood Cliffs, NJ: Prentice Hall.

Chow, V. T. (1985). *Open Channel Hydraulics*. New York: McGraw-Hill.

Hwang, N. H. C., and Hita, C. E. (1987). *Fundamentals of Hydraulic Engineering Systems* (2nd ed.). Englewood Cliffs, NJ: Prentice Hall.

Merritt, F. S. (2004). *Standard Handbook for Civil Engineers* (5th ed.). New York: McGraw-Hill.

Nalluri, C., and Featherstone, R. E. (2001). *Civil Engineering Hydraulics* (4th ed.). London: Blackwell Science.

Simon, A. L., and Korom, S. F. (1996). *Hydraulics*. Englewood Cliffs, NJ: Prentice Hall.

Strum, T. W. (2001). *Open Channel Hydraulics*. New York: McGraw-Hill.

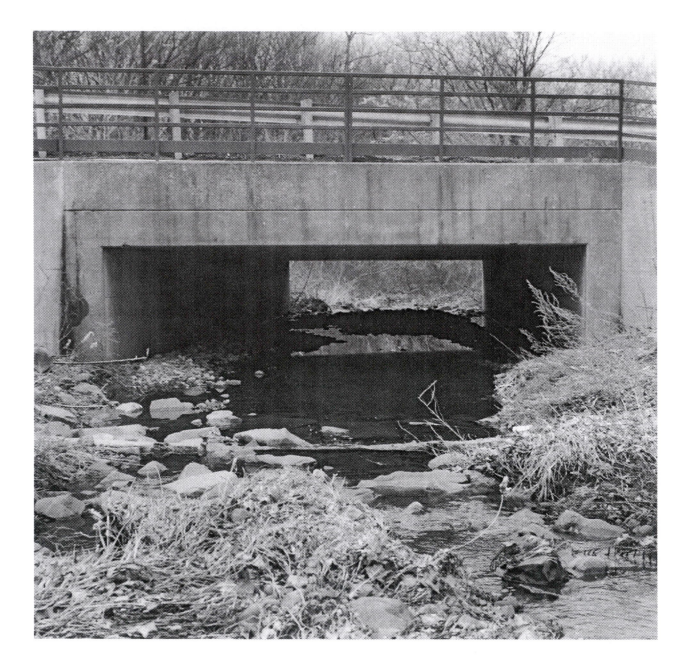

9

CULVERT HYDRAULICS

Culverts are structures intended to convey a stream or channel through an obstruction such as a road or railroad embankment. The culvert essentially is a tube placed in the embankment, allowing water to flow under the road or railroad with no interference between the two. Figure 9-1 shows a typical culvert/embankment arrangement. Headwalls or wingwalls generally are placed at the upstream and downstream ends to assist grading and hydraulic efficiency. Culverts are made in several cross sections, some of which are shown in Figure 9-2.

OBJECTIVES

After completing this chapter, the reader should be able to:

- Identify the type of flow pattern in a culvert: inlet control or outlet control
- Analyze an existing culvert for adequacy using inlet and outlet control
- Choose an adequate culvert size for a given discharge
- Assess the need for increased inlet efficiency for a culvert

9.1 FUNDAMENTAL CONCEPTS

When flow in a stream (or channel) encounters a culvert, it experiences a constriction that causes a change in flow depth. The flow of water in this case can be likened to the flow of traffic from a four-lane highway into a two-lane tunnel. As the traffic enters the tunnel, it must squeeze together, thus causing a slowdown that affects the cars approaching the tunnel, not the cars traveling through the tunnel. As soon as each car gets into the tunnel, traveling is much easier, and traffic speeds up. When the traffic emerges from the other end, traveling is usually even easier and speeds up a little more.

Generally, the hydraulics of a culvert behave in a similar way. Water backs up as it is waiting to get into the culvert; once inside, it speeds up. Because of the continuity equation (Equation 4-10), the slow-moving water upstream of the culvert

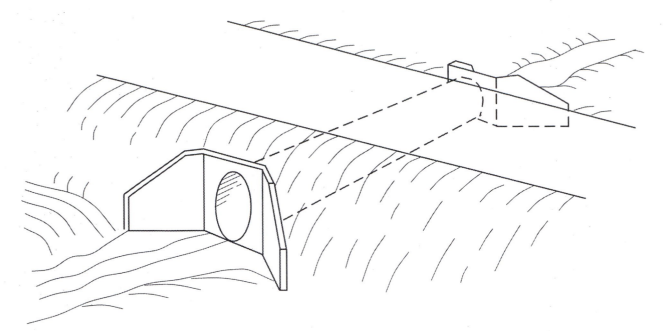

FIGURE 9-1 Typical culvert through a road embankment.

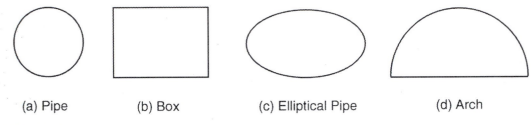

(a) Pipe   (b) Box   (c) Elliptical Pipe   (d) Arch

FIGURE 9-2 Typical culvert cross sections.

has an increased depth, and the faster water in the culvert is shallower. Figure 9-3 shows a typical pattern of flow through a culvert. It also serves to define many of the specialized terms used in culvert analysis.

Figure 9-4 depicts the principal hydraulic components of culvert flow. Reference will be made to the diagrams in Figure 9-4 later as culvert flow is described in more mathematical terms.

Although culvert flow generally behaves as described above, there are several variations of the flow pattern due to specific circumstances. The following factors affect the flow through a culvert:

1. The size of the opening (cross-sectional area)
2. Entrance geometry
3. Length of the culvert
4. Roughness of the culvert
5. Slope
6. Downstream depth of flow (tailwater)

Downstream depth, also called **tailwater depth**, can be very important in determining the flow pattern. Tailwater depth depends in general on the characteristics

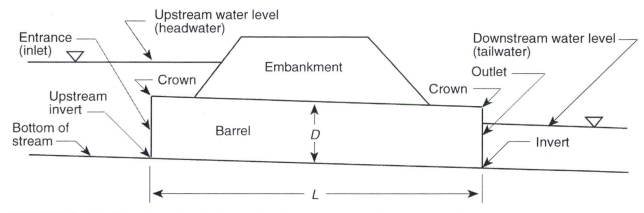

FIGURE 9-3   Profile of a typical culvert showing terms used in culvert analysis.

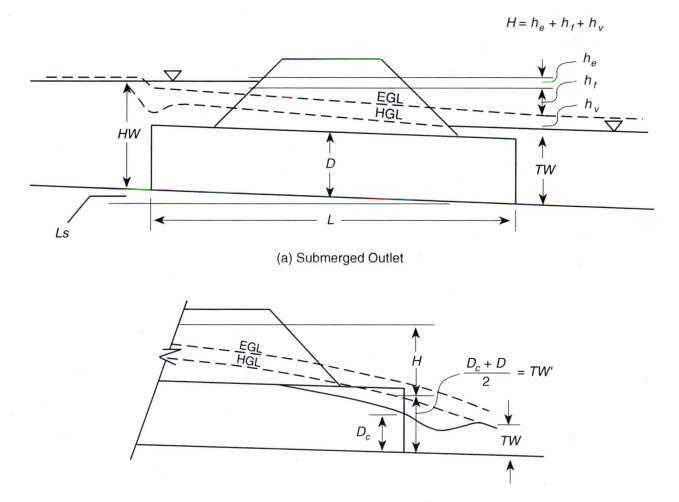

$$H = h_e + h_f + h_v$$

(a) Submerged Outlet

(b) Unsubmerged Outlet

FIGURE 9-4   Hydraulic components of culvert flow.

of the stream and is usually independent of the culvert. Tailwater depth generally is determined by computing normal depth for the stream as it exists downstream of the culvert.

Several types of culvert flow have been identified by varying the factors listed above. For instance, tailwater depth might be above or below the crown of the culvert. Also, the culvert might be relatively short or long; a long culvert exerts more friction loss on the flow. Furthermore, the culvert slope might be subcritical or supercritical. We can see that many combinations of conditions are possible, and each combination results in a different flow pattern through the culvert.

However, regardless of the details of the flow pattern, only one part of the pattern is of primary concern in culvert analysis: upstream depth.

It is the upstream water depth, called **headwater depth**, that provides the potential energy to drive the water through the culvert, and we will see that this depth becomes a measure of the capacity or adequacy of a given culvert. Downstream (tailwater) depth is determined by the stream, while upstream (headwater) depth is determined by the culvert. In this section, we will learn how to compute headwater depth for a variety of flow and culvert factors.

When water flows through a culvert, the headwater depth is greater than the tailwater depth. The increase in upstream depth is caused by the constriction inherent in the culvert, as we have seen already. However, experimentation has shown that the constriction can take place at either the entrance (upstream end) of the culvert or the outlet (downstream end) depending on which of the previously listed factors prevails. If constriction occurs more at the entrance than the outlet, the culvert is said to be operating under *inlet control,* whereas if the outlet end creates the greater constriction, the culvert is operating under *outlet control.*

9.2 TYPES OF FLOW

The water profile through a culvert varies greatly depending on the conditions mentioned above. The simplest type of flow occurs when the culvert cross section matches the upstream and downstream channels and the culvert acts as an open channel. In this case, shown in Figure 9-5, when tailwater is below the crown, the water surface profile is unchanged through the culvert, and tailwater depth equals headwater depth. We will call this type of flow Type A flow. Type A flow typically may be seen during low-flow conditions but rarely during flood conditions.

The next type of flow, which we will call Type B flow, occurs when headwater depth rises above the inlet crown and tailwater depth is relatively low and the culvert barrel is relatively short. For this type of flow, shown in Figure 9-6, the inlet becomes submerged, and the culvert acts like an orifice. Culverts with Type B flow usually operate in inlet control.

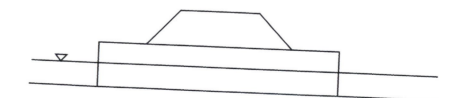

FIGURE 9-5 Type A flow: Culvert acting like an open channel.

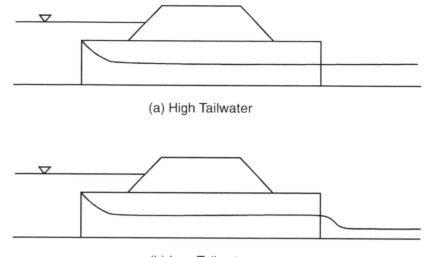

(a) High Tailwater

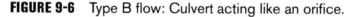

(b) Low Tailwater

FIGURE 9-6 Type B flow: Culvert acting like an orifice.

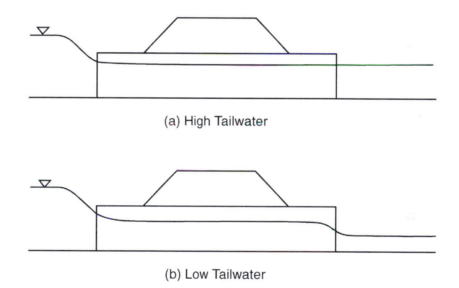

(a) High Tailwater

(b) Low Tailwater

FIGURE 9-7 Type C flow: Culvert acting like a weir.

Type C flow occurs when conditions are similar to Type B flow but the culvert is relatively long or otherwise restrictive to flow. Shown in Figure 9-7, Type C flow does not submerge the inlet but drops into the culvert just upstream, thus creating a weir-like effect. Culverts with Type C flow usually operate in outlet control.

Type D flow occurs when the tailwater is above the culvert crown and tailwater is relatively high, as shown in Figure 9-8. In this case, the culvert acts as a pipe flowing full, and control is at the outlet.

The flow in culverts can be complicated by factors such as culvert slope, which can produce supercritical flow under certain circumstances. The descriptions assumed subcritical flow conditions, which is the case for the majority of culvert analyses.

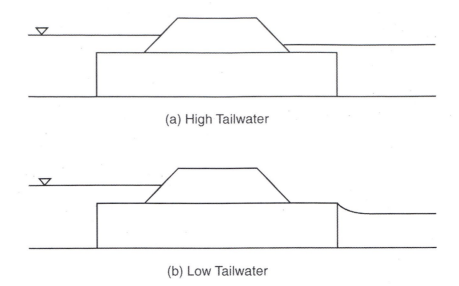

(a) High Tailwater

(b) Low Tailwater

FIGURE 9-8   Type D flow: Culvert acting like a pipe flowing full.

9.3   INLET CONTROL

Inlet control occurs when it is harder for the stream flow to get through the entrance of the culvert than it is to flow through the remainder of the culvert and out again into the stream. Critical factors in inlet control are cross-sectional area of the inlet and inlet geometry.

To compute the headwater depth for a culvert operating under inlet control, only the flow rate Q and the entrance size and shape must be taken into consideration. All other factors such as barrel length, roughness, slope, and tailwater depth are not important. We will see later how to determine whether the given culvert is operating under inlet or outlet control.

Figure 9-9 shows examples of culverts operating under inlet control. In each case, the value HW represents the depth of the headwater measured from the invert (lowest point) of the entrance to the water level. It is HW that we seek to determine in evaluating a culvert operating under inlet control. (HW actually represents the vertical distance from the entrance invert to the energy grade line of the headwater, but in most cases the energy grade line is so close to the water surface that the two lines may be taken as being the same.)

Design charts are used to determine HW in order to avoid the difficult mathematics involved. The charts, reproduced in Appendix B-1 and B-2, have been developed through research and testing. To use the charts, you must know the stream flow (also called discharge), the size and shape of the culvert entrance cross section, and the geometry of the entrance end of the culvert barrel.

The entrance cross section generally is circular, box, elliptical, or arch, as shown in Figure 9-2. Entrance geometry relates to the shape of the end of the barrel at the entrance. Figure 9-10 depicts the four usual types of entrance geometry used for circular and oval pipe culverts.

Entrance geometry has a significant effect on culvert capacity for culverts operating under inlet control despite its minor appearance. The ease with which water can flow past the entrance edge and into the pipe determines the entrance head loss. The smaller the entrance loss, the greater is the overall capacity.

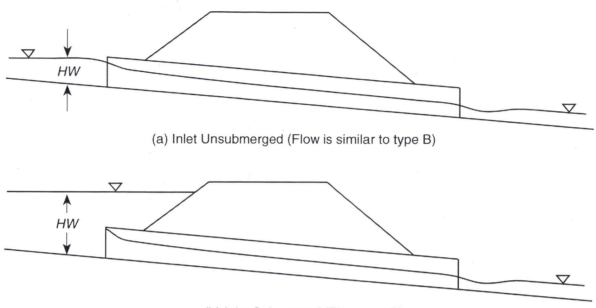

(a) Inlet Unsubmerged (Flow is similar to type B)

(b) Inlet Submerged (Flow type B)

FIGURE 9-9   Examples of culverts under inlet control. The inlet can be either unsubmerged or submerged, but the outlet is always unsubmerged. *(Courtesy of Federal Highway Administration, Hydraulic Charts for the Selection of Highway Culverts.)*

Example 9-1

Problem

Determine the headwater depth *HW* of a 36-inch-diameter concrete pipe culvert operating under inlet control with a stream flow of 65 cfs. The culvert has a headwall and grooved edge.

Solution

Select Chart 2 (Concrete Pipe Culverts with Inlet Control) in Appendix B-1. Find the pipe diameter on the left-hand scale and the discharge on the middle scale. Using a straight-edge, connect the two points just determined and extend the line to the left-hand scale of the group of three scales on the right. This is Scale (1). Finally, project the line horizontally from Scale (1) to Scale (2) and read a value of *HW/D* of 1.57. Then:

$$HW = (1.57)D$$
$$= (1.57)(3)$$
$$= 4.71 \text{ ft}   \text{(Answer)}$$

Thus, the headwater depth is 4.71 feet, which is above the crown of the culvert pipe.

The cross-section geometry of the stream was not needed in this case. Neither was the slope, length, or roughness of the pipe. Why?

If the elevation of the headwater is desired, you would just add *HW* to the elevation of the entrance invert. Thus, if the entrance invert is 450.00, then the headwater elevation is 454.71.

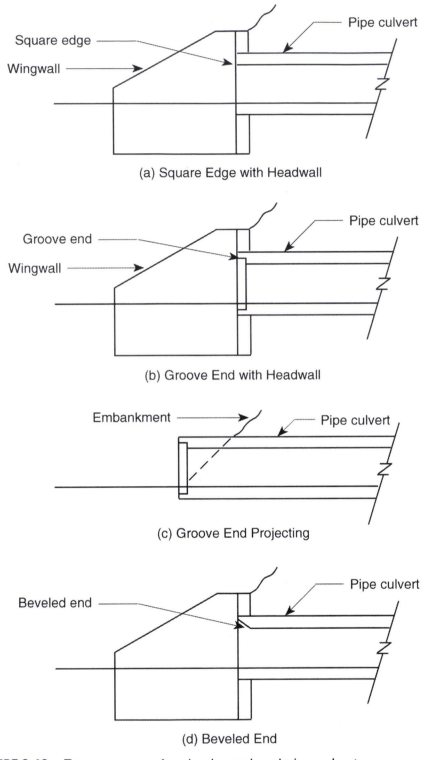

(a) Square Edge with Headwall

(b) Groove End with Headwall

(c) Groove End Projecting

(d) Beveled End

FIGURE 9-10   Entrance types for circular and oval pipe culverts.

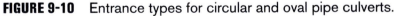

Example 9-2

Problem

Determine the headwater depth of a 3 foot by 6 foot concrete box culvert operating under inlet control with a stream flow of 80 cfs. The culvert has wingwalls at 45 degree flare.

Solution

Select Chart 1 (Box Culverts with Inlet Control) in Appendix B-1. Find the height of the box (3 feet) on the left-hand scale. Next, compute the value Q/B:

$$\frac{Q}{B} = \frac{80}{6}$$
$$= 13.3 \text{ cfs/ft}$$

Find 13.3 cfs/ft on the middle scale and connect the two points just determined and extend the line to Scale (1) of the three scales on the right side of the chart. Since the wingwall flare falls between 30 degree and 75 degree, use Scale (1) and read the value HW/D of 0.91. Then

$$HW = (.91)D$$
$$= (.91)(3)$$
$$= 2.73 \text{ ft} \quad \text{(Answer)}$$

Thus, the headwater depth is 2.73 feet, which is below the crown of the box culvert. If the elevation of the inlet invert is 450.00, then the elevation of the headwater is 452.73.

9.4   OUTLET CONTROL

Outlet control is a different and more complex procedure. Outlet control occurs when it is harder for the stream flow to negotiate the length of the culvert than it is to get through the entrance in the first place. To compute the headwater depth, the barrel size, shape, slope, and roughness, as well as tailwater depth, must be known. Figure 9-11 shows examples of culverts operating under outlet control. In each case, the headwater elevation is determined by adding total head H to the hydraulic grade line elevation at the outlet end of the culvert.

As shown in Figure 9-4, total head H includes velocity head, h_v, entrance loss, h_e, and friction loss, h_f. It does not include pressure head because usually pressure head is zero at the outlet and the hydraulic grade line is at the water surface. This is in accordance with Bernoulli's principle, described in Chapter 4.

But close inspection of Figure 9-4(b) reveals that the hydraulic grade line can sometimes be above the tailwater surface. In such a case, water exiting from the culvert is still under some pressure, and its depth is critical depth, D_c. Then, the position of the hydraulic grade line at the outlet is called TW', as shown in Figure 9-4(b). The exact value of TW' is difficult to compute, but a reliable estimate is that TW' lies halfway between critical depth and the culvert crown. Thus,

$$TW' = \frac{D_c + D}{2} \tag{9-1}$$

When tailwater depth is above the crown of the culvert, the hydraulic grade line is at the water level, and to find headwater depth, HW, add H to TW and subtract Ls_o, which is the rise of the culvert invert from outlet end to invert end. Thus,

$$HW = TW + H - Ls_o \tag{9-2a}$$

When the hydraulic grade line is located a distance TW' above the invert, HW is computed as

$$HW = TW' + H - Ls_o \tag{9-2b}$$

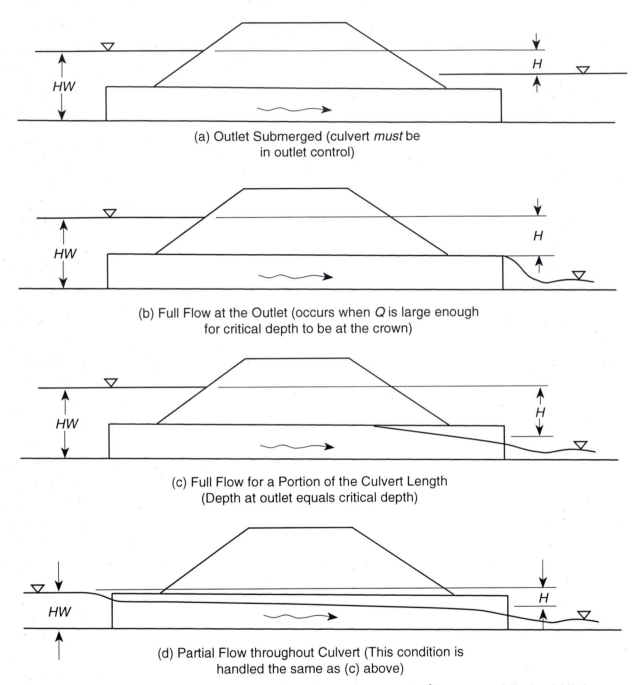

(a) Outlet Submerged (culvert *must* be
in outlet control)

(b) Full Flow at the Outlet (occurs when *Q* is large enough
for critical depth to be at the crown)

(c) Full Flow for a Portion of the Culvert Length
(Depth at outlet equals critical depth)

(d) Partial Flow throughout Culvert (This condition is
handled the same as (c) above)

FIGURE 9-11   Examples of culverts operating under outlet control. *(Courtesy of Federal Highway Administration, Hydraulic Charts for the Selection of Highway Culverts.)*

The problem is to determine the position of the hydraulic grade line. As shown in Figure 9-11, tailwater can be at various depths for various reasons. The stream can be flat or steep, discharge can be great or small, or the culvert barrel can be short or long, and so on. Therefore, when tailwater is below the culvert crown, the hydraulic grade line may be either at the water level or above the water level. If it is at the water level, it is located a distance *TW* above the invert. If it is above the water level, it is located a distance *TW′* above the invert. The practical solution to the problem is to compute both *TW* and *TW′* and choose the larger of the two. Therefore, if *TW* > *TW′*, use Equation 9-2a to compute *HW* and if *TW* < *TW′*, use Equation 9-2b.

Design charts are used to determine H in order to avoid the difficult mathematics involved. The charts reproduced in Appendix B-2 and B-3 have been developed through research. To use the charts, you must know the discharge, the culvert size, shape, roughness, and entrance conditions.

Example 9-3

Problem

Determine the headwater depth of a 3 foot by 6 foot concrete box culvert operating under outlet control with a stream flow of 80 cfs. The culvert is 100 feet long and has wingwalls at 45 degree flare and a square edge at the crown. The slope of both the stream and the culvert is 0.250 percent, and the elevation of the upstream invert is 450.00. Tailwater depth is 3.20 feet.

Solution

Because the culvert is in outlet control, analysis begins at the outlet end. First, determine tailwater depth. Normally, this is done by using Manning's equation, as in Example 7-8. In this case, tailwater depth is given as 3.20 feet.

Since tailwater depth is above the culvert crown, it is not necessary to determine critical depth.

Next, choose Chart 8 in Appendix B-2 to determine the value of H as illustrated in Figure 9-4(a). However, before using the chart, determine entrance loss, k_e. Appendix B-3 indicates $k_e = 0.4$ for the culvert in question.

Now, locate the cross-sectional area of 18 ft^2 on the area scale. Next, locate the length of 100 feet on the length scale, and connect the two points just determined. Note the point where the connecting line crosses the turning line.

Next, locate the discharge of 80 cfs on the discharge scale. Draw a line from the discharge point to the turning line point, and extend the line to the head scale and read the head value H, which in this case is 0.57 foot. Therefore, $H = 0.57$ foot.

Finally, calculate headwater elevation from equation 9-2a:

$$HW = TW + H - Ls_o$$
$$= 3.20 + 0.57 - (100)(0.0025)$$
$$= 3.52 \text{ ft} \quad \text{(Answer)}$$

Example 9-4

Problem

Determine the headwater depth of a 3 foot by 6 foot concrete box culvert operating under outlet control with a stream flow of 80.0 cfs, as in Example 9-3, except that tailwater depth is below the culvert crown ($TW = 1.00$ foot). All other parameters are identical to those in Example 9-3.

Solution

Since tailwater depth is below the culvert crown, critical depth must be determined.

Note: To find critical depth in a box culvert, use the channel charts in Appendix A-3, choosing a rectangular channel with the same width as the culvert.

Using Chart 5 in Appendix A-3, critical depth is found to be $D_c = 1.8$ feet. The position of the hydraulic grade line (TW') is then computed as

$$TW' = \frac{(D_c + D)}{2}$$
$$= \frac{(1.8 + 3)}{2}$$
$$= 2.4 \text{ ft}$$

Since TW' is greater than TW, TW' will be used to compute headwater elevation. Total head H is determined to be 0.63 ft using Chart 8 of Appendix B-2, as in Example 9-3.

Using equation 9-2b, we have

$$HW = TW' + H - Ls_o$$
$$= 2.4 + 0.63 - (100)(0.002)$$
$$= 2.83 \text{ ft} \quad \text{(Answer)}$$

In analyzing a given culvert, we usually do not know whether it operates in inlet or outlet control. Various mathematical methods can be used to determine the type of control based on the specific parameters involved. However, an easier method is available: Calculate upstream depth HW assuming inlet control, then calculate HW assuming outlet control, and compare the two answers. Whichever value of HW is greater indicates the prevailing control and becomes the answer to the analysis.

The proper method used to determine headwater depth for any culvert problem is to analyze separately both inlet and outlet control and then choose as the answer the greater value of HW from the two values determined.

In calculating tailwater depth, TW, it is important to know whether the downstream channel is flowing with normal depth or is influenced by an obstruction resulting in backwater (higher than normal depth). Examples presented in this text assume normal depth in the downstream channel. If obstructions are located downstream, tailwater depth could be higher than normal depth. In such cases, a different method of analysis must be used. Tailwater depth must be computed by using a backwater computation as discussed in Section 8.2. The usual method used when backwater computations are needed is the computer program HEC-RAS developed by the U.S. Army Corps of Engineers. Refer to Appendix E for a list of applicable computer software.

9.5 ENTRANCE EFFICIENCY

When a culvert operates under inlet control, it is harder for water to get into the culvert than it is to pass through the rest of the barrel and out the end. This means that perhaps a smaller barrel could be used if there were some way to get the water in initially.

Such a problem can be solved by changing the geometry of the culvert entrance. Simply adding a beveled edge to the entrance can somewhat increase entrance capacity. In addition, special inlet designs called *side-tapered* and *slope-tapered* inlets can be employed to increase entrance capacity significantly.

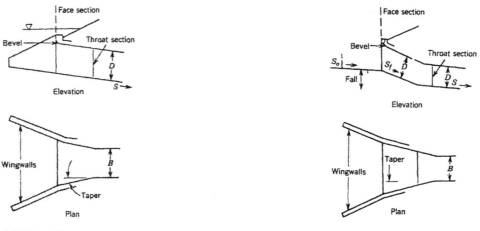

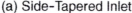

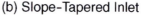

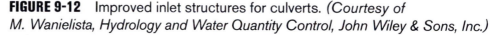

(a) Side-Tapered Inlet   (b) Slope-Tapered Inlet

FIGURE 9-12   Improved inlet structures for culverts. *(Courtesy of M. Wanielista, Hydrology and Water Quantity Control, John Wiley & Sons, Inc.)*

Figure 9-12 shows sketches of the essential features of side-tapered and slope-tapered inlets. These are concrete structures constructed at the entrance to a culvert and have the effect of reducing entrance head loss. Slope-tapered inlets are the more effective, but they require a vertical distance from the culvert invert to the stream invert, which often is not available. If vertical room is not available, a side-tapered design may be considered.

An improved inlet can, under the right conditions, realize a significant saving in the cost of a culvert. Consider, for example, a 6 foot by 16 foot box culvert, 100 feet long, operating under inlet control. The size of the opening (6 feet by 16 feet) serves only the purpose of letting enough water into the culvert. Once inside, the water may require a much smaller barrel (say, 4 feet by 12 feet) to convey it to the other end. So the entire 100-foot length is sized at 6 feet by 16 feet simply because the entrance must be that large. The cost saving in reducing 100 feet of culvert from 6 feet by 16 feet to 4 feet by 12 feet is probably well worth the cost of constructing an improved inlet structure.

The actual design of improved inlet structures is beyond the scope of this text, but the designer should be aware of this option. Various design manuals include procedures for such a design. Examples are included in the Further Reading at the end of this chapter.

PROBLEMS

1. A 24-inch concrete pipe culvert conveying a discharge of 20 cfs operates under inlet control. The culvert has a square edge with headwall. Find the headwater depth.

2. A 30-inch concrete pipe culvert conveying a discharge of 45 cfs operates under inlet control. The culvert is installed with its groove end projecting from the embankment. Find the headwater depth.

3. A culvert is constructed with twin 48-inch pipes with their groove ends built into a headwall. The culvert conveys a discharge of 285 cfs and operates under inlet control. Find the headwater depth.

4. A concrete box culvert 3 feet by 6 feet conveying a discharge of 125 cfs operates under inlet control. The culvert has 45 degree wingwalls. Find the headwater depth.

5. A concrete box culvert 4 feet by 8 feet ($n = 0.012$) conveying a discharge of 225 cfs operates under outlet control. The culvert has a length of 80 feet, slope of 0.60 percent, and 45 degree wingwalls with square edge. Tailwater depth is 2.75 ft. Find the headwater depth.

6. A triple concrete box culvert 5 feet by 12 feet ($n = 0.012$) conveying a discharge of 1620 cfs operates under outlet control. The culvert has a length of 105 feet, slope of 0.75 percent, and 45 degree wingwalls with square edge. Tailwater depth is 4.1 feet. Find the headwater depth.

7. A 60-inch concrete pipe culvert ($n = 0.012$) conveying a discharge of 100 cfs operates under outlet control. The culvert has a length of 250 feet, slope of 0.55 percent, and 45 degree wingwalls with square edge. Tailwater depth is 3.33 feet. Find the headwater depth.

8. A twin 18-inch concrete pipe culvert ($n = 0.012$) conveying a discharge of 25 cfs operates under outlet control. The culvert has a length of 50 feet, slope of 0.88 percent, and 45 degree wingwalls with square edge. Tailwater depth is 3.33 feet. Find the headwater depth.

9. Find the headwater elevation for a stream flow of 65 cfs for the culvert shown below. Tailwater depth is 2.00 feet. The culvert has wingwalls with 45 degree flare and a square edge.

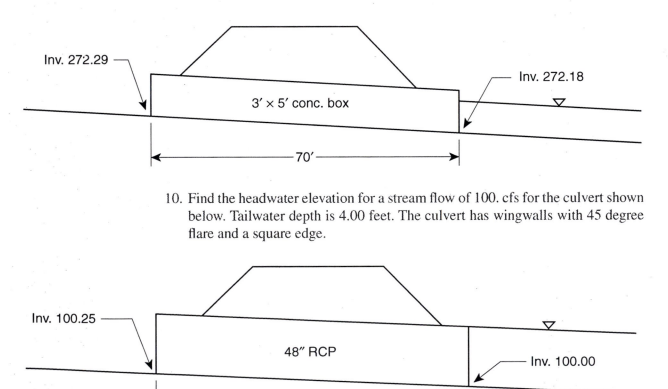

10. Find the headwater elevation for a stream flow of 100. cfs for the culvert shown below. Tailwater depth is 4.00 feet. The culvert has wingwalls with 45 degree flare and a square edge.

11. Find the headwater elevation for a stream flow of 140 cfs for the culvert shown below. Tailwater depth is 2.50 feet. The culvert has no wingwalls and has a groove edge.

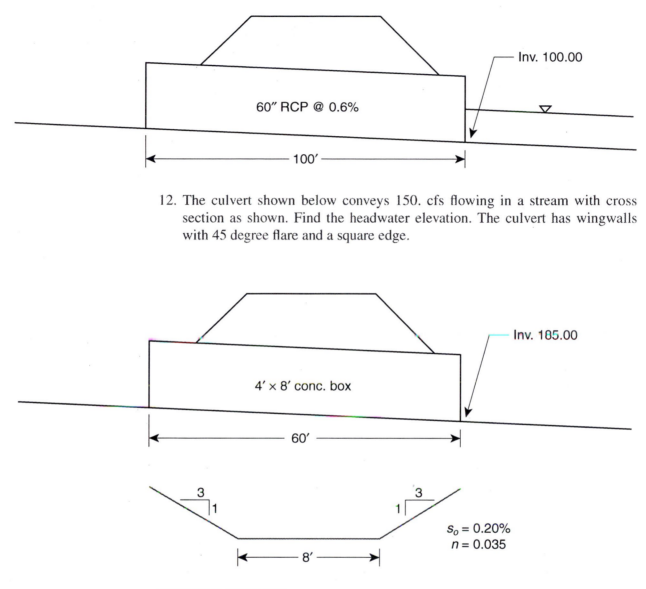

12. The culvert shown below conveys 150. cfs flowing in a stream with cross section as shown. Find the headwater elevation. The culvert has wingwalls with 45 degree flare and a square edge.

FURTHER READING

Brater, E. F., and King, H. (1976). *Handbook of Hydraulics.* New York: McGraw-Hill.

Chow, V. T. (1985). *Open Channel Hydraulics.* New York: McGraw-Hill.

Herr, L. (1965 revision). *Hydraulic Charts for the Selection of Highway Culverts.* Hydraulic Engineering Circular No. 5. Washington, DC: U.S. Department of Commerce, Bureau of Public Roads.

Linsley, R. K., and Franzini, J. B. (1992). *Water Resources Engineering* (4th ed.). New York: McGraw-Hill.

U.S. Department of Transportation. Federal Highway Administration. (1967). *Use of Riprap for Bank Protection.* Hydraulic Engineering Circular No. 11. Washington, DC: Department of Transportation.

U.S. Department of Transportation. Federal Highway Administration. (1972). *Hydraulic Design of Improved Inlets for Culverts.* Hydraulic Engineering Circular No. 13. Washington, DC: Department of Transportation.

U.S. Department of Transportation. Federal Highway Administration. (1975). *Design of Stable Channels with Flexible Linings.* Hydraulic Engineering Circular No. 15. Washington, DC: Department of Transportation.

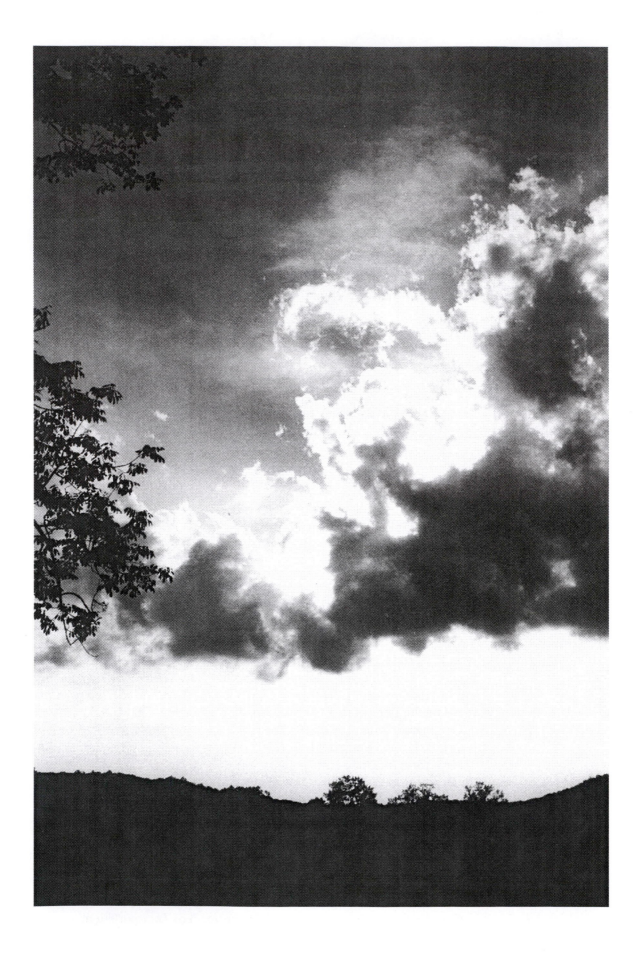

10

FUNDAMENTAL HYDROLOGY

Before rainwater can flow in a stream or channel, as described in Chapter 7, or a culvert, as described in Chapter 9, it must first descend from the sky, make its way across the surface of the land, and accumulate into a concentrated form.

In this chapter, we will see how to calculate the quantity of flow, Q, that results from the rainfall and must be conveyed by the hydraulic structure to be designed. The value of Q resulting from rainfall is called **runoff** and depends on several factors, including the amount of rainfall, the size of the area on which the rainfall lands, and the nature of the ground over which the rainwater flows. Each of these factors will be discussed in detail in the sections that follow.

OBJECTIVES

After completing this chapter, the reader should be able to:

- Describe the hydrologic cycle
- Delineate a drainage basin on a topographic map
- Calculate time of concentration for a drainage basin
- Estimate storm frequency for a given rainfall intensity
- Calculate a runoff hydrograph using a unit hydrograph

10.1 HYDROLOGIC CYCLE

Nature is a great recycler, and water is a prime example. The water that flows in streams comes from the ocean and is returned again in a constant cycle called the **hydrologic cycle**. Although complex in its functioning, the hydrologic cycle can be simply explained as the following steps:

1. Water evaporates from the oceans and lakes of the earth.
2. The evaporated water vapor forms into clouds.
3. The clouds move through the atmosphere in global weather patterns.

4. The water vapor condenses and precipitates in the form of rain, snow, or hail.
5. The rain lands on the ground and flows overland to the streams.
6. The streams flow to rivers and eventually into the oceans and lakes.

A schematic diagram of the hydrologic cycle is shown in Figure 10-1.

One aspect of stream flow is not explained by the oversimplified description of the hydrologic cycle: the constancy of the flow we observe in rivers and large streams. You might think that streams would flow only when it rains, but experience contradicts this notion.

In fact, streams and rivers are fed by rainfall in three ways. Figure 10-2 shows a typical stream cross section and illustrates what happens to rainwater when it lands on ground near the stream. Some of the rain is lost immediately to evaporation and **evapotranspiration** (the loss of water vapor from plants to the atmosphere), some flows by gravity over the surface of the ground and eventually into the stream, and the remainder infiltrates into the ground. Of the infiltrated water, some flows in

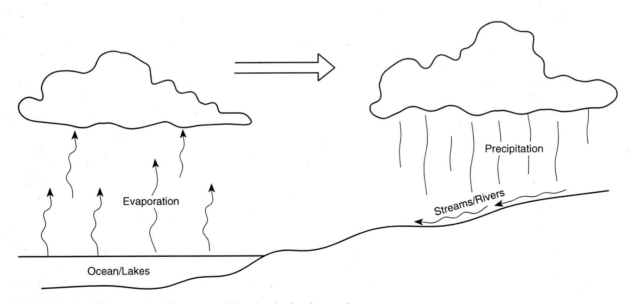

FIGURE 10-1   Schematic diagram of the hydrologic cycle.

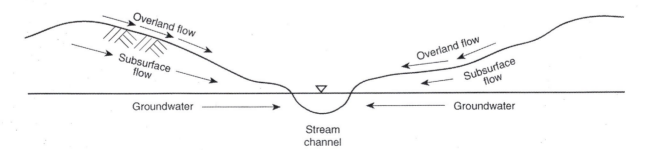

FIGURE 10-2   Typical stream cross section showing three ways in which stormwater reaches the stream.

underground or subsurface flow by gravity to the stream, and some percolates to the stored underground water body called groundwater. Although the overland flow is relatively quick, reaching the stream in minutes or, at most, hours, the subsurface flow and groundwater flow are much slower, lasting many days. Therefore, after an initial quick surge of overland flow when it rains, streams receive a constant feed of subsurface water throughout the days between rainfalls.

The constant low-level flow in streams due to the subsurface feed is called **base flow**, and the quick surge due to overland flow is called **direct runoff**. It is direct runoff that we are concerned with in the design of hydraulic structures because direct runoff represents the greatest volume of water that the structure must handle.

In relatively small streams, following any normal rainfall event, direct runoff peaks and begins to diminish before subsurface and groundwater flows have a chance to make a significant contribution to the stream. Therefore, the flow rate that we call runoff will be assumed to consist entirely of direct runoff.

10.2   DRAINAGE AREA

In calculating the rate of runoff in a stream resulting from a rainfall event, we must first determine the size of the area over which the rain falls. For every stream, a well-defined area of land intercepts the rainfall and transports it to the stream. The area of land is called the **catchment area**, **watershed**, or **drainage basin**. These three terms generally are used interchangeably. Figure 10-3 shows a typical drainage basin for a stream. All rainwater that lands within the drainage basin makes its way to the stream, while all rain landing outside the drainage basin makes its way away from the stream and into some other stream.

The imaginary line that outlines the boundary of the drainage basin is called the **basin divide** and is determined by the topography of the land. Delineating the basin divide is done on a contour map of the land surrounding the stream and is the first step in computing runoff.

Figure 10-4 shows a simplified contour map with a drainage area delineated upon it. The first step in delineating the drainage basin is deciding the point on the stream where the basin starts. The starting point is called the **point of analysis** (also called the **point of concentration**) and can be anywhere along the stream. Normally, the point of analysis is chosen at the location of a proposed hydraulic structure, such as a culvert.

The basin divide in Figure 10-5 illustrates the major principles in delineating a drainage basin:

1. Draw the divide perpendicular to contour lines (when the contour lines represent a slope).
2. Draw the divide along a ridge and across a saddle.
3. Never draw the divide along or across a swale.
4. Draw the divide between and parallel to two contour lines of the same elevation.
5. When in doubt about your line, test it by imagining a drop of rain landing near the line; then trace the runoff path taken by the drop. If the drop flows toward the point of analysis, it landed inside the basin. (When water runs downhill, it travels perpendicular to the contour lines.)

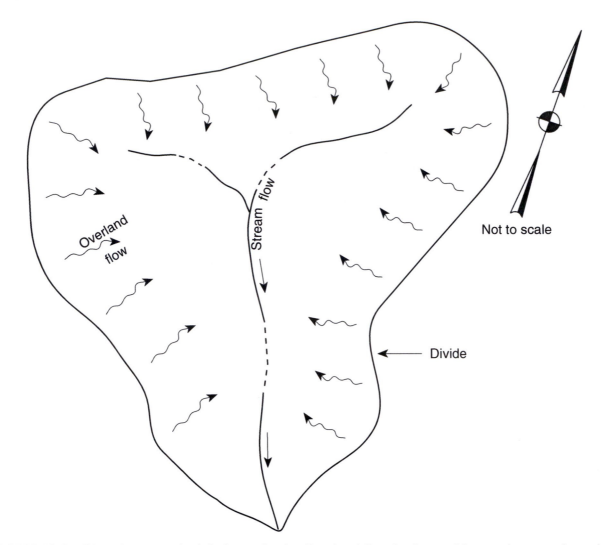

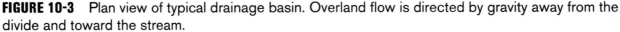

FIGURE 10-3   Plan view of typical drainage basin. Overland flow is directed by gravity away from the divide and toward the stream.

The principal land features in basin delineation are shown in Figure 10-6. A **swale** is characterized by bent contour lines that point uphill; a **ridge** is the opposite: the contour lines point downhill. A **saddle** is the transition between two ridges and two swales.

After you have delineated the drainage basin, your next step is to measure the area of the basin. The units normally are acres in the English system and square meters in the SI system. The area measurement is of the horizontal plane contained within the delineation, not the actual surface of the ground.

Measure the area using one of three methods: (1) planimeter, (2) approximate geometric shapes, or (3) computer software. When using a planimeter, always measure the area three times, and then compute an average. Figure 10-7 shows a typical drainage area computed by both planimeter and geometric shapes.

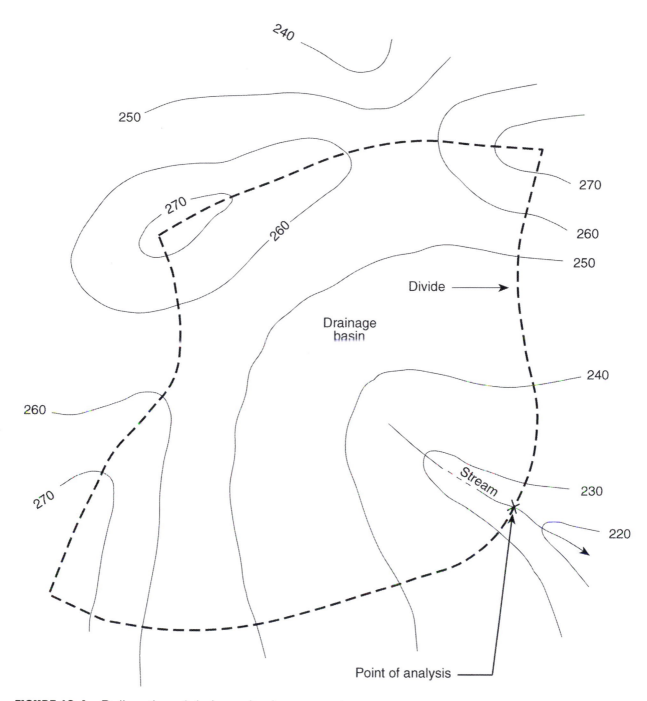

FIGURE 10-4   Delineation of drainage basin on a contour map.

Geometric shapes can be either triangles, as shown in Figure 10-7, or grid squares superimposed over the drainage basin. If the area is within 5 percent of the actual area, it is accurate enough for design. This is because delineating a drainage area is from the outset an approximation; the actual area can never be known with absolute precision.

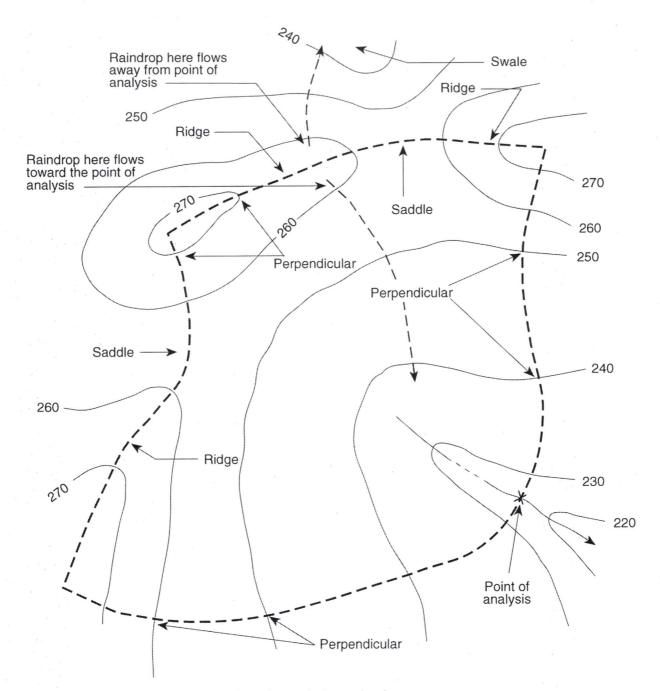

FIGURE 10-5 Principles used in delineating a drainage basin.

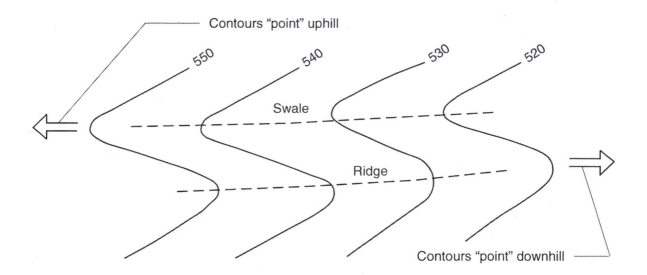

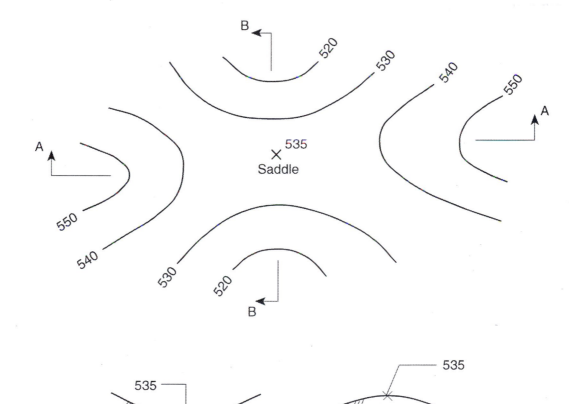

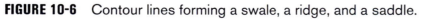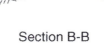

FIGURE 10-6   Contour lines forming a swale, a ridge, and a saddle.

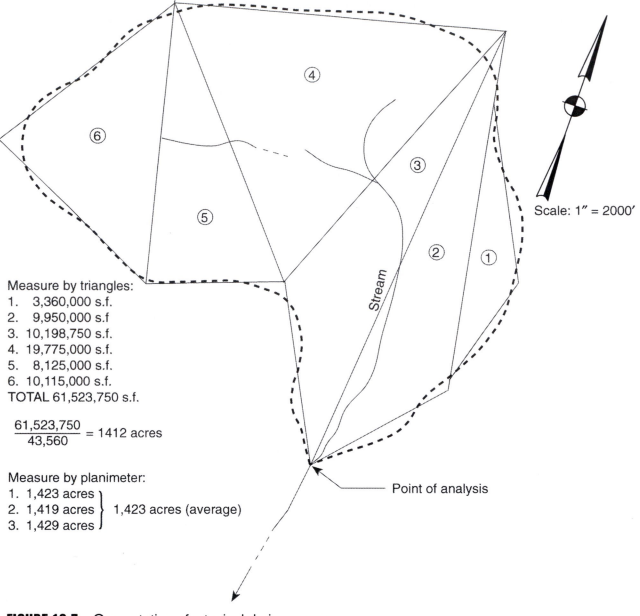

Measure by triangles:
1. 3,360,000 s.f.
2. 9,950,000 s.f
3. 10,198,750 s.f.
4. 19,775,000 s.f.
5. 8,125,000 s.f.
6. 10,115,000 s.f.
TOTAL 61,523,750 s.f.

$$\frac{61,523,750}{43,560} = 1412 \text{ acres}$$

Measure by planimeter:
1. 1,423 acres ⎫
2. 1,419 acres ⎬ 1,423 acres (average)
3. 1,429 acres ⎭

Scale: 1″ = 2000′

Point of analysis

FIGURE 10-7   Computation of a typical drainage area.

10.3   TIME OF CONCENTRATION

When the size of the drainage basin has been determined, the next step in finding Q is to compute the **time of concentration**, t_c: the amount of time needed for runoff to flow from the most hydraulically remote point in the drainage basin to the point of analysis. The path or route taken by the most remote drop is called the **hydraulic path** and is illustrated in Figure 10-8.

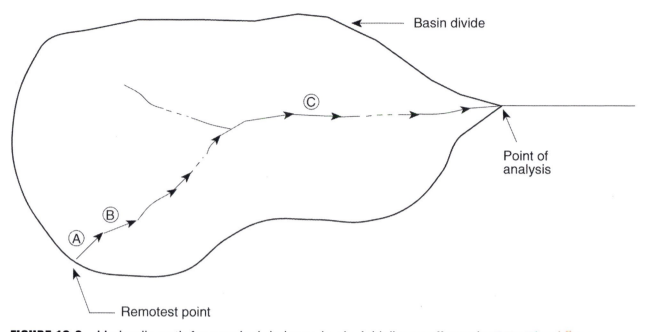

FIGURE 10-8   Hydraulic path for a typical drainage basin. Initially, runoff travels as overland flow (segment A), then as shallow concentrated flow (segment B), and finally as stream flow (segment C).

The hydraulic path might not cover the greatest distance, but it takes the greatest time compared to the routes of all other drops in the drainage basin. The time is determined by adding all the individual flow times for the different types of flow as the drop makes its way toward the point of analysis. Therefore,

$$t_c = t_1 + t_2 + t_3 + \cdots + t_n$$

where $t_1, \ldots, t_n$ represent the travel times for overland flow, shallow concentrated flow, stream flow, and any other type of flow encountered.

Overland flow is usually the first type of flow as the drop starts from the remotest point. It is characterized by sheet flow down a relatively featureless slope similar to the manner in which water flows across pavement. This is the slowest of all types of flow and is computed by either a nomograph (see Example 10-1) or empirical formula. Typically, overland flow cannot travel more than 100 feet before consolidating into a more concentrated flow.

Shallow concentrated flow occurs when the natural indentations of terrain cause the runoff to form into small rivulets. Since the rivulets are more concentrated, the flow efficiency is increased, and therefore the velocity is also increased. Time for shallow concentrated flow is determined by empirical nomograph, such as that shown in Figure 10-9. (See Example 10-1.)

Stream flow is usually the last (and the fastest) flow to occur along the hydraulic path. Time for stream flow can be computed by using Manning's equation. (See Example 10-1.)

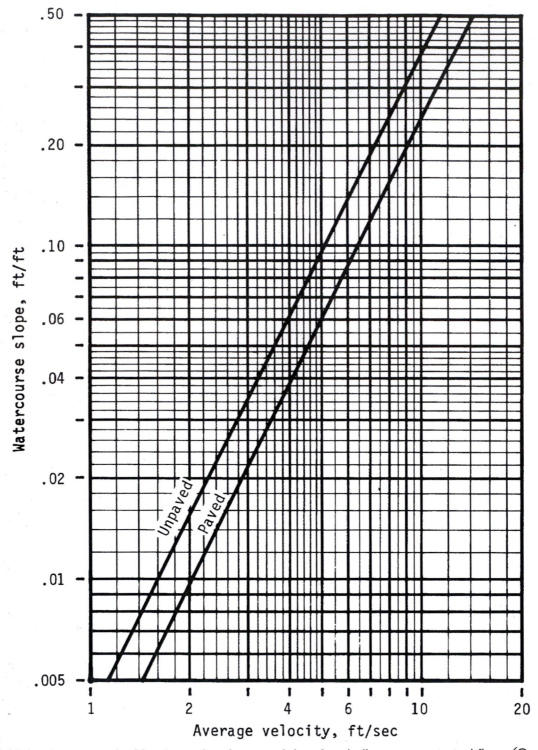

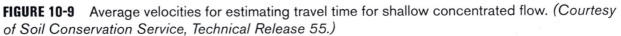

FIGURE 10-9 Average velocities for estimating travel time for shallow concentrated flow. *(Courtesy of Soil Conservation Service, Technical Release 55.)*

Example 10-1

Problem

Determine the time of concentration for the drainage basin shown in Figure 10-8 having the following conditions:

A. Overland flow: 100′ @ 2.5%, average cover
B. Shallow concentrated flow: 600′ @ 4.0%
C. Stream flow: 4700′ @ 0.3%, average cross section as shown:

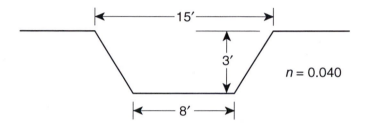

Solution

A. Overland flow—By using the nomograph in Appendix C-2, overland flow time is found to be 19 minutes. Therefore, $t_1 = 12$ minutes.

B. Shallow concentrated flow—Using the graph in Figure 10-9 for unpaved surface, velocity = 3.2 ft/s.

$$t_2 = \frac{d}{v} = \frac{600}{3.2}$$
$$= 187.5\,\text{s} = 3.1\,\text{min}$$

C. Stream flow—Since our ultimate goal in finding t_c is to find Q for flood conditions, assume that the stream is filled up to its top of bank. (This assumption is made valid by the fact that as water level rises onto the overbanks, channel velocity does not appreciably increase.)

$$a = 34.5\,\text{ft}^2$$
$$p = 17.2\,\text{ft}$$
$$R = 2.01\,\text{ft}$$
$$v = \frac{1.49}{n} R^{2/3} s_o^{1/2}$$
$$= \frac{1.49}{0.040}(2.01)^{2/3}(0.003)^{1/2}$$
$$= 3.25\,\text{ft/s}$$

Therefore,

$$t_3 = \frac{d}{v} = \frac{4700}{3.25}$$
$$= 1.446\,\text{s} = 24.1\,\text{min}$$

Finally, t_c is found as the sum of the three individual flow times:

$$t_c = t_1 + t_2 + t_3$$
$$t_c = 12 + 3.1 + 24.1$$
$$t_c = 39 \text{ min} \quad \text{(Answer)}$$

It is important to remember that not all drainage basins have the same three types of flow along the hydraulic path. For instance, we will see later that some basins have no stream but may have pavement, pipes, or drainage ditches.

Also, in Example 10-1, the implicit assumption was made that all three grades used were uniform. Although such an assumption usually can be made, conditions in the field rarely are so simple. If, for instance, the stream grade was steep for a portion of its length and flatter for the remainder, two separate times might have to be computed to determine total flow time in the stream. This concept also applies to all other flow types.

10.4 RAINFALL

Rainfall occurs in haphazard patterns, making it very difficult to quantify for design purposes. However, over the past hundred years, reams of data have been compiled on rainfall in the United States. A statistical analysis of this information leads to the determination of an average or typical rainfall.

The result of the statistical analysis is a series of synthetic or theoretical storms categorized by total inches of rainfall and the time it takes for the rain to fall. These categories of storms have been determined for each area of the country. The U.S. Weather Bureau published *Rainfall Frequency Atlas of the United States* (Technical Paper 40), which shows, through a series of maps, the expected size of storms throughout the country. The report covers rainfall durations of 30 minutes to 24 hours and return periods from 1 to 100 years. Later, it was realized that the study did not show enough detail in the mountainous regions west of 103°W longitude. So a follow-up study was prepared by the National Oceanic and Atmospheric Administration (NOAA) to depict more detailed precipitation data for the eleven western states of the continental United States. The study, called *NOAA Atlas 2*, is bound in eleven volumes, one for each state, each containing a series of maps depicting the precipitation data. However, both TP40 and *Atlas 2* have been superceded by *NOAA Atlas 14*, which is available in electronic form only. *NOAA Atlas 14* can be accessed at http://hdsc.nws.noaa.gov. A selection of these maps for eastern and western states is reproduced in Appendix D-3 for use in determining rainfall at various locations in the continental United States.

The size of a storm is described by the number of inches of rainfall together with the duration of the rainfall. Thus, a rainfall event of 5.0 inches over 12 hours is in one category, and a rainfall of 5.0 inches over 24 hours is in another. Although both events produced the same rainfall, one is more intense, and intensity of rainfall is very important in computing runoff.

Rainfall Frequency

Probability of occurrence is described by the term **return period**, which is the average number of years between two rainfall events that equal or exceed a given number of inches over a given duration. For example, a rainfall of 5.0 inches in 24 hours in western Texas has a return period of 10 years, and a rainfall of 5.0 inches in 12 hours has a return period of 25 years. This is because the latter storm is much more intense and therefore rarer.

In describing the 5-inch, 24-hour storm in western Texas, one would say that it is a 10-year frequency storm, or simply a 10-year storm. Another description would be that it has a 10-year return period. This means that *on average* over a long period of time, one would expect a storm of this intensity or greater to occur only once in 10 years.

However, it is important to caution against incorrect interpretations of storm frequency. For example, it does *not* mean that if a 10-year frequency storm occurs today that there would be no more such storms for 10 years. Storm intensity is a random phenomenon. A 10-year storm could occur in one location in successive years as long as the long-time average is one every 10 years.

Another incorrect interpretation of storm frequency involves geography. The western Texas example storm may have covered two or three counties. If another 10-year storm occurs the following year several counties away from the first storm, that storm is independent of the first and should not be counted in its frequency pattern. Storm frequency evaluation is different for each location in the United States.

Another incorrect interpretation of storm frequency involves storm duration. In the western Texas example, if a 5-inch, 24-hour storm (10-year frequency) occurs one year and a 3-inch, 12-hour storm (also 10-year frequency) occurs the next year, the second storm, despite being labeled a 10-year storm, is independent of the first and should not be counted in its frequency pattern.

The statistical analysis used to determine storm frequency is based in part on a graph of historic data similar to that in Figure 10-10. The actual analysis is more complex than that presented here, but a simplified description will suffice to convey

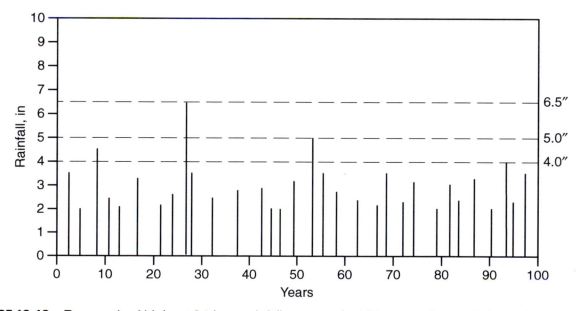

FIGURE 10-10 Bar graph of highest 24-hour rainfall amounts in 100 years of records for a given location.

the fundamental concept of storm frequency. If you examine Figure 10-10, you will see that only one storm of a 24-hour duration reached the 6.5-inch level in 100 years of data. So a 6.5-inch, 24-hour storm is said to be a 100-year storm. Also, you will see that in 100 years, two storms equaled or exceeded 5.0 inches. So a 5.0-inch, 24-hour storm is called a 50-year storm. What is a 25-year storm in this example?

Note that in Figure 10-10, the data are compiled in such a way that some years are not represented, since only the most severe storms are included. This type of data arrangement is called the *partial-duration series*. Other analyses compile the data differently. For example, the *annual series* uses the greatest single rainfall of each year. This series includes more storms but may exclude an extreme event if two major storms occur in one year. Analysis that was used to prepare *NOAA Atlas 14* used a combination of data series.

If 200 years of data are kept in the example of Figure 10-10, it might turn out that an 8-inch, 24-hour storm occurs. In this case, the number of inches of a 100-year storm would probably be adjusted by statistical analysis to be between 6.5 inches and 8.0 inches.

After compiling rainfall data for a number of years, meteorologists have also been able to establish average patterns of rainfall *within* a typical storm. Figure 10-11(a) shows a typical pattern of intensity throughout a 24-hour storm. Our common experience reveals that rainfall intensity fluctuates throughout each storm and that each storm is different. However, a long-term average produces a single pattern, as illustrated in Figure 10-11(b).

You might imagine that for a given location in the United States, a series of such patterns could be drawn, one for each rainfall amount—that is, 1-inch, 24-hour; 2-inch, 24-hour; and so on. For each graph thus drawn, the area under the curve would represent the total inches of rainfall for that storm.

Analysis of intensity and duration for an average storm pattern reveals that the storm has one very intense period near the halfway point and less intense periods before and after. If you study Figure 10-11(b), you will see that you could arbitrarily select a period (or duration) of 3 hours in the most intense portion of the storm during which 2.7 inches fall. The intensity during this period is 0.90 inch/hour. Similarly, if you look at the most intense 2 hours of the storm, you would find that 2.5 inches fall, giving an intensity of 1.25 inches/hour. Finally, if you look at the most intense 1 hour of the storm, you would find that 2.0 inches fall, giving an intensity of 2.0 inches/hour.

These examples suggest a principle: For smaller durations of time in the most intense portion of a storm, the rainfall intensity increases.

The relationship between rainfall intensity and duration for various return periods for a given location in the United States is shown on **intensity-duration-frequency (I-D-F) curves** developed by various governmental agencies based on data from Weather Bureau records. Selected examples of I-D-F curves for various locations in the United States are reproduced in Appendix C-3 for use in solving runoff problems by the Rational Method.

The intensity-duration relationship is central to the Rational Method for determining peak runoff, which is presented in Chapter 11. Therefore, it is important that you study it carefully and thoroughly.

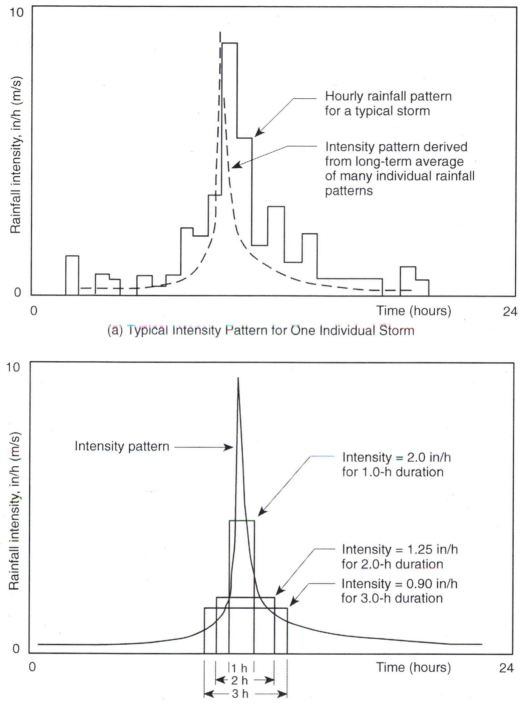

(a) Typical Intensity Pattern for One Individual Storm

(b) Intensity Pattern Based Upon Long-Term Average

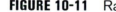

FIGURE 10-11   Rainfall intensity pattern for a 5.0-inch, 24-hour storm in New Jersey.

Example 10-2

Problem

In a rainfall event occurring in New Jersey, 1.33 inches of rain falls over a duration of 20 minutes. What is the return period of this storm?

Solution

A rainfall depth of 1.33 inches over a duration of 0.33 hour represents a rainfall intensity of 4.0 in/h. Using the I-D-F curves for New Jersey in Appendix C-3, enter the graph at a duration of 20 minutes and project a line upward. Then enter the graph at 4.0 inches, project a line across to the right, and locate the intersection of the two lines.

The intersection falls on the curve representing the 10-year frequency storm. Therefore, this rainfall event has an approximate return period of 10 years and is referred to as a 10-year storm.   (Answer)

10.5 RUNOFF HYDROGRAPHS

Sometimes, it is useful to know the entire relationship between runoff and time for a given rainfall event. This relationship, when graphed, is called a **hydrograph** and is shown in general form in Figure 10-12.

A close inspection of Figure 10-12 reveals that, in general, the slope of the rising portion of the hydrograph is steeper than the falling portion. This is characteristic of all hydrographs. In streams that carry significant discharge before the storm event, a distinction is made between the prior stream flow, called *base flow,* and runoff from the storm, called *direct runoff.* Figure 10-13 shows the relationship between base flow and direct runoff. The area above the base flow line constitutes the direct runoff hydrograph. Generally, in projects involving small streams, base

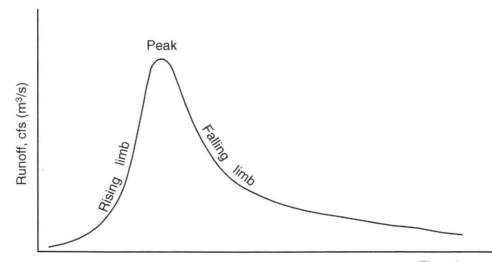

FIGURE 10-12 Typical hydrograph.

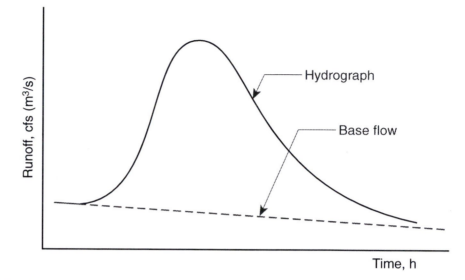

FIGURE 10-13   Typical hydrograph including base flow.

flow is negligible in comparison to direct runoff. In all our subsequent discussion of hydrographs, we will assume direct runoff hydrographs.

Runoff represented in the hydrograph consists of the water that has fallen on the drainage basin in the form of rainfall. However, not all of the rainfall becomes runoff. Some of the rainfall is lost to the runoff process through infiltration, evaporation, surface ponding, and even evapotranspiration. The remainder of the rainfall (that which is not lost) is called **rainfall excess** and becomes runoff.

Generally, rainfall is lost in two processes: initial losses and infiltration. In the beginning of the rainfall event, the first rainfall to hit the ground is lost to ponding and surface absorption. Thus, no runoff begins until the initial ponding and absorption—that is, initial losses—are completed. Then, as runoff proceeds, some of the water running over the ground is absorbed and infiltrates into the ground. This infiltration process continues throughout the rainfall event. However, the infiltration rate decreases in the later hours of the rainfall because as the ground becomes more saturated, less infiltration can take place. Figure 10-14 shows a typical rainfall pattern with the relationship between rainfall losses and rainfall excess.

Although all runoff hydrographs have the same general shape, they differ in details depending on several factors, including the following:

1. Amount of rainfall
2. Rainfall pattern
3. Time of concentration
4. Physical characteristics of the drainage basin

Thus, the peak could be located at various positions along the time axis, or the peak could be of various magnitudes, or the slope of the rising or falling limbs could be steep or moderate.

Although many methods have been developed to calculate hydrographs for a given drainage basin and storm, they fall into two general categories:

1. Direct measurement hydrograph
2. Synthetic hydrograph

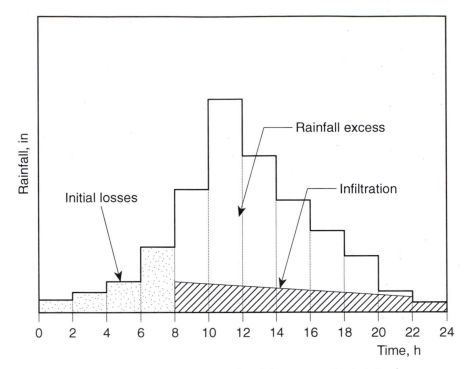

FIGURE 10-14 Relationship between rainfall losses and rainfall excess.

Direct measurement is used for large river basins in which one or more measuring stations are used to record actual hydrographs for every major storm over a number of years. These data, together with related rainfall data, are analyzed statistically to develop a generalized hydrograph that can be applied to any anticipated rainfall in the future. Synthetic hydrographs are used for small drainage basins where no measured runoff data are available. In these cases, a method must be devised to reasonably predict the hydrograph resulting from a given rainfall event without ever having experienced actual runoff at the site. Hydrograph calculations discussed in Chapter 11 are limited to synthetic hydrographs.

Unit Hydrograph

Both synthetic hydrographs and direct measurement hydrographs are constructed by the use of a concept called the **unit hydrograph**. Introduced in 1932 by L. K. Sherman, the unit hydrograph is defined as a hydrograph resulting from one unit of rainfall excess falling over the drainage basin in one unit of time. The unit of rainfall excess is 1 inch in the English system of units and 1 millimeter in the SI system. For simplicity, we will limit our discussion of unit hydrographs to the English system. The unit of time is variable but is usually taken as a fraction of the time of concentration, typically one-fifth.

The principal elements of a unit hydrograph are shown in Figure 10-15. Inspection of Figure 10-15 reveals several factors related to the rainfall-runoff process. First, note that rainfall is plotted in inches at the top of the graph and inverted for convenience. Runoff is plotted in cfs/in, and the two plottings share the same time axis.

The exact shape of the graph depends on the characteristics of the particular drainage basin being considered. So for each drainage basin encountered, a

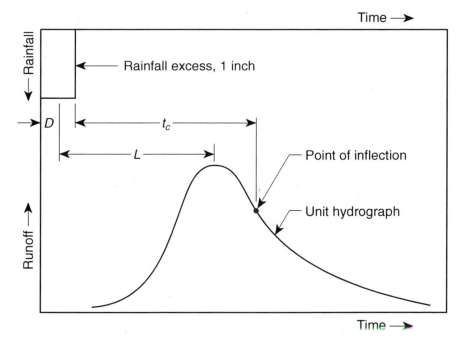

FIGURE 10-15 Principal elements of a unit hydrograph.

different unit hydrograph exists. But all unit hydrographs have one attribute in common: that the area under the curve represents the total runoff volume, which in turn is equal to 1 inch multiplied by the area of the drainage basin.

Various methods for constructing the unit hydrograph have been published over the years. Factors used in the construction include time of concentration, t_c, and basin lag, L. Lag is related empirically to time of concentration by

$$L = 0.6t_c$$

Figure 10-16 shows how these parameters relate to the shape of the unit hydrograph. But other characteristics of the drainage basin are also used to refine the shape. Some of the important methodologies bear the names of their authors and include the Clark Method, the Snyder Method, and the NRCS Dimensionless Unit Hydrograph. The last is named for the Natural Resources Conservation Service (NRCS), an agency of the U.S. Department of Agriculture and the successor to the Soil Conservation Service (SCS).

Assumptions made in the use of unit hydrographs include the following:

1. Rainfall is constant throughout the unit time. Although rainfall intensity varies constantly with time, we can assume constant rainfall for a short period of time without compromising the validity of the analysis. This simplifies the analysis.
2. Rainfall is uniformly distributed over the drainage basin. Actual rainfall varies over a drainage basin; but for relatively small basins, variations are not extreme, and uniform distribution can be assumed to simplify the computations. If a drainage basin is too large to assume uniform distribution of rainfall, the basin should be divided into subbasins.

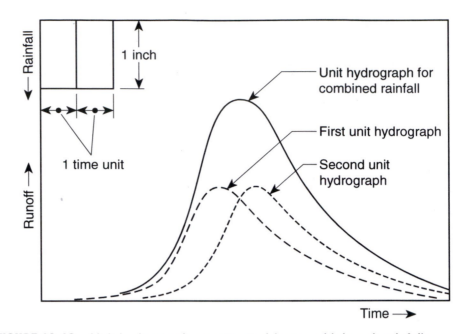

FIGURE 10-16 Unit hydrograph constructed from multiple unit rainfalls.

3. Two or more unit hydrographs plotted on the same time axis can be combined to form a resultant hydrograph that has ordinates equal to the sum of the ordinates of the plotted hydrographs at each point on the time axis. This is the principal of superposition.

By using the superposition principle, a hydrograph can be constructed for rainfall events greater than the unit rainfall by dividing the rainfall excess into a number of components, each equal to the unit rainfall. Since each unit rainfall produces a unit hydrograph, all the resulting hydrographs can be combined to create one resultant hydrograph. For example, in Figure 10-16, two unit rainfalls occur one after the other. Each unit rainfall produces a unit hydrograph of equal magnitude and shape but separated by a time value equal to the unit time. The resultant hydrograph is constructed by plotting each of its ordinates as the sum of the ordinates of the two unit hydrographs at each point along the time axis.

In this way, once the unit hydrograph has been constructed for a given drainage basin, a hydrograph can be developed for any rainfall pattern longer than the unit time. Thus, if the generalized pattern of rain is known for a particular drainage basin, a unit hydrograph can be constructed for the drainage basin and for the rainfall pattern. Then a runoff hydrograph for that drainage basin can be computed for any rainfall amount by multiplying the number of inches of rainfall excess by the unit hydrograph.

Example 10-3

Problem

The unit hydrograph for a 24-hour storm for a drainage basin is shown in tabular form in Table 10-1. Sketch the hydrograph for the basin resulting from a 6.0-inch, 24-hour storm. Initial rainfall losses for this storm equal 0.5 inch. Also, estimate the area of the basin.

TABLE 10-1   Unit Hydrograph for Example 10-3

Time (h)	Discharge (cfs/in)	Time (h)	Discharge (cfs/in)
1	0.086	13	1.7
2	0.19	14	1.4
3	0.38	15	1.2
4	0.71	16	1.0
5	2.3	17	0.84
6	5.5	18	0.69
7	6.4	19	0.54
8	5.8	20	0.45
9	4.4	21	0.36
10	3.2	22	0.25
11	2.5	23	0.19
12	2.1	24	0.15

Solution

The unit hydrograph is shown in graphical form in Figure 10-17. Because it is a *unit* hydrograph, it results from a rainfall excess of 1 inch. Rainfall excess for the storm in question is 6.0 inches minus 0.5 inch, or 5.5 inches. Therefore, the resultant hydrograph will have ordinates equal to 5.5 times the ordinates of the unit hydrograph. The resultant hydrograph is shown in Figure 10-17.

The area of the drainage basin can be estimated by recalling that the volume of runoff is computed in two ways: (1) depth of rainfall excess multiplied by the area and (2) area under the hydrograph.

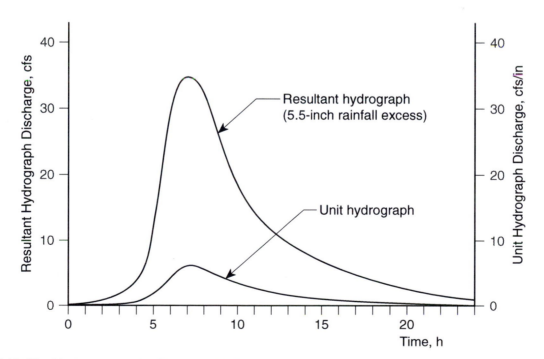

FIGURE 10-17   Hydrographs for Example 10-3.

Area under the resultant hydrograph in Figure 10-17 is 198,000 cubic feet.

$$\text{Volume} = \text{Area} \times \text{Depth} \qquad \text{or}$$

$$\text{Area} = \frac{\text{Volume}}{\text{Depth}}$$

$$\text{Area} = \frac{198,000}{\dfrac{5.5}{12}} = 432,000 \text{ s.f.}$$

$$\text{Area} = 9.92 \text{ acres} \quad \text{(Answer)}$$

10.6 ROUTING

When runoff from a rainfall event travels down a stream, it is considered a flood wave even though the "crest" of such a wave would not be discernible to casual observers. As the flood wave moves down the stream, it decreases in height and spreads out in the direction of the stream. The reduction of the flood wave height or magnitude is called **attenuation**, and the procedure for computing the reduction is called **routing**. (The term *routing* describes a mathematical procedure, not the mapping of a course of movement.)

A stone thrown into a pond causes ripples to move across the surface. Each ripple is a wave, and as it moves away from the center, it decreases in magnitude. This is an attenuation process similar to a flood wave in a stream, except that the stream example is one-dimensional in contrast to the two-dimensional ripple.

To further describe stream attenuation, consider the drainage basin tributary to the stream in Figure 10-18. If observers were placed at stations 1, 2, and 3 and were able to measure the hydrograph resulting from the runoff, they would record very different results. As the location becomes farther from the point of analysis, the height of the hydrograph (peak Q), drops, and the location of the peak shifts to the right on the time axis. The entire hydrograph flattens and becomes longer, although the total area under the curve remains constant.

The flattening and elongating of the hydrograph demonstrate the classical characteristics of attenuation. The area under the curve remains constant because the total amount or volume of runoff is not increased or decreased. (It must be noted that the hydrographs at Stations 2 and 3 in Figure 10-18 ignore any additional runoff entering the stream along its length.)

Computation of the hydrographs at Stations 2 and 3 is performed by routing the hydrograph at Station 1. The routing concept is based on the fact that as runoff enters a section of the stream, called a *reach*, some of the water is temporarily stored in the reach and then released at the downstream end.

A similar process occurs in a detention basin except to a more dramatic degree. Water enters one end of the basin, is stored temporarily, and then exits the other end at a reduced rate. This type of routing is described in detail in Chapter 14.

Flood routing for streams is difficult because the hydraulic process is complex. However, the U.S. Army Corps of Engineers has developed a procedure for estimating a stream routing, called the Muskingum Method. It was first conceived for the Muskingum River in Ohio and then made universal for streams in general.

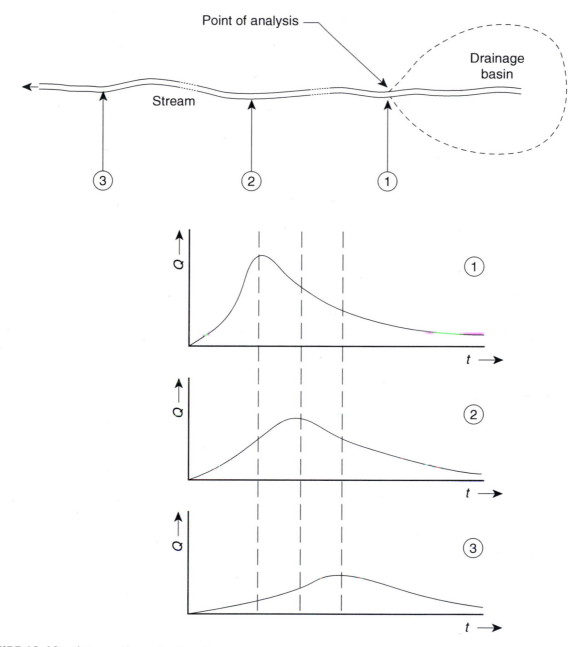

FIGURE 10-18   Attenuation of a flood wave.

Therefore, it is important to realize that as runoff flows down a stream, its peak discharge value does not remain constant but inevitably decreases. Actual computations by the Muskingum Method are beyond the scope of this book. However, we will see the effects of stream routing in Chapter 11 and of reservoir routing in Chapter 14.

10.7   SUBBASINS

In computing a runoff hydrograph, if the delineated drainage basin is too large or not sufficiently homogeneous, it must be subdivided into smaller units called subareas or **subbasins**. We must remember that one of the underlying assumptions

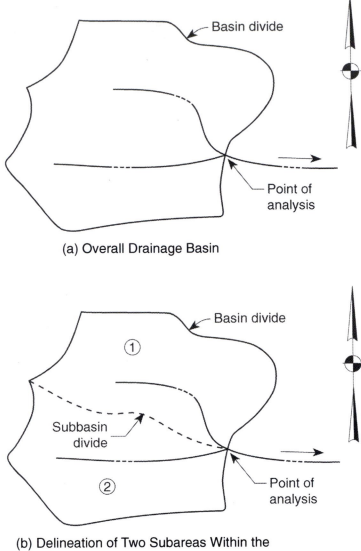

(a) Overall Drainage Basin

(b) Delineation of Two Subareas Within the
Overall Basin

FIGURE 10-19   Drainage basin divided into subbasins.

of hydrograph construction is a drainage basin with relatively uniform characteristics throughout. These characteristics include cover conditions, average slope, and soil types.

Figure 10-19(a) shows the outline of a drainage basin with a stream branched into two areas of differing characteristics. Figure 10-19(b) shows how the basin can be subdivided into two subareas for computation purposes. The point of analysis for the overall basin is at the **confluence** of the two branches of the stream.

The hydrograph for the entire basin at the point of analysis is the sum of the hydrographs generated by each of the subareas. Each subarea produces a hydrograph just as any single watershed does.

To compute the total runoff hydrograph for the drainage basin in Figure 10-19, compute the hydrographs for the two subareas and add them together. Hydrographs

TABLE 10-2   Hydrographs Used in Example 10-4

(1) Time (h)	(2) Hydrograph Subbasin 1 (cfs)	(3) Hydrograph Subbasin 2 (cfs)	(4) Hydrograph Total Basin (cfs)
0	0	0	0
1	0.4	0.7	1.1
2	0.8	1.9	2.7
3	1.5	6.0	7.5
4	2.6	13.8	16.4
5	4.5	21.7	26.2
6	6.0	18.8	24.8
8	10.0	10.0	20.0
10	11.5	7.5	19.0
12	9.8	5.1	14.9
18	3.1	1.5	4.6
24	1.3	1.0	2.3

are added by using the principle of superposition, in which each ordinate of the resulting hydrograph is the sum of the ordinates of the subarea hydrographs for each point along the time axis. The following example illustrates this concept.

Example 10-4

Problem

Find the runoff hydrograph for the drainage basin depicted in Figure 10-19 for a 25-year storm. Runoff hydrographs for the two subbasins are shown in tabular form in Columns 2 and 3 in Table 10-2.

Solution

The overall runoff hydrograph is shown in Column 4 of Table 10-2. Column 4 is determined by adding the values in Columns 2 and 3 for each time value in Column 1. A graphical depiction of the hydrograph is shown in Figure 10-20.

Scrutiny of Figure 10-20 and Table 10-2 reveals that the peak runoff for the resulting hydrograph is less than the sum of the peaks of the subarea hydrographs. This is a very important attribute of hydrograph analysis. Because of the timing of the peaks, the summation of the hydrograph is smaller than one might expect.

Also, notice in Figure 10-20 that the shape of the resulting hydrograph is different from the generalized shapes of the individual subbasins resulting from unit hydrographs for those subbasins. If the overall drainage basin had been modeled as a whole, the resulting unit hydrograph, and therefore the derived hydrograph, would not reflect the shape shown.

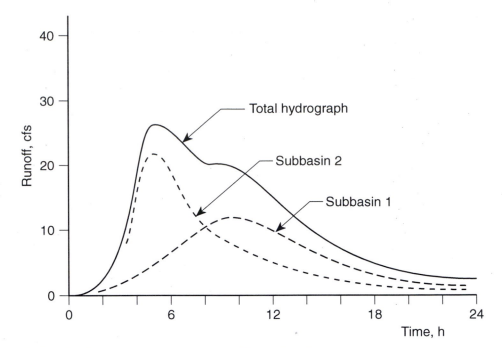

FIGURE 10-20   Hydrographs used in Example 10-4.

PROBLEMS

1. Carefully trace the following delineated drainage area onto tracing paper, and then determine the drainage area in (a) acres and (b) square meters.

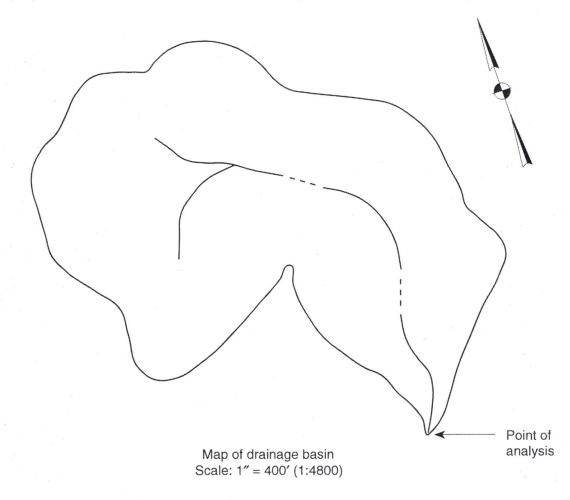

Map of drainage basin
Scale: 1″ = 400′ (1:4800)

Point of analysis

2. Trace the delineated drainage area shown in Figure 10-21 onto tracing paper, and then determine the drainage area in (a) acres and (b) square meters.
3. Measure the area of the drainage basin shown in Figure 10-22. Express the area in (a) acres and (b) square meters.
4. Measure the area of the drainage basin shown in Figure 10-23. Express the area in (a) acres and (b) square meters.
5. Delineate the catchment area tributary to the point of analysis shown in Figure 10-24. Measure the area in acres.
6. Delineate the catchment area tributary to the point of analysis shown in Figure 10-25. Measure the area in acres. Assume that all roads have crowns and gutter flow on both sides.
7. Delineate the watershed tributary to the point of analysis shown in Figure 10-26. Measure the area in acres.
8. Delineate the watershed's tributary to the two points of analysis, A and B, shown in Figure 10-27. Measure the areas in acres.

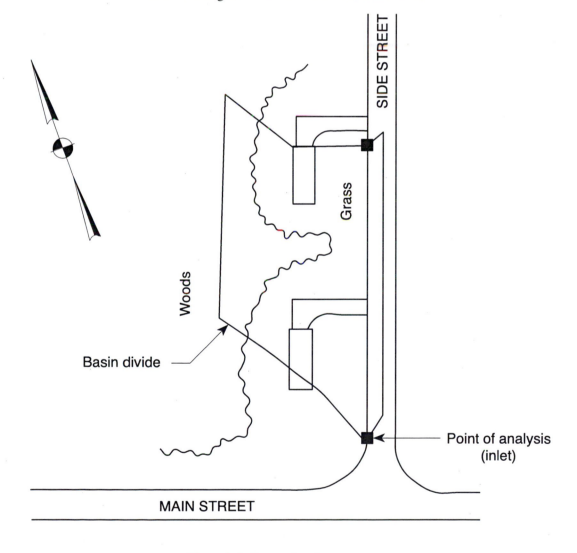

Map of drainage basin
Scale: 1″ = 100′ (1:1200)

FIGURE 10-21   Delineation of the drainage basin for problem 2.

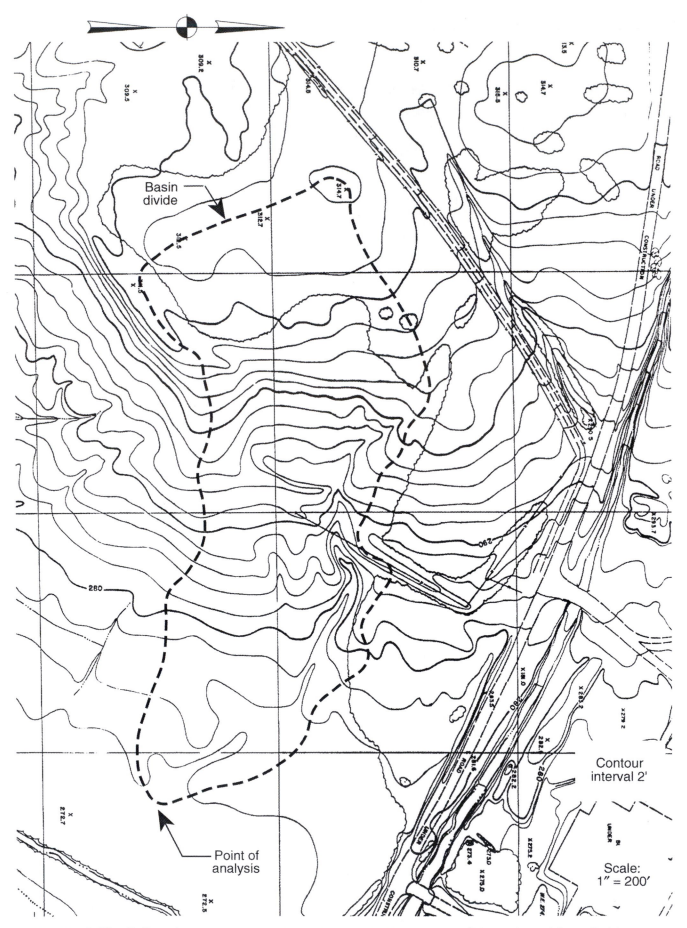

FIGURE 10-22 Delineation of a drainage basin located in New Jersey. *(Map adapted from Robinson Aerial.)*

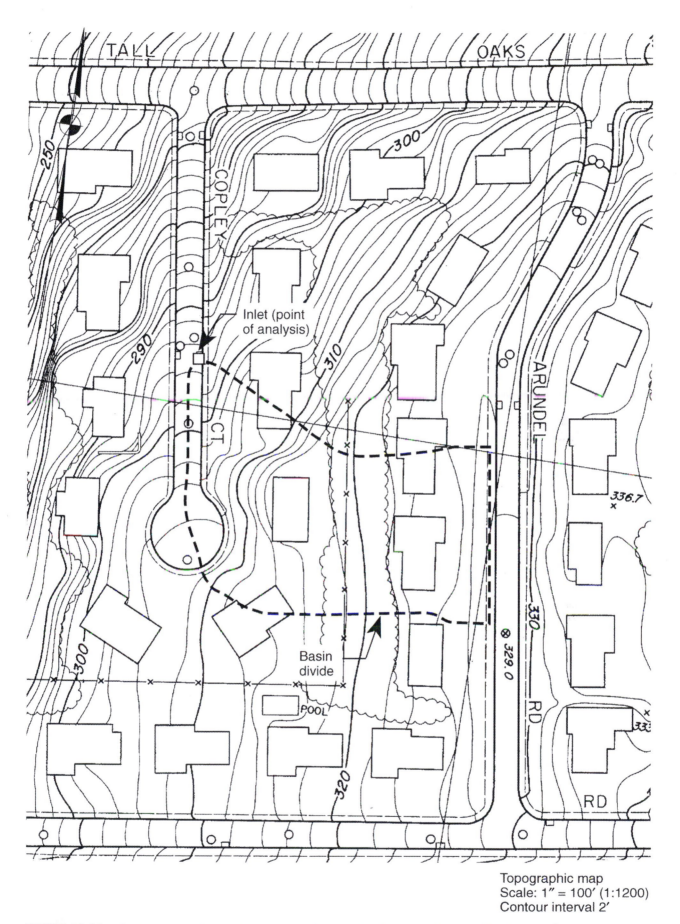

FIGURE 10-23 Delineation of a drainage basin located in Orange County, California. *(Map adapted from Aero Service.)*

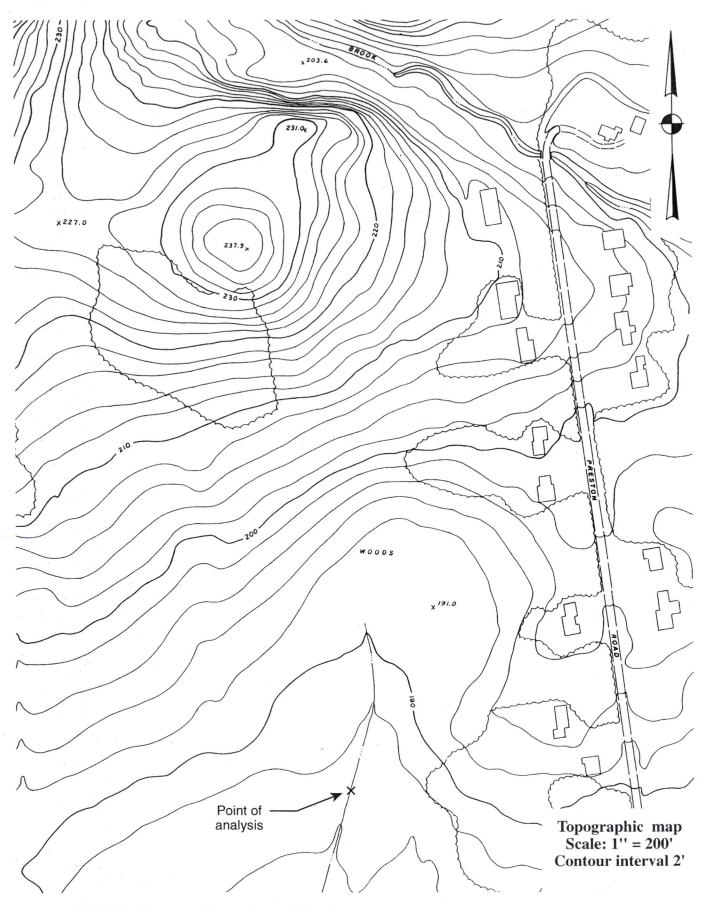

Point of analysis

Topographic map
Scale: 1'' = 200'
Contour interval 2'

FIGURE 10-24 Topographic map for problem 5.

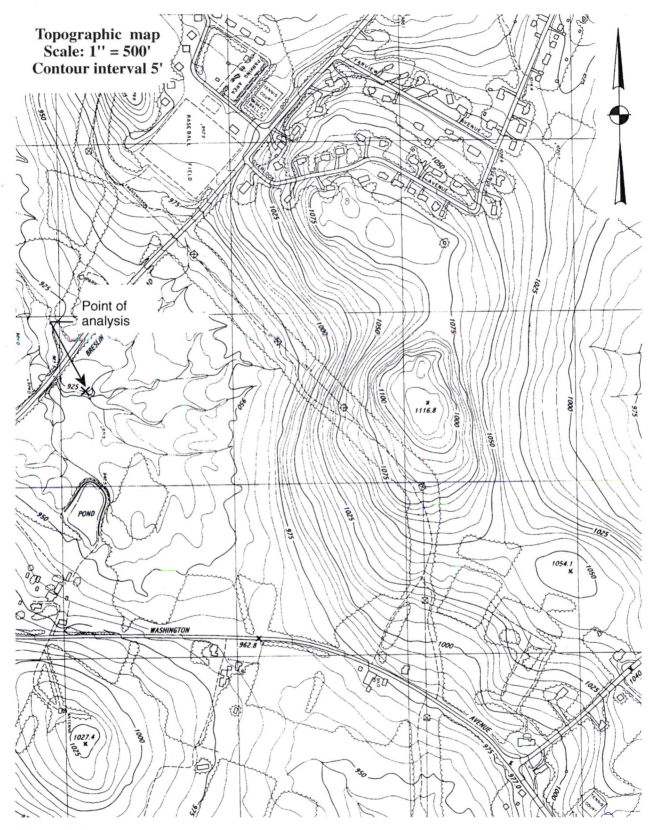

FIGURE 10-25   Topographic map for problem 6.

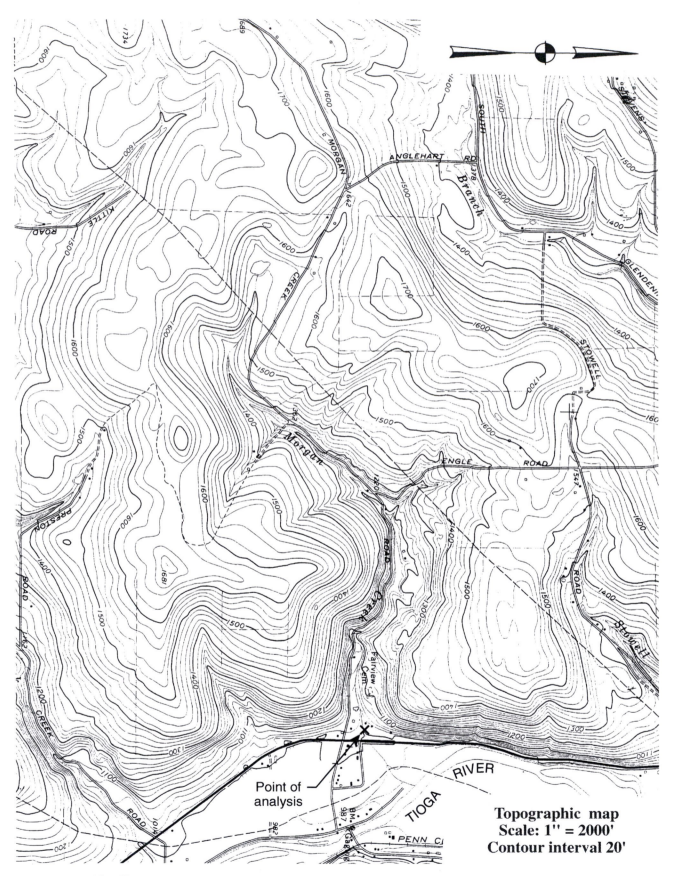

Point of analysis

Topographic map
Scale: 1'' = 2000'
Contour interval 20'

FIGURE 10-26 Topographic map for problem 7.

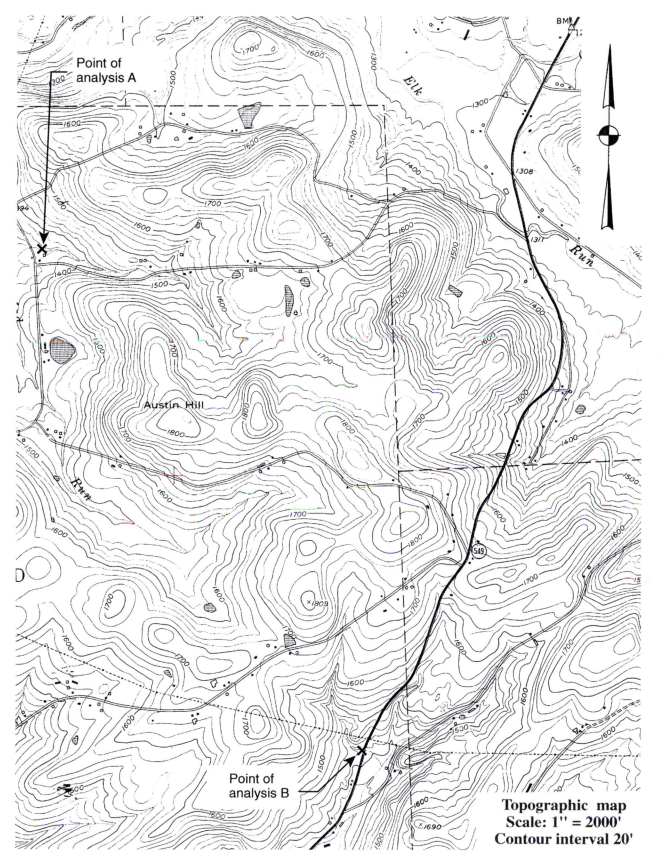

FIGURE 10-27   Topographic map for problem 8.

9. Trace the hydraulic path and determine the time of concentration for the drainage basin in problem 3. For overland flow, use Appendix C-2. The average cross section is shown below.

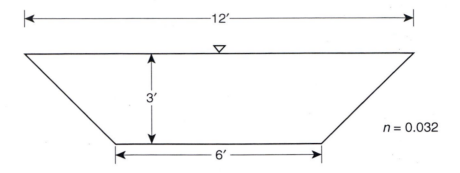

10. Trace the hydraulic path and determine the time of concentration for the drainage basin in problem 4. For overland flow, use Appendix C-2.

11. Trace the hydraulic path and determine the time of concentration for the drainage basin in problem 5. For overland flow, use Appendix C-2. For an average stream cross section, use that in problem 9.

12. Trace the hydraulic path and determine the time of concentration for the drainage basin in problem 6. For overland flow, use Appendix C-2. For an average stream cross section, use that in problem 9.

13. Trace the hydraulic path for the watershed in problem 7.

14. Copy the unit hydrograph shown below. Then sketch the hydrograph resulting from a rainfall excess of 4.2 inches. Estimate the watershed area in acres.

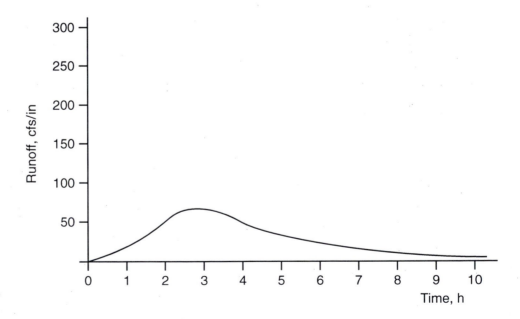

15. Runoff hydrographs for two watersheds are shown in Figure 10-28. Draw the hydrograph resulting from the sum of the two hydrographs at the confluence of the two watersheds. What is the peak runoff for each of the watersheds, and what is the peak runoff for the combined watersheds?

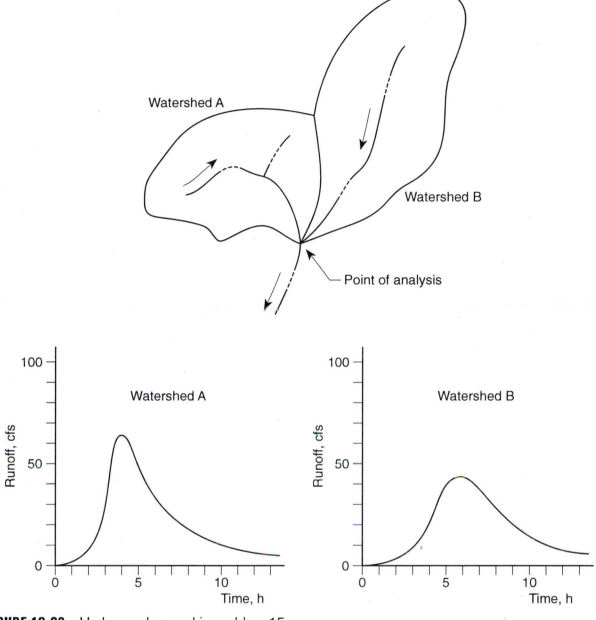

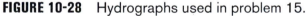

FIGURE 10-28   Hydrographs used in problem 15.

FURTHER READING

Chow, V. T., Maidment, D. R., and Mays, L. R. (1988). *Applied Hydrology.* New York: McGraw-Hill.

Hershfield, D. M. (1961). *Rainfall Frequency Atlas of the United States for Durations from 30 Minutes to 24 Hours and Return Periods of 1 to 100 Years* (Tech. Paper 40). Silver Spring, MD: U.S. National Weather Service.

Ponce, V. M. (1989). *Engineering Hydrology: Principles and Practices.* Englewood Cliffs, NJ: Prentice Hall.

U.S. Soil Conservation Service. (1972). *National Engineering Handbook.* Springfield, VA: U.S. Department of Agriculture.

Viessman, W., Jr., Lewis, G. L., and Knapp, J. W. (1989). *Introduction to Hydrology.* (3rd ed.). New York: Harper and Row.

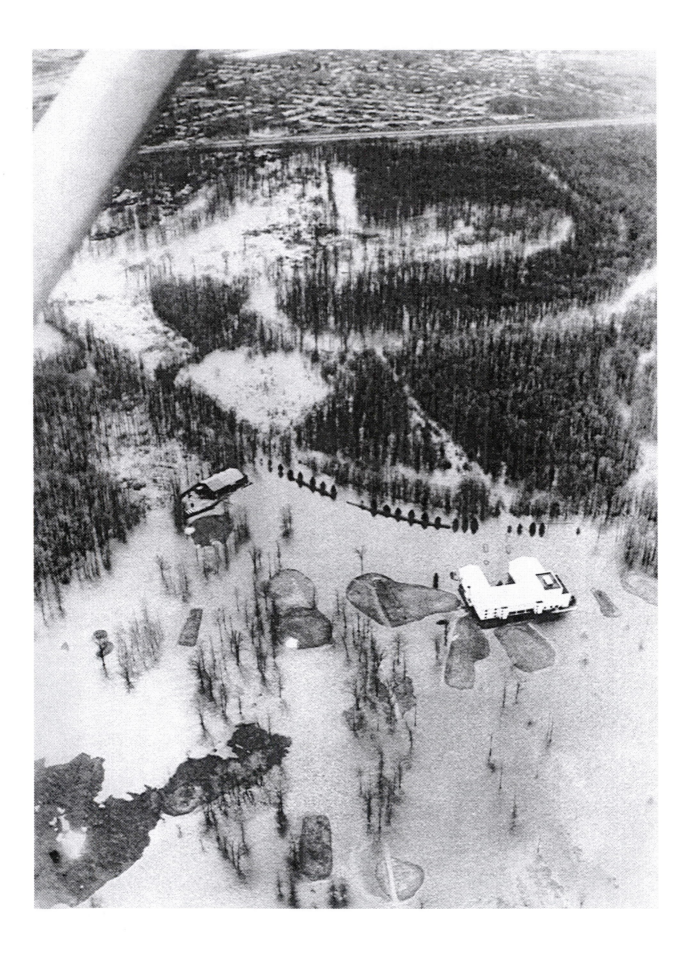

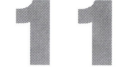

RUNOFF CALCULATIONS

The process in which rainfall accumulates on the ground and runs toward streams and rivers is complicated. As we saw in Chapter 10, great variations occur in rainfall intensity and rainfall patterns. Add to this the infinite variety in ground topography, soil types, vegetation, and human-made features.

It is no wonder that many mathematical methods have been devised to calculate runoff, both peak values and hydrographs, over the years. The design of a hydraulic structure such as a culvert or storm sewer or grass swale requires estimating the quantity of runoff it must convey. In this chapter, we will examine two methods used to calculate runoff in wide use today by engineers working in stormwater management: the Rational Method and the NRCS Method.

OBJECTIVES

After completing this chapter, the reader should be able to:

- Calculate peak runoff by the Rational Method
- Calculate peak runoff by the NRCS Method
- Calculate a runoff hydrograph by the Modified Rational Method
- Calculate a runoff hydrograph by the NRCS Method

11.1 RATIONAL METHOD

Many methods to compute runoff have been developed over the years, and the first and most enduring of these is the Rational Method. Most methods are based on empirical relationships among drainage area, time of concentration, rainfall, and other factors. However, the Rational Method, introduced in England in 1889, has its genesis in pure reasoning, from which it received its name.

The Rational Method is used to compute the peak runoff, Q_p, following a rainfall event. It makes no attempt to estimate runoff before or after the peak but simply estimates the one quantity of flow that is greatest.

Originally, the Rational Method formula for peak runoff was given as

$$Q_p = Ai \tag{11-1}$$

where Q_p = peak runoff, cfs
$\quad\quad A$ = drainage area, acres
$\quad\quad i$ = rainfall intensity, in/h

This was based on a completely impervious drainage basin in which all rainfall is converted to runoff. Later, a proportionality factor, c, called the **runoff coefficient**, was added in an attempt to account for infiltration into the ground and for evapotranspiration. So the formula became

$$Q_p = Aci \tag{11-2}$$

where c is the dimensionless runoff coefficient. Values of c vary between 0.0 and 1.0.

Equations 11-1 and 11-2 are consistent with SI units. So, for example, if A is given in m^2 and i in m/s, the resulting Q_p will have units m^3/s.

The original reasoning expressed in the Rational Method is described as follows:

1. Consider a drainage basin with area A that is rained on at a constant intensity i for a duration equal to t_c. Assume that no rain falls before or after the downpour of intensity i and duration t_c. Figure 11-1 shows a graphic representation of the rainfall.

Note: To help understand the idea above, remember that in the intensity pattern shown in Figure 10-11, a duration of any length can be considered and then idealized into a constant intensity over that duration. In this case, we are picking a duration that happens to be the same time as t_c.

2. Now picture yourself at the point of analysis watching the runoff flowing by. As soon as the rainfall starts, some runoff flows by. This early runoff comes from rainfall that landed near the point of analysis. As time goes by, runoff increases as raindrops from farther away reach the point of analysis. (But even as these farther raindrops arrive, the close raindrops are still arriving because it is still raining.)
3. Finally, when a time equal to t_c has elapsed, the remotest raindrop arrives at the point of analysis, and at this moment, the rainfall stops. This then marks the maximum runoff rate, and the rate begins declining immediately. After another period equal to t_c, all the water in the drainage basin has run off.
4. To quantify peak runoff Q_p, examine Figure 11-1. The total volume of runoff equals the area under the graph of runoff versus time. Thus, volume computed in cubic feet is

$$\text{Volume} = \frac{1}{2}(2)(60t_c)Q_p$$
$$= 60t_c Q_p$$

But remember that because the drainage basin is hypothetically completely impervious, total runoff equals total rainfall. Total rainfall is computed simply as the depth of rainfall times the area over which the rainfall occurred. Depth of rainfall in feet is the rainfall intensity converted to feet per second times the duration converted to seconds. Thus,

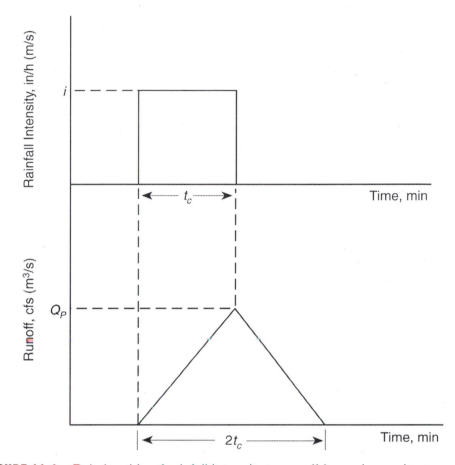

FIGURE 11-1   Relationship of rainfall intensity to runoff for an impervious drainage basin according to the Rational Method.

$$\text{Depth} = \frac{i}{(12)(3600)}\left(60t_c\right)$$

$$= \frac{it_c}{720}$$

and rainfall volume is

$$\text{Volume} = \text{Depth} \times \text{area}$$

$$= \frac{it_c}{720}(43560A)$$

$$= 60.5it_cA$$

Finally, equating the volumes gives

$$60t_cQ_p = 60.5it_cA$$

or

$$Q_p = 1.0083Ai$$

TABLE 11-1   Typical Runoff Coefficients for Use with the Rational Method

Surface Type	Runoff Coefficient	
	Range of Values	**Typical Design**
Impervious (pavement, roofs)	0.75–0.95	0.95
Lawns	0.05–0.35	0.30
Unimproved (woods, brush)	0.10–0.30	0.20

Note: *These values of c are typical for lower-intensity storms (up to 25-year return period). Higher values are appropriate for larger design storms. A more extensive list of c values is presented in Appendix C-1.*

which is approximated to

$$Q_p = Ai$$

which represents the Rational Method for a hypothetical drainage basin that is totally impervious.

5. To account for infiltration and evapotranspiration of runoff, a proportionality constant c was added to the equation. Values of c are empirically determined and correspond to various surface conditions within the drainage basin. Table 11-1 lists some common c values in use today.

6. The fact that rain is falling on the catchment area before and after the duration t_c does not change the derived value of Q_p. The only effect is to change the shape of the graph of runoff versus time.

7. Keep in mind that the actual rainfall covers a period of several hours. We have chosen to focus on the most intense portion of the rainfall having a duration of t_c. Any other duration would result in a smaller value of Q_p. If we chose a duration less than t_c, the intensity would be greater, but we would not include runoff from the entire drainage basin. If we chose a duration greater than t_c, the intensity would be less, thus reducing mathematically the amount of rainfall.

Example 11-1

Problem

Compute the peak runoff, Q_p, for a 25-year storm using the Rational Method for a drainage basin located in Pennsylvania (Region 1) and having the following parameters:

1. Area: $A = 24$ acres
2. Time of concentration:

   Overland: average grass surface
   Length = 100 ft
   Slope = 2.0%

   Shallow concentrated flow:
   Length = 750 ft
   Slope = 4.0%

Stream:
    Length = 1000 ft
    Slope = 0.4%
    Average cross section:

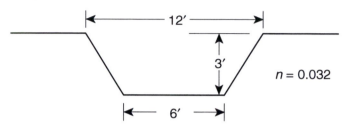

3. Runoff coefficient:
    Impervious, 0.5 acre @ $c = 0.90$
    Grass, 11.5 acres @ $c = 0.35$
    Wooded, 12 acres @ $c = 0.25$

Solution

To compute Q_p, the values of A, i, and c must be determined. In this case, A is known to be 24 acres. To find rainfall intensity, i, we first find time of concentration, t_c.

Time for overland flow, t_1, is found from the nomograph in Appendix C-2:

$$t_1 = 12.5 \text{ min}$$

Time for shallow concentrated flow, t_2, is found from Figure 10-9, using the line marked "Unpaved":

$$v = 3.2 \text{ ft/s}$$
$$t_2 = \frac{d}{v} = \frac{750}{3.2} = 234 \text{ s}$$
$$= 3.9 \text{ min}$$

Time for stream flow, t_3, is found by using Manning's equation. Assume that the stream is flowing bank full. First, find cross-sectional area, a, and wetted perimeter, p, using the average cross section given:

$$a = 27 \text{ ft}^2$$
$$p = 14.5 \text{ ft}$$

Next, find hydraulic radius, R:

$$R = \frac{a}{p}$$
$$= \frac{27}{14.5} = 1.86 \text{ ft}$$

Next, find v from Manning's equation:

$$v = \frac{1.49}{n} R^{2/3} s_o^{1/2}$$
$$= \frac{1.49}{0.032}(1.86)^{2/3}(0.004)^{1/2}$$
$$= 4.45 \text{ ft/s}$$

Finally, find t_3:

$$t_3 = \frac{d}{v} = \frac{1000}{4.45} = 225 \text{ s}$$
$$= 3.7 \text{ min}$$

Therefore, time of concentration is

$$t_c = t_1 + t_2 + t_3$$
$$= 12.5 + 3.9 + 3.7$$
$$= 20.1 \text{ min}$$

The time of concentration, 20.1 min, is taken as the duration of rainfall in determining rainfall intensity, i:

Duration = 20.1 min

Rainfall intensity is found by using the I-D-F curves for Pennsylvania (Region 1) shown in Appendix C-3. Use the 25-year curve.

$$i = 3.1 \text{ in/h}$$

Now, find the composite runoff coefficient, using the c-values given:

$$c = \frac{(0.5)(0.9) + (11.5)(0.35) + (12)(0.25)}{24}$$
$$= 0.31$$

Finally, compute peak runoff, Q_p, using Equation 11-2:

$$Q_p = Aci$$
$$= (24)(0.31)(3.1)$$
$$= 23 \text{ cfs} \quad \text{(Answer)}$$

Example 11-2

Problem

Suppose a lawn drain is designed for a location in Orange County, California, as shown in Figure 11-2. Compute peak runoff, Q_p, using the Rational Method for a 15-year storm using the proposed lawn drain as the point of analysis. The grate elevation is 377.0.

Solution

For an actual design, a site visit is essential. However, in this case, we will do our best, using the aerial topography shown in Figure 11-2.

Begin by delineating the drainage area as depicted in Figure 11-3. Notice that the basin divide cuts through the dwelling at the southerly end of the basin. The divide was drawn by following the contour lines and ignoring the dwelling. If a site visit reveals a different drainage pattern at the house, the delineation should be altered.

Next, the drainage basin area is measured by planimeter to be 2.10 acres. At the same time, areas of the various surface types are measured. The area of woods is

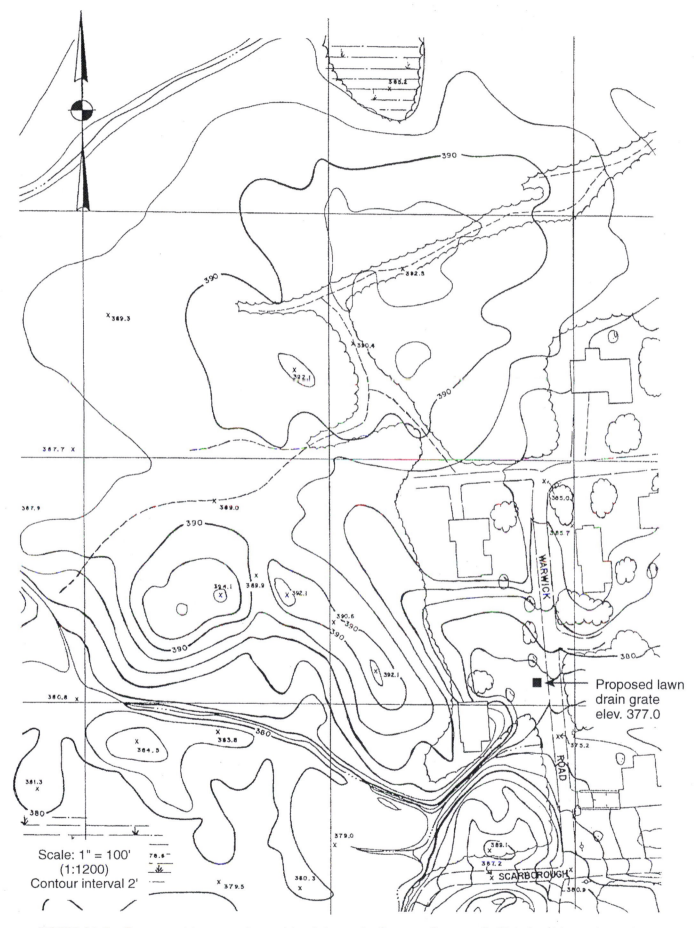

FIGURE 11-2 Topographic map of a residential area in Orange County, California. (*Map adapted from Robinson Aerial.*)

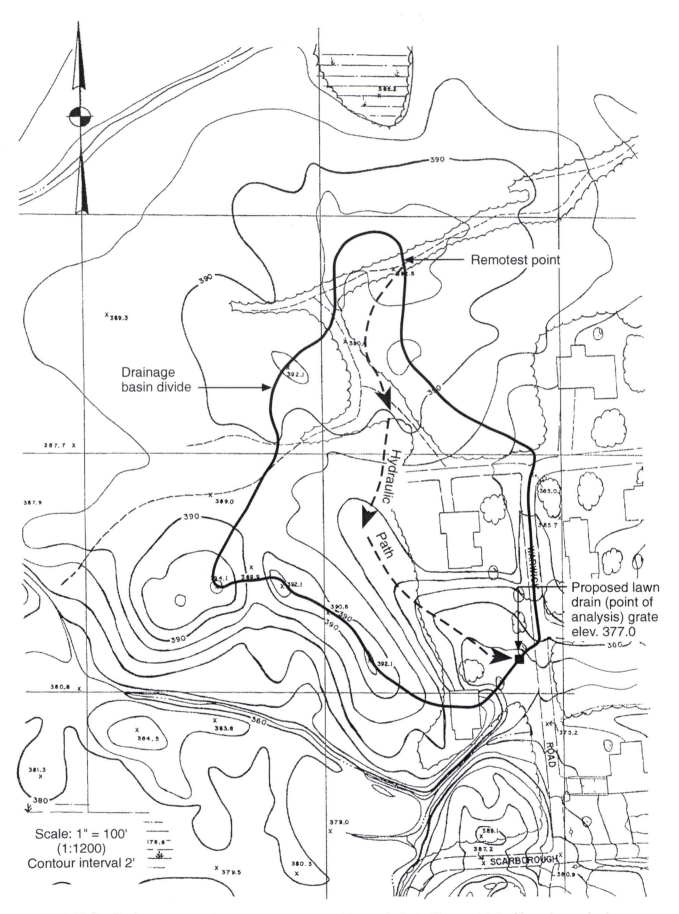

FIGURE 11-3   Drainage area tributary to a proposed lawn drain in Figure 11-2. Also shown is the hydraulic path. (*Map adapted from Robinson Aerial.*)

1.22 acres, and the impervious area is 0.14 acre. The remaining area of 0.74 acre is considered grass.

Runoff coefficients for the three surface types are taken from Table 11-1. Therefore, the composite c value is computed as follows:

Impervious, 0.14 acres @ $c = 0.90$
Grass,   0.74 acres @ $c = 0.30$
Woods,   1.22 acres @ $c = 0.20$

$$c = \frac{(0.14)(0.90)+(0.74)(0.30)+(1.22)(0.20)}{2.10} = 0.28$$

Next, delineate the hydraulic path, as shown in Figure 11-3. Starting at the remotest point, runoff flows as overland flow for 100 feet. Shallow concentrated flow then continues all the way to the point of analysis, a measured distance of 410 feet.

To find the time for overland flow, t_1, first find the slope:

$$\text{slope} = \frac{392.5 - 390.4}{100} \times 100\% = 2.1\%$$

Time is found from the nomograph in Appendix C-2 using average grass surface:

$t_1 = 12.5$ min

To find the time for shallow concentrated flow, t_2, first find the slope:

$$\text{slope} = \frac{390.4 - 377.0}{410} \times 100\% = 3.3\%$$

Velocity is found from Figure 10-9 by using the line marked "Unpaved":

$v = 2.9$ ft/s

Time is then computed as

$$t_2 = \frac{d}{v} = \frac{410}{2.9} = 141 \text{ s}$$
$$= 2.4 \text{ min}$$

Therefore, time of concentration is

$$t_c = t_1 + t_2$$
$$= 12.5 + 2.4$$
$$= 14.9 \text{ min}$$

The time of concentration, 14.9 min, is taken as the duration of rainfall in determining rainfall intensity, i:

Duration = 14.9 min

Rainfall intensity is found by using the I-D-F curves for Orange County, California, in Appendix C-3. For a 15-year storm, interpolate between the 10-year and 25-year curves:

$i = 2.0$ in/h

Finally, compute peak runoff, Q_p, using Equation 11-2:

$$Q_p = Aci$$
$$= (2.10)(0.28)(2.0)$$
$$= 1.2 \text{ cfs} \quad \text{(Answer)}$$

The primary application of the Rational Method is in estimating peak runoff for small drainage basins—those that are tributary to minor drainage structures such as storm sewers and small drainage swales. The usual basin size is less than 15 acres, and the Rational Method should not be used for drainage areas larger than 100–200 acres.

In addition to size of drainage area, some other important limitations to the Rational Method should be understood. First, the drainage basin surface characteristics should be homogeneous. Although, ideally, one c-value should predominate the basin, in practical application, this is not possible. This is why a composite c is computed. However, grossly disproportional surface types should be avoided if possible. For example, if a 2.0-acre drainage basin consists of 1.9 acres of paved parking and 0.1 acre of woods at one edge, the hydraulic path would undoubtedly run through the wooded area, producing a time of concentration too large to be representative of the vast majority of the basin.

Another drainage basin characteristic to be avoided is any significant ponding within the basin, which might affect the peak discharge. Although this condition usually does not occur, another method of computing peak runoff should be considered when it does.

Finally, it should be remembered that the Rational Method is intended for peak runoff computation, not for the entire hydrograph of a rainfall event. Many methods have been devised to stretch the computation into a hydrograph, giving the full relationship of runoff to time following the rainfall. Such computational procedures are loosely referred to as the Modified Rational Method. Although valid results can be obtained for small applications, such as minor detention basins, care should be taken when employing the method. Always be aware of the basis of Modified Rational Method you may be using, and keep in mind that such procedures tend to stretch the Rational Method beyond the task for which it was intended.

11.2 MODIFIED RATIONAL METHOD

As was described in Section 11.1, the Rational Method is a procedure for computing peak discharge for a small drainage basin. For the design of storm sewers and swales, peak discharge suffices, but for detention basin design, a runoff hydrograph is required for use in the routing procedure. Therefore, the Modified Rational Method was devised.

The **Modified Rational Method** expands the original Rational Method to yield a hydrograph for use in detention basin design. First adopted in the 1970s, the method remains in wide use today, although many variations have been created. A few of the variations are described below.

In its simplest form, the Modified Rational Method consists of a simple triangular hydrograph, as shown in Figure 11-4. Peak discharge is Q_p as computed by the basic Rational Method, $Q_p = ciA$. The time base of the hydrograph is $2t_c$, which is consistent with the theory supporting the basic Rational Method. (See Figure 11-1.)

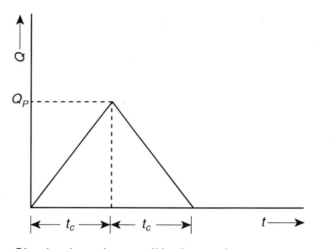

FIGURE 11-4   Simple triangular runoff hydrograph.

The hydrograph shown in Figure 11-4 makes no allowance for ground storage in the runoff process, which in actual conditions results in a longer time base. Therefore, the general hydrograph shape is a simple approximation of that shown in Figure 10-12, which is more consistent with that found in real runoff experience.

Taking the simple triangular hydrograph one step further, a method was devised to estimate the required storage volume of small detention basins having a single outlet. Although detention basin design is discussed in Chapters 14 and 15, a brief explanation of the method follows.

The procedure starts with a triangular runoff hydrograph similar to the one shown in Figure 11-4 for a given drainage area, time of concentration, and runoff coefficient and then considers a series of additional hydrographs that would result from longer rainfall durations than t_c. According to the Rational Method, the greatest peak discharge occurs when the rainfall duration equals t_c. When the rainfall duration is greater than t_c, peak discharge is reduced, but total runoff volume is increased, and greater volume can increase the required size of a detention basin.

Shown in Figure 11-5, curve 1 depicts the triangular hydrograph, while curve 2 shows a trapezoidal hydrograph resulting from a rainfall having a duration equal to $2t_c$. This hydrograph has a lower peak, Q_{p2}, because on the appropriate I-D-F curve, a longer duration corresponds to a smaller rainfall intensity. It has a trapezoidal shape because, according to the Rational Method, if rainfall continues beyond the time of concentration, runoff remains constant because no additional water arrives at the point of analysis. The hydrograph has a receding limb covering a time equal to t_c, the same as curve 1. Curves 3 and 4 are described similarly.

The series of curves shown in Figure 11-5 represents various possibilities of runoff hydrograph resulting from a storm of a given frequency, depending on the rainfall duration within the storm. According to the method, each hydrograph would be routed through a detention basin having a predefined outlet, and the one resulting in the greatest storage volume would determine the required size of the detention basin. This method is probably known to more engineers as the Modified Rational Method than is any other.

The method is intended as a simple approximation for small detention basins with simple outlet structures. It has all the limitations of the Rational Method, such

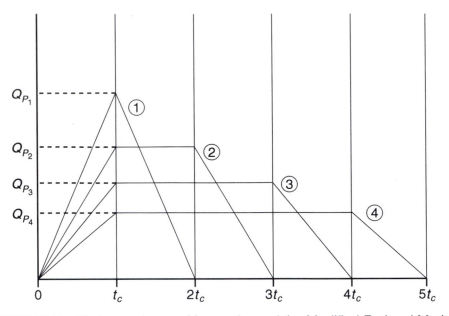

FIGURE 11-5   Hydrographs used in one form of the Modified Rational Method.

as the assumption that rainfall is constant over the rainfall duration and no ground storage occurs during runoff. It has been estimated that the method is appropriate for catchment areas less than 20 acres.

Another hydrograph construction, shown in Figure 11-6, is often used for small watersheds. This hydrograph, which could also be called the Modified Rational Method, starts with the simple triangle of Figure 11-4 and expands the time base to $2.67t_c$. Peak discharge remains Q_p as computed by the Rational Method. By stretching the receding limb of the triangular hydrograph, the shape more closely resembles that of a true runoff hydrograph. However, the resulting runoff volume becomes 33 percent greater than the rainfall excess that contributes to the hydrograph. This discrepancy adds a conservative safety factor to the method.

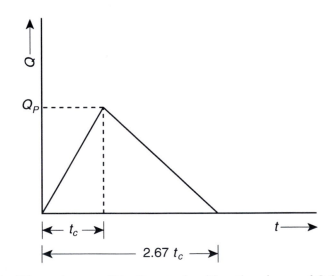

FIGURE 11-6   Triangular runoff hydrograph with a time base of $2.67t_c$.

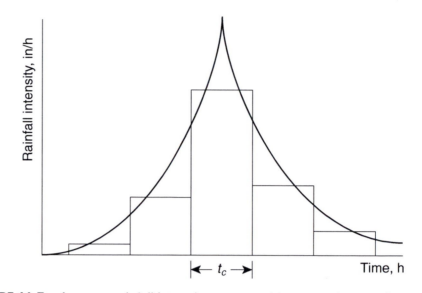

FIGURE 11-7   Average rainfall intensity pattern with a superimposed step graph based on durations equal to t_c.

In detention basin design, the hydrograph would be used alone in routing through a proposed detention basin. Alternate hydrographs based on different rainfall durations would not be used as in the previously described method.

Finally, another variation of the Modified Rational Method, published by Baumgardner and Morris in 1982, is of interest. This method attempts to consider a runoff hydrograph from an entire rainfall event (storm), and not just a short duration within the event.

Starting with the triangle concept shown in Figure 11-4, the method then considers other durations (of length t_c) throughout the rainfall, each with its characteristic runoff hydrograph. To illustrate this, consider a typical storm (for a given frequency) as shown in Figure 11-7. Peak rainfall over a duration equal to t_c is drawn as a constant rainfall intensity; then additional time durations equal to t_c are measured on each side of the peak. For each duration, the average rainfall intensity is expressed as a constant over the duration. This procedure results in a step graph, first ascending and then descending throughout the rainfall event.

Each step in Figure 11-7 results in a triangular runoff hydrograph as shown in Figure 11-8. The graph of runoff versus time contains five hydrographs, one for each of the five rainfall intensities in the associated intensity versus time graph. In practice, the number of intensity steps can vary depending on the time of concentration and the overall duration of rainfall considered. For small watersheds, an overall storm duration of 3 hours is considered adequate. This results in five to ten steps in the intensity versus time graph.

It should be noted that a storm duration of 3 hours does not imply that the entire storm was completed in 3 hours. (Some storms last 3 hours; some last longer.) Instead, it means that of the entire storm duration, a 3-hour segment having the greatest intensity is used.

Finally, to complete the runoff hydrograph, the individual triangular hydrographs are added by the principle of superposition to yield the hydrograph shown in Figure 11-9. This hydrograph can then be used to route through a proposed detention basin.

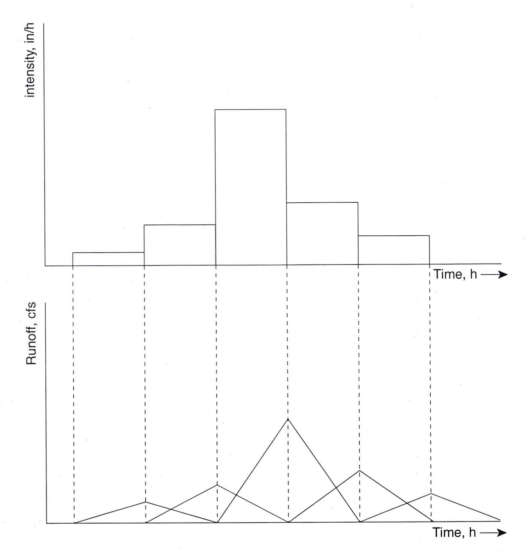

FIGURE 11-8 Rainfall intensity step graph with an associated triangular runoff hydrograph for each duration.

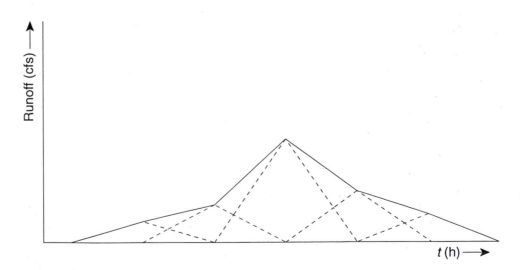

FIGURE 11-9 Finished runoff hydrograph computed by superposition of individual triangular hydrographs.

This method results in a hydrograph with a peak equal to Q_p as computed by the basic Rational Method but with a shape and time base more consistent with an overall rainfall event and not just one intense downpour within the rainfall event. Use of this method requires the routing of just one hydrograph and not a series of trapezoidal hydrographs, as described above.

All variations of the Modified Rational Method are intended for small watersheds and are limited by the assumptions of the original Rational Method.

11.3 NRCS METHOD

The NRCS Method is a procedure for computing a synthetic hydrograph based on empirically determined factors developed by the Soil Conservation Service (SCS). Originally called the SCS Method, it is now named for the Natural Resources Conservation Service (NRCS), which is descended from the SCS.

The method was first published by SCS in 1975 in a design manual titled *Urban Hydrology for Small Watersheds,* Technical Release 55, also known as TR-55. The manual underwent major revisions in 1986. As a design manual, TR-55 contains charts and graphs that allow the user to compute peak runoff and runoff hydrographs for watersheds located within the United States.

In 2002, TR-55 was replaced by WinTR-55, which is a software version of the paper manual. WinTR-55 is designed to be used interactively on a PC and has eliminated the charts and graphs of the paper version.

Presentation of the NRCS Method in this text utilizes many of the charts and graphs of TR-55 (1986) for illustration purposes. Actual use of the method should be done by using WinTR-55 or one of the commercial software packages containing the NRCS Method. Data used by NRCS in the WinTR-55 software have, in many cases, superseded data found in TR-55 (1986).

WinTR-55 is available on-line at http://www.wcc.nrcs.usda.gov/hydro.

The NRCS Method is widely used in the design of hydraulic structures such as culverts, detention basins, stream relocation, and large drainage ditches. These structures generally have tributary drainage areas ranging from a few acres to about 25 square miles. For drainage areas larger than a few square miles, the validity of the NRCS Method, or of any synthetic hydrograph method, diminishes because the variety of basin characteristics becomes too diverse and because the rainfall pattern might not cover the entire drainage area.

Because WinTR-55 has not yet been converted to SI units, our discussion of the NRCS Method will be presented entirely in English units.

At the core of the NRCS Method is the dimensionless unit hydrograph described in the *National Engineering Handbook, Part 630, Hydrology,* published originally by SCS and now by NRCS. The NRCS dimensionless unit hydrograph is shown in Figure 11-10. Notice that the time axis is calibrated not in time units but as t/T_p, where T_p is the time to the peak of the hydrograph. Therefore, the time axis units are h/h, or dimensionless. In this way, each point on the time axis represents a percentage, or fraction, of the time to peak. Similarly, notice that the runoff axis is calibrated not in cfs but as q/q_p, where q_p is the peak runoff. Therefore, each point on the runoff axis represents a percentage of the peak discharge. The dimensionless unit hydrograph has proportions relative to the unit rainfall excess that simulate almost all drainage areas. The rising limb contains 38 percent of the hydrograph, and the falling limb contains 62 percent. The time of concentration is the time elapsed from the end of the unit rainfall excess to the point of inflection of the falling limb.

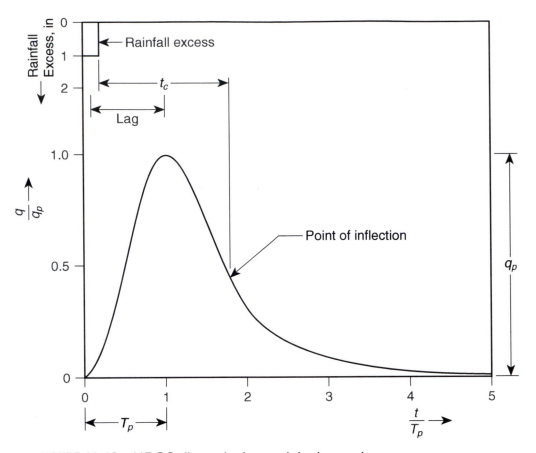

FIGURE 11-10 NRCS dimensionless unit hydrograph.

By using the unit hydrograph shown in Figure 11-10, a resultant hydrograph can be constructed for any rainfall distribution by dividing the distribution into a number of unit rainfall excess elements and drawing the unit hydrograph for each. The resultant hydrograph would then be the summation of all the unit hydrographs. The NRCS has developed a database of unit hydrographs based on parameters describing the characteristics of watersheds as well as rainfall patterns for specific geographical locations. So for a watershed located in the United States, the following parameters must be specified to define a hydrograph:

1. Location
2. Cover characteristics
3. Time of concentration

Specifying these parameters defines a unit hydrograph with ordinate units cfs/s.m./in. Thus, if the ordinates are multiplied by the area of the watershed in square miles and by the rainfall excess in inches, a resultant, or derived, hydrograph results. Therefore, in addition to the above three parameters, the size of the watershed and the precipitation must be specified. Following is a discussion of the parameters outlined above:

- **Location:** The geographic location of the watershed is specified by indicating the county and state in which it is located. This is important because NRCS has identified four different general rainfall patterns occurring throughout the country, and different rainfall patterns result in different unit hydrographs. A map showing the locations of the four rainfall patterns is reproduced from TR-55 in Appendix D-4. Also, the location determines the 24-hour rainfall amount. Rainfall maps based on TP40 and *Atlas 2* are shown in Appendix D-3. (These maps are shown for instructional purposes. Actual runoff computations should be based on *NOAA Atlas 14*, as discussed in Section 10.4.)

- **Cover characteristics:** To determine the amount of rainfall losses, both initial losses and infiltration, cover characteristics must be known. This is specified by a curve number (CN), which is a function of soil type and surface cover, such as impervious cover or vegetative cover. A table of CN values corresponding to various cover conditions and soil types is shown in Appendix D-1.
- **Time of concentration:** Time of concentration, t_c, is a major factor in determining the shape of the unit hydrograph. It is computed as the sum of all travel times along the hydraulic path as in the Rational Method. However, travel time for overland flow is computed by a special empirical formula developed by NRCS.
- **Drainage area:** Drainage area, A_m, is the area in square miles enclosed by the watershed divide, which is delineated as in the Rational Method.
- **Precipitation:** Precipitation, P, is the total depth of rainfall in inches, not intensity as in the Rational Method. All rainfall events are assumed to be 24-hour duration.

The WinTR-55 software has the capability to compute the runoff hydrograph for a watershed for a rainfall event of specified frequency. WinTR-55 can also route the hydrograph downstream along a stream or through a reservoir. It can also combine hydrographs.

Computations

To compute a runoff hydrograph (or only the peak runoff) using the NRCS Method, first determine the design storm frequency. This usually depends on the size of the structure to be designed. Next, follow the steps described below. The steps shown here are based on the charts and graphs of TR-55 (1986), but use of WinTR-55 is similar.

Step 1: Delineate and measure the drainage area tributary to the point of analysis. This is done in the same manner as for the Rational Method.

Step 2: Determine the cover number, CN, for the watershed. If the watershed consists of a variety of CNs, which is nearly always the case, compute a composite CN, which is a weighted average of the individual CN values. A table of CN values is shown in Appendix D. In computing CN, first determine the "hydrologic soil group" that describes the soils in the drainage basin. Generally, this is done by use of an NRCS Soil Survey of the local region, usually the county within which the drainage area is situated. Each soil type is assigned a hydrologic soil group of A, B, C, or D, depending on its characteristics of infiltration and antecedent moisture condition. Hydrologic soil group A represents the highest rate of infiltration (sandy soil), while D represents the lowest rate (clay soil or rock outcrops). A list of selected soil types together with their respective hydrologic soil group designation is shown in Appendix D-2. These should be referred to in computing runoff by the NRCS Method.

Example 11-3

Problem

A 400-acre drainage basin contains the following soils:

Soil Type	Hydrologic Soil Group
Boonton gravely loam	B
Parker gravely sandy loam	B
Washington loam	B

Cover conditions within the drainage basin are as follows:

Cover	Area (acres)
Impervious	5.0
Wooded (good cover)	225
Meadow (good condition)	55
Residential ($\frac{1}{4}$-acre lots)	115

Compute the composite CN.

Solution

Use hydrologic soil group B, since it predominates. Next, determine CN for each cover condition, using Appendix D-1. Create a table as follows:

Cover	Area (acres)	CN	Product
Impervious	5.0	98	490
Wooded	225	55	12,375
Meadow	55	58	3,190
Residential	115	75	8,625
	400		24,680

$$\text{Weighted CN} = \frac{24,680}{400} = 61.7$$

Use CN = 62   (Answer)

Example 11-4

Problem

A 250-acre drainage basin contains the following soils:

Soil Type	Area (acres)	Hydrologic Soil Group
Califon Loam	100	C
Netcong Loam	150	B

Cover conditions are as follows:

Cover	Area (acres)
Residential ($\frac{1}{2}$-acre lots)	190
Wooded (fair condition)	25
Open space (fair condition)	35

Compute the composite CN.

Solution

Since hydrologic soil group is mixed, determine the percentage of each type: B, 60 percent, and C, 40 percent.

Next, determine CN for each cover condition by interpolating between B and C values using Appendix D-1:

Cover	CN B (60%)	C (40%)	Interpolated CN
Residential	70	80	74.0
Wooded	65	76	69.4
Open space	69	79	73.0

Finally, create a table as follows:

Cover	Area (acres)	CN	Product
Residential	190	74.0	14,060
Wooded	25	69.4	1,735
Open space	35	73.0	2,555
	250		18,350

$$\text{Weighted CN} = \frac{18{,}350}{250} = 73.4$$

Use CN = 73   (Answer)

Step 3: Determine the rainfall excess, measured in inches. It is the amount of rainfall available for runoff after subtracting initial losses and infiltration and is computed from the following empirical formula:

$$Q = \frac{(P - I_a)^2}{(P - I_a) + S} \tag{11-3}$$

where Q = runoff, in
P = rainfall, in
S = potential maximum retention after runoff begins, in
I_a = initial losses, in

Note: The symbol Q is used for runoff depth in inches to be consistent with symbols used in TR-55. Be sure not to confuse this parameter with Q used for runoff rate in the Rational Method.

Initial losses are related directly to CN in Table 11-2. Also, S is related directly to CN by the relation

$$S = \frac{1000}{CN} - 10 \tag{11-4}$$

However, Q can be determined without the use of formulas by referring to Figure 11-11.

TABLE 11-2 I_a Values for Runoff Curve Numbers

Curve Number	I_a (in)	Curve Number	I_a (in)
40	3.000	70	0.857
41	2.878	71	0.817
42	2.762	72	0.778
43	2.651	73	0.740
44	2.545	74	0.703
45	2.444	75	0.667
46	2.348	76	0.632
47	2.255	77	0.597
48	2.167	78	0.564
49	2.082	79	0.532
50	2.000	80	0.500
51	1.922	81	0.469
52	1.846	82	0.439
53	1.774	83	0.410
54	1.704	84	0.381
55	1.636	85	0.353
56	1.571	86	0.326
57	1.509	87	0.299
58	1.448	88	0.273
59	1.390	89	0.247
60	1.333	90	0.222
61	1.279	91	0.198
62	1.226	92	0.174
63	1.175	93	0.151
64	1.125	94	0.128
65	1.077	95	0.105
66	1.030	96	0.083
67	0.985	97	0.062
68	0.941	98	0.041
69	0.899		

(Courtesy of Soil Conservation Service, Technical Release 55.)

Example 11-5

Problem

Find the runoff depth, Q, for a drainage basin with CN of 78 using the NRCS Method. Design rainfall is 6.5 inches.

Solution

By using Table 11-2, I_a is found to be 0.564 in. Next, by using Equation 11-4,

$$S = \frac{1000}{CN} - 10$$
$$= \frac{1000}{78} - 10$$
$$= 2.28 \text{ in}$$

Solution for runoff equation

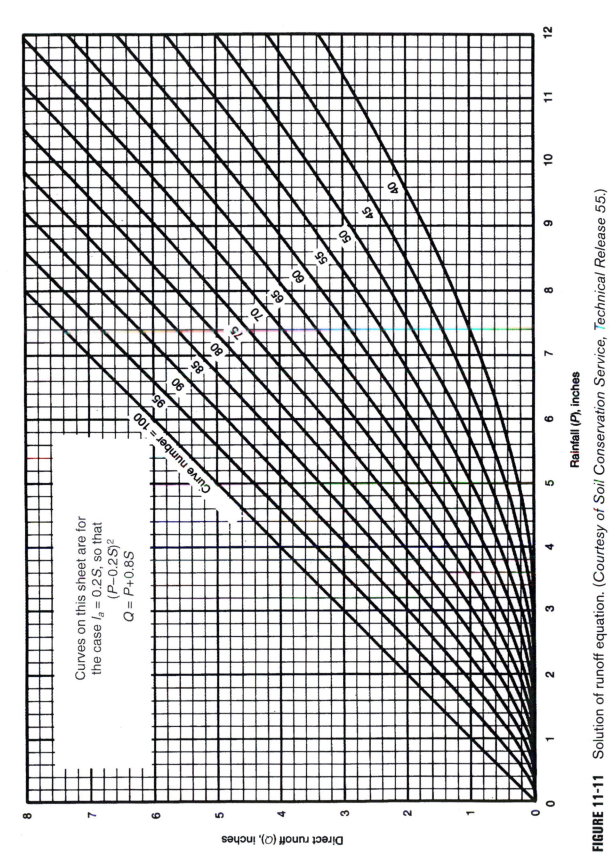

FIGURE 11-11 Solution of runoff equation. (*Courtesy of Soil Conservation Service, Technical Release 55.*)

Finally, using Equation 9-3, we have

$$Q = \frac{(P-I_a)^2}{(P-I_a)+S}$$
$$= \frac{(6.5-0.564)^2}{(6.5-0.564)+2.82}$$
$$= 4.0 \text{ in}\quad (\text{Answer})$$

As an alternative, use Figure 11-11. Enter the graph at a rainfall of 6.5 inches, and trace upward until you reach CN = 78, which is interpolated between the curves for 75 and 80, respectively. Then trace to the left and read the value of Q to be 4.0 in. (Answer)

Step 4: Compute time of concentration. All travel times are determined as explained in Section 10.3 except overland flow, which is computed by the following empirical formula:

$$T_t = \frac{0.007(nL)^{0.8}}{(P_2)^{0.5} s^{0.4}} \tag{11-5}$$

where T_t = overland travel time, h
   n = roughness coefficient (see Table 11-3)
   L = length of flow, ft
   P_2 = 2-year precipitation, in
   s = gradient, ft/ft

Note: The term s is used to denote the slope of the ground for computation of overland flow and shallow concentrated flow. This should not be confused with the term for slope of the EGL in open channel flow.

TABLE 11-3   Roughness Coefficients, *n*, for Computing Overland Flow.

Surface Description	n^1
Smooth surfaces (concrete, asphalt, gravel, or bare soil)	0.011
Fallow (no residue)	0.05
Cultivated soils:	
Residue cover ≤ 20%	0.06
Residue cover >20%	0.17
Grass:	
Short grass prairie	0.15
Dense grasses[2]	0.24
Bermudagrass	0.41
Range (natural)	0.13
Woods:[3]	
Light underbrush	0.40
Dense underbrush	0.80

[1]*The n-values are a composite of information compiled by Engman (1986).*

[2]*Includes species such as weeping lovegrass, bluegrass, buffalo grass, blue grama grass, and native grass mixtures.*

[3]*When selecting n, consider cover to a height of about 0.1 foot. This is the only part of the plant cover that will obstruct sheet flow.*

(Courtesy of Soil Conservation Service, Technical Release 55.)

The maximum value of L, based on NRCS research, is 100 feet. After this distance has been reached, sheet flow usually becomes shallow concentrated flow. If overland flow encounters a swale before reaching a distance of 100 feet, then flow type changes to shallow concentrated flow at that point.

When selecting an n-value from Table 11-3, remember that the relevant surface condition is that which prevails within 1 inch of the ground because that is where the water flows. Therefore, thick underbrush growing several inches above the ground should not influence the selection of n. Most field conditions yield an n-value between 0.15 and 0.40.

Example 11-6

Problem

Find the overland travel time T_t for the drainage basin shown in Figure 11-12, located in St. Louis, Missouri.

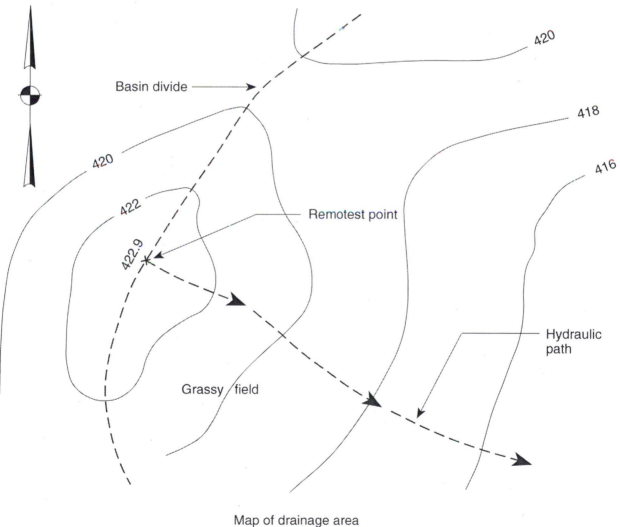

Map of drainage area
Scale: 1″ = 50′

FIGURE 11-12   Portion of a drainage basin showing beginning of hydraulic path.

Solution

From inspection of the map shown in Figure 11-12, assume that the length of overland flow is 100 feet. This is because the contour lines do not indicate a swale and the length cannot be greater than 100 feet.

Next, find the slope. The elevation of the remotest point is 422.9 feet. From the contour lines, the elevation at the end of 100 feet is 419.2. Therefore, the slope is

$$s = \frac{422.9 - 419.2}{100}$$
$$= 0.037 \text{ ft/ft}$$

Next, estimate the *n*-value. From Table 11-3, $n = 0.15$.

Two-year precipitation, P_2, is taken from Appendix D-3 (using the 2-year, 24-hour rainfall map) and interpolating between the lines of equal rainfall amount. In this case, for St. Louis, $P_2 = 3.5$ inches.

Then, from Equation 11-5,

$$T_t = \frac{0.007(nL)^{0.8}}{(P_2)^{0.5} s^{0.4}}$$
$$= \frac{0.007\{(0.15)(100)\}^{0.8}}{(3.5)^{0.5}(0.037)^{0.4}}$$
$$= 0.12 \text{ h} \quad \text{(Answer)}$$

Step 5: Compute the hydrograph or the peak runoff.

Peak Runoff

Peak runoff is computed by

$$q_p = q_u A_m Q \tag{11-6}$$

where q_p = peak runoff, cfs
$\quad q_u$ = unit peak discharge, csm/in
$\quad A_m$ = drainage area, mi^2
$\quad Q$ = runoff, in

Unit peak discharge, q_u, is another empirical parameter that depends on rainfall pattern, time of concentration, rainfall, and initial losses. The unit "csm/in" is an abbreviation meaning cfs per square mile per inch of runoff. Values of q_u can be found by using the graphs shown in Appendix D-5. When using Appendix D-5, be sure to choose the correct rainfall distribution type, which is determined from the map in Appendix D-4.

Example 11-7

Problem

Using the NRCS Method, find the peak runoff for a 250-acre watershed located in Cook County, Illinois (Chicago), for a 100-year storm. The watershed has the following characteristics:

Composite CN = 72
Time of concentration = 1.5 h

Solution

Step 1: Find the drainage area, A_m:

$$A_m = 250 \text{ acres} \times \frac{1 \text{ s.m.}}{640 \text{ acres}} = 0.391 \text{ s.m.}$$

Step 2: Determine CN:

CN = 72   (Given)

Step 3: Determine runoff depth (rainfall excess), Q.

First, find the 24-hour, 100-year precipitation for Cook County. According to Appendix D-3, $P = 5.7$ inches. Then by entering 5.7 inches in Figure 11-11 and projecting up to a CN value of 72, Q is found to be 2.7 inches.

Step 4: Compute time of concentration, t_c:

$t_c = 1.5$ h   (Given)

Step 5: Compute peak runoff, q_p.

First, determine unit peak discharge, q_u. From Appendix D-4, the rainfall distribution is Type II. From Table 11-2, $I_a = 0.778$ inch. Therefore, $I_a/P = 0.778/5.7 = 0.14$. Then, using Appendix D-5, Chart 3, enter the time of concentration at 1.5 hours, project up to $I_a/P = 0.14$, and read $q_u = 260$ csm/in. Then

$$\begin{aligned} q_p &= q_u A_m Q \\ &= (260)(0.391)(2.7) \\ &= 274 \text{ cfs}   \text{(Answer)} \end{aligned}$$

Runoff Hydrograph

The runoff hydrograph is computed by selecting the appropriate unit hydrograph and multiplying each ordinate by the rainfall excess and the drainage area. Selected unit hydrographs for Type II rainfall distribution are shown in Appendix D-6. This is expressed in equation form as

$$q = q_t A_m Q \tag{11-7}$$

where q = derived hydrograph ordinate at time t, cfs
  q_t = unit discharge at time t, csm/in
  A_m = drainage area, s.m.
  Q = rainfall excess (runoff depth), in

To select the appropriate unit hydrograph, determine rainfall distribution type, time of concentration, and I_a/P.

A close inspection of Appendix D-6 reveals that the unit hydrographs are shown on six pages, each page corresponding to a different time of concentration. Within each page are 36 hydrographs corresponding to different values of I_a/P and travel time. Travel time is used to compute a routed hydrograph at a point downstream from the point of analysis. If we are interested only in the runoff hydrograph and not a routed hydrograph, we would choose a travel time of 0.0 hour. Each hydrograph consists of a series of ordinates, q_t, each corresponding to a time, t.

The NRCS database contains many more hydrographs than the ones shown in Appendix D-6. For example, Appendix D-6 does not include rainfall distribution Types I, IA, and III. It also does not include times of concentration or I_a/P values between the ones shown. Use of WinTR-55 enables access to all of the unit hydrographs.

After selecting the appropriate unit hydrograph, the resultant, or derived, hydrograph is computed using Equation 11-7 for each of the q_t values.

Example 11-8

Problem

Compute the 50-year runoff hydrograph for a watershed located in Milwaukee County, Wisconsin, having the following characteristics:

  Drainage area = 90 acres
  Composite CN = 80
  Time of concentration = 1.0 h

Solution

Step 1: Find area, A_m:

$$A_m = 90 \text{ acres} \times \frac{1 \text{ s.m.}}{640 \text{ acres}} = 0.141 \text{ s.m.}$$

Step 2: Determine CN:

  CN = 80   (Given)

Step 3: Determine runoff depth (rainfall excess), Q. First, find the 24-hour, 50-year precipitation for Milwaukee County. According to Appendix D-3, P = 5.0 inches. Then by entering 5.0 inches in Figure 11-11 and projecting up to a CN value of 80, Q is found to be 2.9 inches.

Step 4: Compute time of concentration, t_c:

  $t_c = 1.0$ h   (Given)

Step 5: Locate the appropriate unit hydrograph in Appendix D-6 using the following values:

1. $t_c = 1.0$ h
2. $I_a/P = 0.50/5.0 = 0.10$
3. Rainfall distribution Type II (from Appendix D-4)
4. $T_t = 0.0$

The unit hydrograph is found in Chart 3, line 1 of Appendix D-6 and is reproduced in the following table as the first two columns. Note that in selecting the appropriate unit hydrograph, if any of the parameters t_c, I_a/P, or T_t does not match those in Appendix D-6, you must round off to the nearest value.

Hydrograph Time (h)	Unit Discharges (csm/in)	Hydrograph Ordinates (cfs)
11.0	11	4
11.3	15	6
11.6	20	8
11.9	29	12
12.0	35	14
12.1	47	19
12.2	72	29
12.3	112	46
12.4	168	69
12.5	231	94
12.6	289	118
12.7	329	135
12.8	357	146
13.0	313	128
13.2	239	98
13.4	175	72
13.6	133	54
13.8	103	42
14.0	83	34
14.3	63	26
14.6	50	20
15.0	40	16
15.5	33	13
16.0	29	12
16.5	26	11
17.0	23	9
17.5	21	9
18.0	20	8
19.0	17	7
20.0	15	6

Step 6: Using Equation 11-7, compute each q-value:

$$q = q_t A_m Q$$
$$= q_t(0.141)(2.9)$$
$$= 0.41\ q_t$$

Each q-value becomes a value in the third column in the table, which is the desired hydrograph and answer to the problem.

Note that the peak discharge, according to the hydrograph, is 146 cfs, occurring at time 12.8 hours.

Subbasins

As was described in Section 10.7, watersheds can be divided into subbasins when they are too large or not sufficiently homogeneous. Subbasin analysis is easily achieved by using the NRCS Method, as illustrated in Example 11-9 below.

In Example 11-9, the watershed depicted in Figure 11-13 is divided into three subbasins, but the overall point of analysis is downstream from the points of analysis for two of the subbasins. To calculate the runoff hydrograph at the overall point of

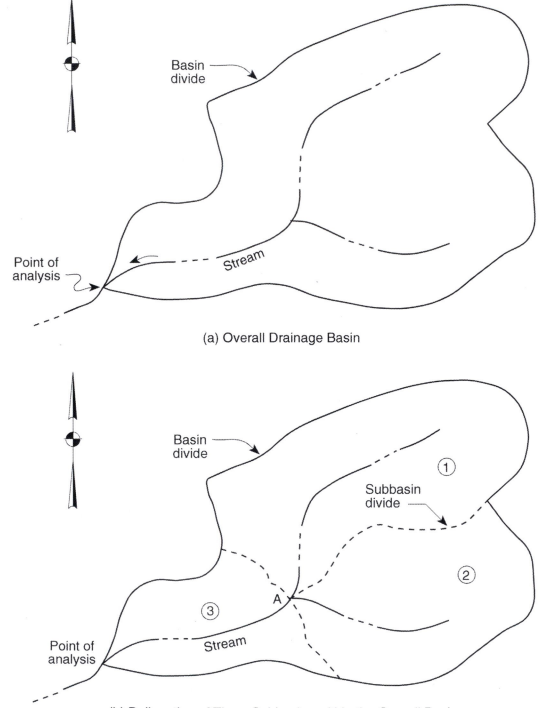

(a) Overall Drainage Basin

(b) Delineation of Three Subbasins within the Overall Basin

FIGURE 11-13   Drainage basin divided into three subbasins.

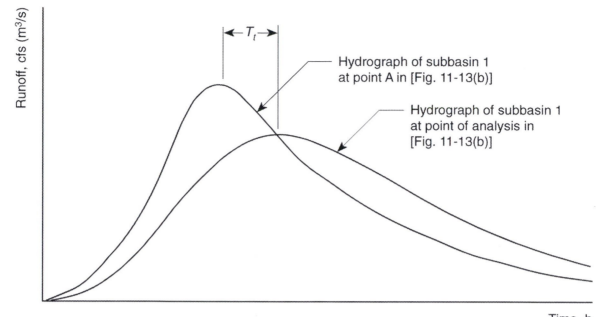

FIGURE 11-14   Attenuation of hydrograph due to travel in stream.

analysis, not only must the three individual hydrographs be combined, but the two up-stream hydrographs must be routed downstream to the overall point of analysis. All three hydrographs must be at the same location before being combined. The stream routing is computed in accordance with the concepts described in Section 10.6.

As the runoff from Subbasins 1 and 2, shown in Figure 11-13, flows downstream toward the point of analysis, the hydrographs describing the runoff change. Figure 11-14 shows the hydrograph for Subbasin 1 at point A and then again at the point of analysis. Routing the hydrograph has resulted in an attenuated hydrograph. (However, the areas under the two hydrographs are equal, since the amount of runoff has not changed.) A similar analysis applies to Subbasin 2.

Figure 11-14 shows that the attenuated hydrograph has a diminished peak runoff and the time of the peak has moved to the right by an amount equal to the travel time, T_t.

It is important to remember in this discussion of attenuation that the hydrographs depicted in Figure 11-14 represent only the runoff from Subbasin 1, even though this runoff becomes mixed with water from the other two subbasins as it moves down the stream.

Example 11-9

Problem

Find the runoff hydrograph for the drainage basin depicted in Figure 11-13 for a 25-year storm. Assume that the basin is located in Green Bay, Wisconsin (Brown County), and has the following list of parameters. The travel time from point A to the point of analysis is 12 minutes (0.20 h).

Subbasin 1

$A_m = 0.250$ s.m.

$CN = 83$

$t_c = 1.0$ h

Subbasin 2

$A_m = 0.190$ s.m.

CN = 62

$t_c = 1.25$ h

Subbasin 3

$A_m = 0.100$ s.m.

CN = 71

$t_c = 0.50$ h

Solution

Step 1: Find area, A_m: (Given)

Step 2: Determine CN: (Given)

Step 3: Determine runoff depth, Q:

First, find the 24-hour, 25-year precipitation for Brown County. According to Appendix D-3, $P = 4.1$ inches. Then, by entering 4.1 inches in Figure 11-11 and projecting up to the CN value, the following Q-values are found:

Subbasin	CN	Q (in)
1	83	2.25
2	62	0.90
3	71	1.50

Step 4: Compute t_c: (Given)

Step 5: Locate the appropriate unit hydrographs in Appendix D-6, using the following values:

Subbasin	t_c (h)	I_a/P	T_t (h)
1	1.0	$\dfrac{0.410}{4.1} = 0.10$	0.20
2	1.25	$\dfrac{1.226}{4.1} = 0.30$	0.20
3	0.50	$\dfrac{0.817}{4.1} = 0.20$	0.00

Unit hydrographs are reproduced in Table 11-4 as Columns 2, 4, and 6. Values of the derived hydrograph ordinates are listed in Columns 3, 5, and 7 and are computed by multiplying by the amount A_mQ. Values of A_mQ are as follows:

Subbasin	A_m (s.m.)	Q (in)	A_mQ (s.m.-in)
1	0.250	2.25	0.563
2	0.190	0.90	0.171
3	0.100	1.50	0.150

TABLE 11-4 Tabular hydrographs for Example 11-9.

(1)	(2)	(3)	(4)	(5)	(6)	(7)	(8)
	Subbasin 1		Subbasin 2		Subbasin 3		
Hydrograph Time (h)	Unit Discharges (csm/in)	Hydrograph Ordinates (cfs)	Unit Discharges (csm/in)	Hydrograph Ordinates (cfs)	Unit Discharges (csm/in)	Hydrograph Ordinates (cfs)	Hydro-graph (cfs)
11.0	10	5.6	0	0	17	2.6	8.2
11.3	13	7.3	0	0	23	3.5	11
11.6	17	9.6	0	0	32	4.8	14
11.9	23	13	0	0	57	8.6	22
12.0	26	15	0	0	94	14	29
12.1	30	17	0	0	170	26	43
12.2	38	21	1	0.2	308	46	67
12.3	54	30	4	0.7	467	70	101
12.4	82	46	14	2.4	529	79	127
12.5	123	69	31	5.3	507	76	150
12.6	176	99	58	9.9	402	60	169
12.7	232	131	93	16	297	45	192
12.8	281	158	133	23	226	34	215
13.0	332	187	202	35	140	21	243
13.2	303	170	239	41	96	14	225
13.4	238	134	231	40	74	11	185
13.6	179	101	199	34	61	9.2	144
13.8	136	77	165	28	53	8.0	113
14.0	105	59	138	24	47	7.1	90
14.3	76	43	108	18	41	6.2	67
14.6	59	33	87	15	36	5.4	53
15.0	45	25	68	12	32	4.8	42
15.5	35	20	55	9.4	29	4.4	34
16.0	30	17	47	8.0	26	3.9	29
16.5	27	15	41	7.0	23	3.5	26
17.0	24	14	37	6.3	21	3.2	24
17.5	22	12	33	5.6	20	3.0	21
18.0	20	11	31	5.3	19	2.9	19
19.0	18	10	28	4.8	16	2.4	17
20.0	16	9	25	4.3	14	2.1	15

Answer

The answer to the problem is the hydrograph shown in Column 8 of Table 11-4, which is computed by adding values in columns 3, 5, and 7 for each time value in column 1. Graphical depiction of the runoff hydrograph is shown in Figure 11-15.

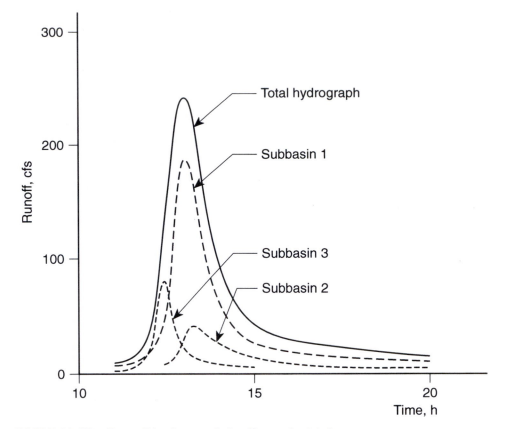

FIGURE 11-15 Runoff hydrograph for Example 11-9.

Careful scrutiny of the runoff hydrograph table reveals an important characteristic of working with subbasins. Peak discharges at the points of analysis for the three subareas are 187 cfs, 41 cfs, and 79 cfs, respectively. However, the total peak discharge is 243 cfs, which is less than the sum of the three individual peaks. This is due to the timing of the peaks. Since they do not occur at the same time, they are not added directly when computing the superposition of the three hydrographs.

11.4 NRCS METHOD VERSUS RATIONAL METHOD

The NRCS Method results in a more realistic depiction of the runoff process than does the Rational Method. It is principally for this reason that the Rational Method tends to be used for small hydraulic structures such as storm sewers, while the NRCS Method is used for larger structures. Generally, the larger the structure, the higher is the cost of failure and therefore the more realistic and conservative should be the design methods.

Among the most distinguishing differences between the two methods is the treatment of rainfall losses. The Rational Method uses a simple multiplier: the runoff coefficient, c. In this way, rainfall losses occur in approximately the same percentage of rainfall for both large storms (100-year storm) and small storms (2-year storm). However, the NRCS Method uses the concept of initial losses based on cover characteristics. Since initial losses remain the same for both large and small storms, they represent a much larger percentage of rainfall for small storms than for large storms. As a result of this difference, if a given watershed has the same 100-year peak runoff for both the Rational and NRCS Methods, then the 2-year peak runoff is much larger for the Rational Method than for the NRCS Method.

Another difference between the methods is the treatment of cover types. Although the CN-value used by NRCS is not directly comparable to the c-value used by the Rational Method, they treat the same concept, namely, infiltration rates due to cover type. CN values specified by the NRCS Method tend to result in higher peak runoff for the more intense storms (above 25-year frequency) than do c-values specified for the Rational Method. For example, the c-value specified for grass cover found in parks is often about 0.25. The CN value for this type of cover ranges from 39 to 80 depending on hydrologic soil group. If we use hydrologic group B, CN = 61. This results in an NRCS peak runoff within 5 percent of the Rational peak runoff for the 25-year storm but 50 percent higher for the 100-year storm. It should be noted, however, that some government agencies are revising c-values for the Rational Method to result in 100-year peak runoff values that are more comparable to those of the NRCS Method.

A third difference between the methods is the treatment of hydrograph construction. The NRCS Method uses a curvilinear hydrograph based on a 24-hour rainfall distribution. An example of an NRCS hydrograph for a specific watershed is shown in Figure 11-16(a). The hydrograph has a peak runoff of 212 cfs and extends over a time of about 17 hours. The Rational Method hydrograph is constructed by one of the methods known as the Modified Rational Method. A well-known method uses a triangular hydrograph with a base equal to $2.67t_c$. Figure 11-16(b) shows such a triangular hydrograph for the same watershed as the NRCS hydrograph. For purpose of comparison, the c-value was adjusted to result in the same peak runoff of 212 cfs. The Modified Rational hydrograph closely approximates the main spike of the NRCS hydrograph, which has virtually the same area under the curve. However, the entire NRCS hydrograph has an area that is about 35 percent greater. Therefore, the NRCS hydrograph represents a greater runoff volume, which can affect, to some extent, routing computations.

It should be noted that the Modified Rational hydrograph was adjusted to give it the same peak runoff value as the NRCS hydrograph. In most cases, the Modified Rational hydrograph would have a smaller peak runoff, making the difference between the hydrographs even more pronounced.

PROBLEMS

1. Find the composite runoff coefficient, c, for a drainage basin having the following cover conditions:

   Pavement: 2500 s.f.
   Roofs: 2000 s.f.
   Driveway: 800 s.f.
   Grassed areas: 0.45 acres
   Woods: 1.21 acres

2. Find the composite runoff coefficient, c, for a drainage basin having the following cover conditions:

   Roof: 700 m^2
   Pavement: 2400 m^2
   Lawns, sandy soil, and average 5% slope: 1.50 hectares
   Unimproved: 2.75 hectares

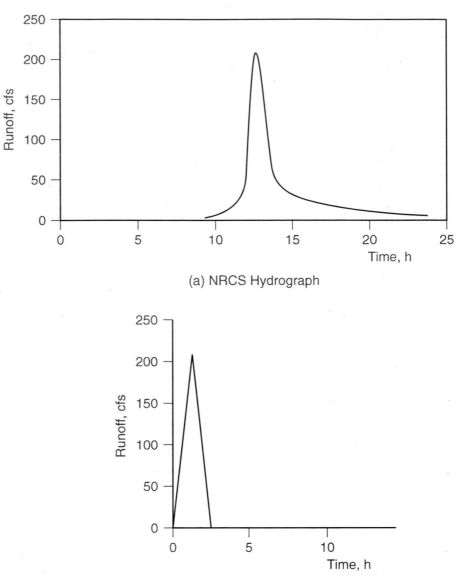

(a) NRCS Hydrograph

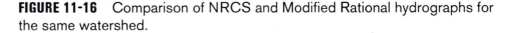

(b) Modified Rational Hydrograph

FIGURE 11-16 Comparison of NRCS and Modified Rational hydrographs for the same watershed.

3. Determine time of concentration, t_c, for use in the Rational Method for a drainage basin having a hydraulic path described as follows:

Overland flow: average grass, 80′ long, 2.5% average slope
Shallow concentrated flow: 450′ long, 4.8% average slope
Gutter flow: 200′ long, 1.9% average slope

4. Determine time of concentration, t_c, for use in the NRCS Method for a drainage basin located near Bismarck, North Dakota, having a hydraulic path described as follows:

Overland flow: average grass, 100′ long, 1.6% average slope
Shallow concentrated flow: 680′ long, 3.2% average slope
Stream flow: 2950′ long, 0.61% average slope

Average cross section:

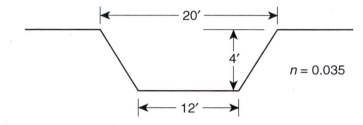

5. A drainage basin located in New Jersey has a time of concentration of 18 minutes. Find the rainfall intensity, i, for use in the Rational Method for a 25-year storm.

6. A drainage basin located in the Atlanta, Georgia, area has a time of concentration of 2.5 hours. Find the rainfall intensity, i, for use in the Rational Method for a 10-year storm.

7. Compute the peak runoff, Q_p, for a 15-year storm using the Rational Method for a drainage basin located in Phoenix, Arizona, and having parameters as follows:

   $A = 14.06$ acres
   Time of concentration
      Overland flow: average grass, 100′ long, 5.0% average slope
      Shallow concentrated flow: 50′ long, 7.0% average slope
   Runoff coefficient
      Impervious: 0.06 acres
      Grass: 6.5 acres
      Woods: 7.5 acres

   Note: In the Arizona I-D-F curves, a 15-year storm is located by the corresponding P_1 value, which for Phoenix is 1.75 inches.

   Express Q_p in (a) cfs and (b) m³/s.

8. Compute the peak runoff, Q_p, for the drainage area in problem 7 for a 50-year storm. Express Q_p in (a) cfs and (b) m³/s.

   Note: In the Arizona I-D-F curves, the P_1 value corresponding to a 50-year storm is 2.25 inches.

9. Compute the composite curve number, CN, for a drainage basin having the following soils and cover conditions:

   Soils

   Bartley Loam: 45 acres
   Parker Loam: 25 acres

   Cover

   Impervious: 2.0 acres
   Residential (⅓-acre lots): 20 acres
   Wooded (fair cover): 28 acres
   Grass (fair condition): 20 acres

10. Compute the composite curve number, CN, for a drainage basin having the following soils and cover conditions:

    Soils

    Maplecrest: 120 acres
    Hamel: 32 acres

Vinsad: 55 acres
Alluvial land: 2 acres

Cover

Impervious: 1.0 acre
Wooded: 100 acres
Disturbed soil (bare): 23 acres
Brush (poor condition): 85 acres

11. A drainage basin located in the Chicago area has a composite CN value of 71.5. Compute the runoff depth, Q, for a 100-year storm.

12. A drainage basin located near Columbus, in central Ohio, has a composite CN value of 66. Compute the runoff depth, Q, for a 25-year storm.

13. Compute the peak runoff, q_p, using the NRCS Method for a 100-year storm for a drainage basin located in the Atlanta, Georgia, area and having the following parameters:

    A_m = 1.413 s.m.
    CN = 68.0
    t_c = 2.35 hours

14. Compute the peak runoff, q_p, using the NRCS Method for a 50-year storm for a drainage basin located at the westernmost end of the Florida Panhandle and having the following parameters:

    A_m = 1.250 s.m.
    CN = 61.2
    t_c = 2.75 hours

15. Calculate peak runoff using the Rational Method for the drainage basin shown in Figure 11-17 for a 5-year storm. The basin is located in Pennsylvania, Region 1.

16. Calculate peak runoff using the NRCS Method for the watershed shown in Figure 11-18 for a 100-year storm. The watershed is located in San Diego, California. For an average stream cross section, use that in problem 4. Assume that the entire watershed is wooded, hydrologic soil group B. Two-year rainfall, P_2, is 1.8 inches.

17. Calculate peak runoff using the NRCS Method for the watershed shown in Figure 11-19 for a 25-year storm. The watershed is located in western Pennsylvania. For an average stream cross section, use that in problem 4. Assume hydrologic soil group C.

18. Calculate peak runoff using the NRCS Method for the watershed shown in Figure 11-20 for a 50-year storm. The watershed is located in central New York State. For an average stream cross section, use that in problem 4. Assume hydrologic soil group B (65 percent), C (25 percent), D (10 percent).

19. Calculate peak runoff using the Rational Method for the drainage basin shown in Figure 10-22 for a 15-year storm. The basin is located in New Jersey. For an average stream cross section, use that in Example 11-1. Assume that the entire basin is wooded.

20. Calculate peak runoff using the Rational Method for the drainage basin shown in Figure 10-23 for a 25-year storm. The basin is located in Orange County, California.

21. Compute the runoff hydrograph for a 50-year storm for a drainage basin located in Tulsa, Oklahoma, having the following parameters:
    A_m = 0.892 s.m.
    CN = 76.0
    t_c = 1.45 hours

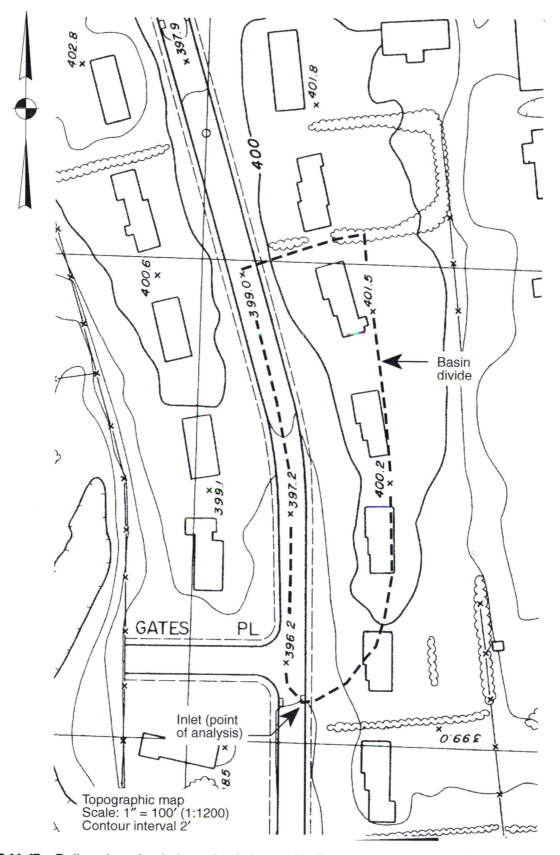

FIGURE 11-17   Delineation of a drainage basin located in Pennsylvania, Region 1. (*Map adapted from Aero Service.*)

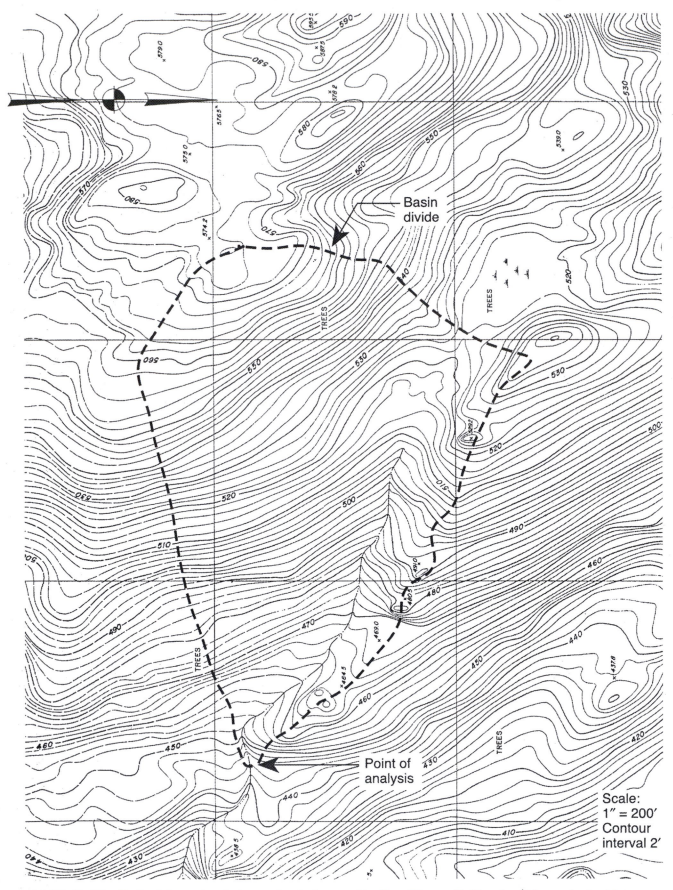

FIGURE 11-18   Delineation of a drainage basin located in San Diego, California. (*Map adapted from Aero Service.*)

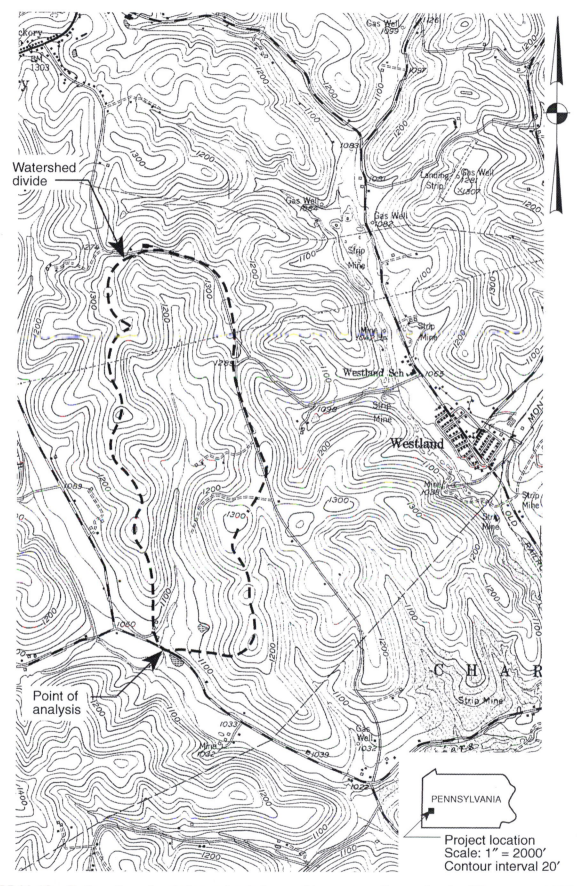

Watershed divide

Point of analysis

Westland

PENNSYLVANIA

Project location
Scale: 1″ = 2000′
Contour interval 20′

FIGURE 11-19   Delineation of a drainage basin located in western Pennsylvania. (*Courtesy of U.S. Geological Survey.*)

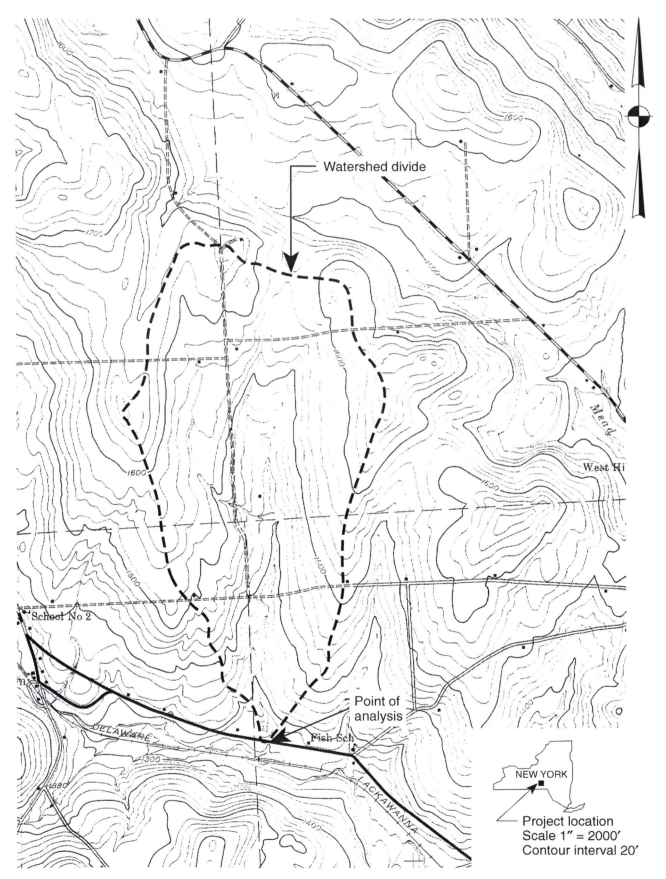

FIGURE 11-20 Delineation of a drainage basin located in central New York. (*Courtesy of U.S. Geological Survey.*)

22. Compute the runoff hydrograph for a 100-year storm for a drainage basin located in the Albany, New York, area (shaped like that shown in Figure 11-13) and having the following parameters:

    Subbasin 1

    $A_m = 1.012$ s.m.

    CN = 82

    $t_c = 1.0$ h

    Subbasin 2

    $A_m = 0.761$ s.m.

    CN = 63

    $t_c = 2.0$ h

    Subbasin 3

    $A_m = 0.550$ s.m.

    CN = 71

    $t_c = 0.50$ h

    Travel time from Point A to Point of Analysis: 0.30 hour.

23. Calculate peak runoff using the Rational Method for the drainage basin shown in Figure 10-24 for a 25-year storm. The basin is located in Atlanta, Georgia. For an average stream cross section, use that in Example 11-1.

24. Calculate peak runoff using the Rational Method for the drainage basin shown in Figure 10-25 for a 25-year storm. The basin is located in New Jersey. For an average stream cross section, use that in Example 11-1. Assume that all roads have crowns and gutter flow on both sides.

25. Calculate peak runoff using the NRCS Method for the watershed shown in Figure 10-26 for the 100-year storm. The watershed is located near Pittsburgh, Pennsylvania. Assume that the soil type is Jonesville and that the entire watershed (except roads) is wooded (fair condition). For an average stream cross section, use that in Example 11-1.

FURTHER READING

Akan, A. O. (1993). *Urban Stormwater Hydrology, A Guide to Engineering Calculations*. Lancaster, PA: Technomic Publishing.

Commonwealth of Pennsylvania, PENNDOT, Bureau of Design. (1990). *Design Manual, Part 2, Highway Design*. Publication 13. Harrisburg, PA: Commonwealth of Pennsylvania.

New Jersey Department of Transportation, Division of Roadway Design, Bureau of Roadway Design Standards. (1994). *Roadway Design Manual*. Trenton, NJ: Department of Transportation.

Urban Water Resources Research Council of ASCE and the Water Environment Federation. (1992). *Design and Construction of Urban Stormwater Management Systems*. New York and Alexandria, VA: ASCE.

U.S. Natural Resources Conservation Service. (2002). WinTR-55. http://www.wcc.nrcs.usda.gov/hydro.

U.S. Soil Conservation Service. (1986). *Urban Hydrology for Small Watersheds*. Technical Release 55. Springfield, VA: U.S. Department of Agriculture.

Viessman, W., Jr., Lewis, G. L., and Knapp, J. W. (1989). *Introduction to Hydrology* (3rd ed.). New York: Harper and Row.

Wanielista, M. P. (1990). *Hydrology and Water Quality Control*. New York: Wiley.

Wanielista, M. P., and Yousef, Y. A. (1993). *Stormwater Management*. New York: Wiley.

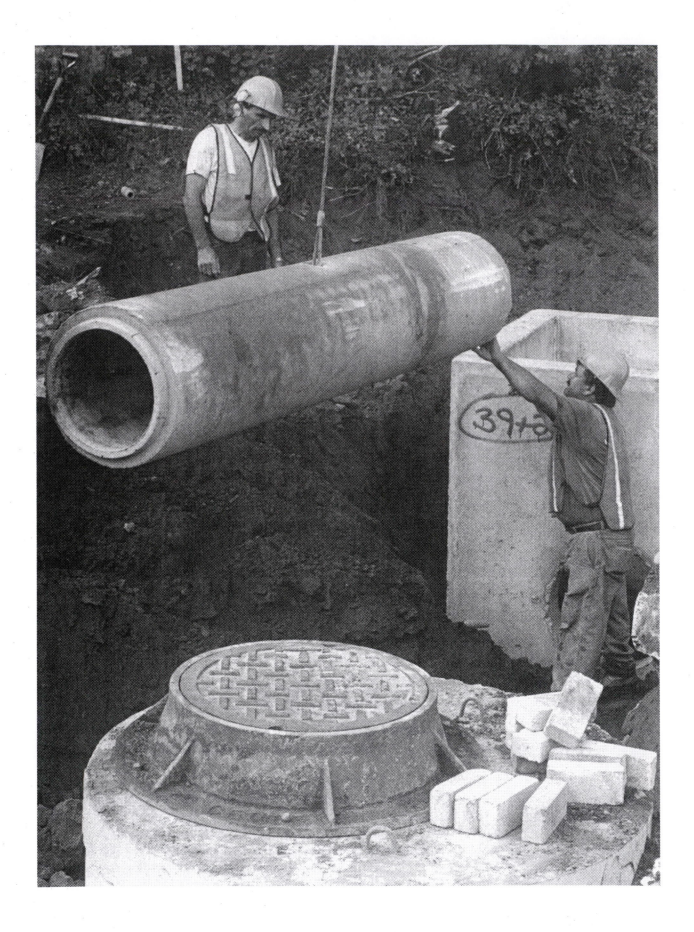

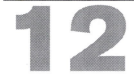
STORM SEWER DESIGN

Storm sewers are underground pipes used to convey stormwater from developed areas safely and conveniently into natural bodies of water such as streams and lakes. They are used typically in roads, parking areas, and sometimes lawns.

Before the development of storm sewers, urban planners managed stormwater by channeling it in a series of swales along streets and alleys and eventually into streams, a practice still in use today in underdeveloped countries. Because the water remained on the ground surface, inconvenience and disease transmission resulted. The introduction of storm sewers allowed for the development of land with modern advancements in transportation virtually unencumbered by stormwater problems.

Throughout the past century, storm sewers have been used in urban settings to convey sewage waste as well as stormwater in the same pipes. Such systems are called **combined sewers** and have now been nearly eliminated in favor of separate storm sewers and sanitary sewers.

In this chapter, we will learn the basic principles in the hydraulic design of storm sewers. Of course, the design of a storm sewer includes many more factors than hydraulics, such as structural stability, construction methods, and cost. Although some of these factors will be mentioned, the principal emphasis will be on hydraulic design.

OBJECTIVES

After completing this chapter, the reader should be able to:

- Lay out a storm sewer system in a road or parking area
- Interpret a storm sewer profile
- Delineate incremental drainage areas in a standard storm sewer design
- Compute pipe sizes in a standard storm sewer design
- Design riprap outfall protection for a storm sewer outlet
- Relate a standard storm sewer design to an actual case study

12.1 FUNDAMENTAL CONCEPTS

The three principal components of a storm sewer system are the inlet, the pipe, and the outflow headwall. The **inlet** is a structure designed to allow stormwater into the system; the **pipe** conveys stormwater toward a receiving stream; and the **headwall** allows stormwater to exit the system. Figure 12-1 depicts these basic elements of a storm sewer system.

Inlets usually are precast concrete square structures placed in the ground and topped with a cast-iron grate at ground level. Inlets are often mistakenly called **catch basins**, which are similar storm sewer structures but have a slightly different purpose. Figure 12-2 depicts a typical inlet. Catch basins are designed with a bottom set lower than the incoming and outgoing pipes to provide a sump, which acts as a sediment trap.

In addition to allowing stormwater into the system, inlets provide access to the pipes for maintenance as well as a point for the pipes to change direction, since pipes must normally be laid straight, without curves.

Pipes are manufactured in a variety of materials, including concrete, reinforced concrete (RCP), corrugated metal, and plastic. In general, the cross sections of pipes

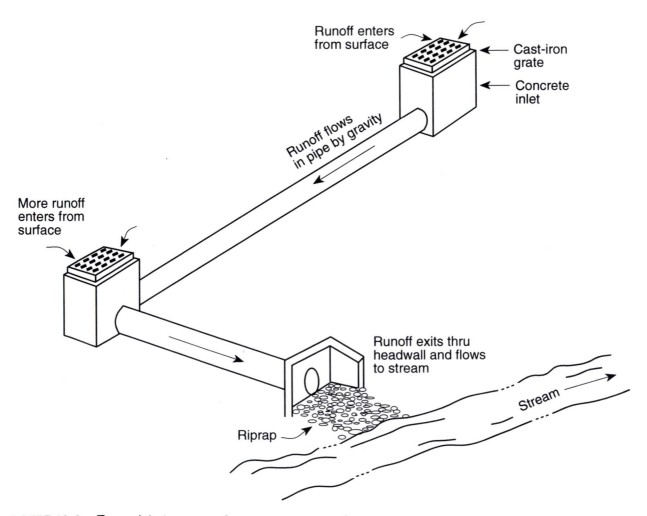

FIGURE 12-1 Essential elements of a storm sewer system.

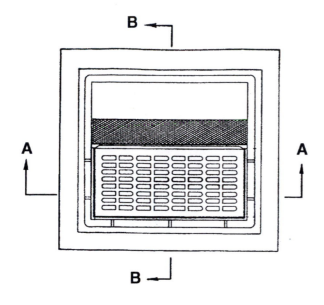

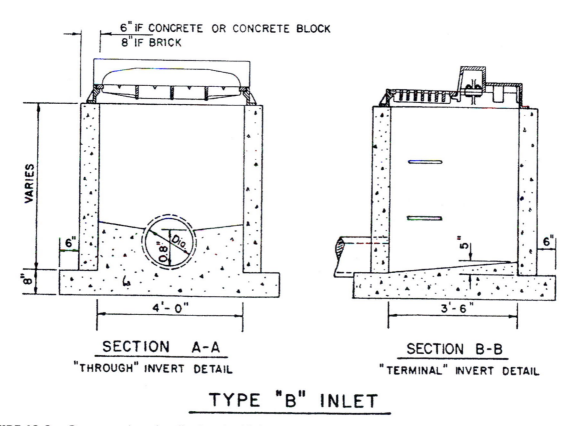

6" IF CONCRETE OR CONCRETE BLOCK
8" IF BRICK

VARIES

6"

8"

0.8" Dia.

4'-0"

SECTION   A-A

"THROUGH" INVERT DETAIL

5"

6"

3'-6"

SECTION B-B

"TERMINAL" INVERT DETAIL

TYPE "B" INLET

FIGURE 12-2   Construction detail of typical inlet.

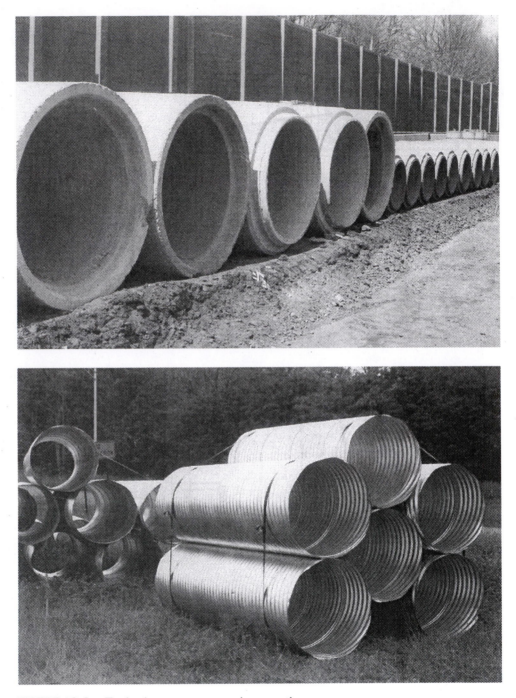

FIGURE 12-3   Typical storm sewer pipe sections.

are round or elliptical, with most pipes being round. Figure 12-3 depicts some typical examples. Pipes are generally laid in trenches in accurate straight alignments and grades. Pipe sections are designed to fit together as the pipe is laid from its downstream end to its upstream end.

The most fundamental element of a storm sewer design is choosing a pipe with sufficient size and grade to convey the design runoff from one inlet to the next. This is accomplished by comparing the capacity in cfs (m^3/s) of the pipe to the design flow in cfs (m^3/s). If the capacity is greater than the flow, the pipe is adequate for use in the storm sewer system.

However, several other factors must also be considered in designing a pipe segment. First, the velocity of flow must be properly controlled. On the one hand, velocity should not be allowed to be too low, or silt and debris could be deposited along the pipe, but on the other hand, excessive velocity should be avoided. The minimum velocity needed to avoid siltation is usually called the **cleansing velocity** and generally is taken as 2.0 ft/s (0.60 m/s). Therefore, the pipe should be designed so that when flowing half full, a minimum velocity of 2.0 ft/s (0.60 m/s) is maintained.

Excessive velocity should be avoided because the result could be damage to the pipe or surcharging of an inlet at a bend point in the system. The choice of a maximum velocity is somewhat elusive because it depends on site-specific conditions. Some municipal ordinances set a design standard of 10 ft/s (3.0 m/s); in such cases, this would become the maximum velocity. In the absence of local regulation, 15 ft/s (4.6 m/s) is a reasonable value for design purposes.

> *Note:* An inlet becomes surcharged when it fills with water due to the inability of the downstream pipe to convey the flow adequately.

To maintain sufficient velocity and keep the storm sewer system flowing smoothly, head losses within the system should be kept to a minimum. This is accomplished principally by streamlining the transitions from one pipe segment to the next.

A few basic rules are generally used in currently accepted engineering practice and are also found in some municipal regulations. First, choose a minimum pipe diameter of 12 inches. (Some municipal regulations require a 15-inch minimum.) This helps to prevent clogging and also facilitates maintenance. Second, throughout a storm sewer system, each pipe segment must be equal to or larger than the segment immediately upstream. This is another measure to prevent clogging. So, for example, if one pipe segment has a diameter of 24 inches and the next downstream segment need only be an 18-inch pipe to convey the design stormwater flow, you must choose a 24-inch pipe size nonetheless. A third rule relates to transitions from one size pipe to a larger size. In making a transition at an inlet, the vertical alignment of the incoming and outgoing pipes should be such that the crowns line up (not the inverts). This promotes smooth flow and helps to prevent a backwater in the upstream pipe. Figure 12-4 illustrates these general rules.

12.2   DESIGN INVESTIGATION

Before you begin a storm sewer design, certain essential data must be acquired through field investigations and other sources:

1. Project meeting
2. Topographic map
3. Site reconnaissance
4. Local land development ordinance
5. Related engineering designs or reports

First, a project meeting must be held with the developer, that is, the person who will be paying for the new storm sewer system. The developer could be an entrepreneur who wishes to build a building for profit or a municipality that wishes to improve the drainage on one of its roads.

At the project meeting, you should determine the scope of the project as clearly as possible. Project scope includes the physical boundaries of the site, the nature of

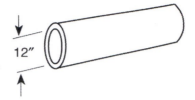

Use a minimum pipe size of 12″ diameter

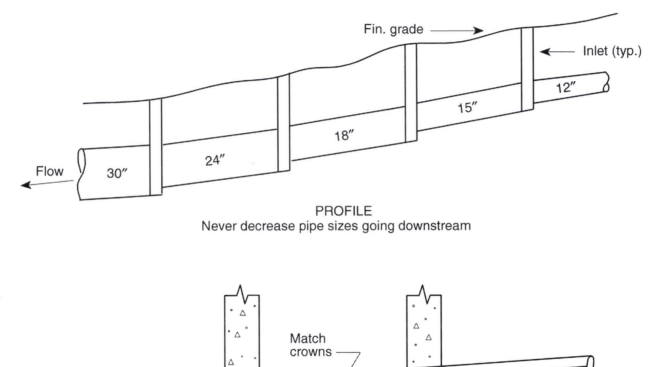

PROFILE
Never decrease pipe sizes going downstream

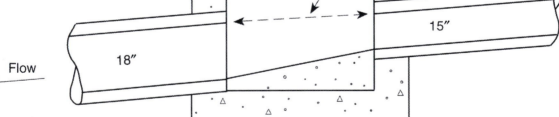

SECTION
When transitioning from smaller to larger pipe, match the crown alignments (not the inverts).

FIGURE 12-4 Some basic rules in storm sewer design.

the development, and whether any off-site improvements will be required. The developer should provide a boundary survey of the land and a sketch showing the proposed project in schematic form. If there is no survey, it should be determined at the meeting whether a boundary survey must be conducted. Also, it should be determined whether a topographic survey must be conducted for the project.

Boundary and topographic surveys, if required, are part of the basic engineering services to be provided for the project.

A topographic survey is almost always needed in order to delineate drainage areas for runoff computation. For most designs, watersheds are relatively small, requiring detailed topography to determine drainage areas adequately. Typically, maps are prepared at a scale of $1'' = 50'$ (1:600) or larger, with contour lines drawn at a 2-foot interval. USGS quadrangle maps drawn at a scale of $1'' = 2000'$ (1:24000) and contour interval of 10 or 20 feet are not sufficiently detailed for storm sewer design.

A useful topographic map can be prepared by one of three usual methods:

1. The map can be based on a ground topographic survey, conducted by a survey crew on the site.
2. The map can be based on an aerial topographic survey, which is drawn from aerial photographs and calibrated by limited ground survey control.
3. A combination of aerial and ground survey can be used.

If the storm sewer system is to be part of a new development where all roads and parking areas will be designed from scratch, aerial topography is adequate. However, if existing roads are involved and the proposed storm sewer must connect to existing pipes, then more precise topography is needed to specify the existing features. In such cases, a combination of aerial and ground topography should be used.

After the topographic map has been obtained, a site visit must be conducted to verify the information on the map and determine certain key information not shown. For instance, the type of ground cover should be noted to help in choosing runoff coefficients. Also, if an existing road has a functioning gutter, it should be noted to help determine the hydraulic path. In addition, if an existing building has a complex drainage pattern not evident in the topographic map, this condition should be noted.

Another purpose of the site visit is to verify any underground utilities, including storm sewers, and investigate irregularities with the topographic map. Any missing utilities should then be added to the map. Applicable local ordinances must be obtained as part of the design investigation. Local ordinances often specify such design parameters as design storm, runoff coefficients, or inlet type and spacing. If any county or state regulations apply, these must be considered as well. Also, the storm intensity-duration-frequency (I-D-F) curves for the project location must be obtained. Finally, if any previous development in the project vicinity has generated design plans or reports, these should be acquired. Existing plans may have a bearing on the proposed project and may also indicate which ideas have already been approved by the local approving agency.

It is also often helpful to schedule a preliminary meeting with the municipal engineer who has jurisdiction over the project. Such a meeting will establish a rapport with the engineer and may reveal problems or project constraints that are not evident in the other materials already gathered.

Armed with all the information gathered in the design investigation, you can now start the design.

12.3   SYSTEM LAYOUT

The first step in storm sewer design is laying out the system. On the site topographic map, find the best location for the system to discharge to a stream or other body of water. You may need more than one discharge point. Next, locate the positions of the inlets, which are placed at low points where they can most efficiently gather runoff. Finally, connect the inlets with pipes and check to confirm that their horizontal and vertical alignments do not interfere with other utilities or site components.

Selection of the discharge point is very important and not always easy. The most important principle guiding this decision is that the stormwater must be transferred from the pipe to the receiving water safely and without causing erosion damage or flooding. So, for instance, a discharge would not be placed in the middle of a field because the concentrated flow leaving the pipe would almost certainly erode the field. If a suitable stream is not available on the project site, you might be forced to extend your system a considerable distance off the site to find a proper discharge point. In Section 12.5, various methods of erosion prevention are discussed.

In many projects, an adjacent or nearby existing storm sewer may be utilized as the receiving body of water, thus eliminating the need to discharge to a stream. In such cases, the proposed storm sewer connects to one of the existing inlets and, in effect, becomes part of the existing system. It might be necessary, however, to check the capacities of the existing pipes to verify that they can accept the additional discharge from the proposed system. Proper selection of the inlet locations is crucial to a good storm sewer design. In addition to choosing low points, many other factors must be considered. The most important of these are summarized below.

1. **Grading.** Obviously, the inlets must be placed where runoff can enter. This is accomplished by coordinating site grading with inlet positioning, that is, by shaping the ground to channel the runoff by gravity into the inlet. The most common way to accomplish this is by use of the curb or gutter along the edge of a road or parking area. Where no curb or gutter is available, such as in the middle of a lawn, the ground is graded into a swale.

2. **Spacing.** Inlets should be placed close enough together to prevent any single inlet from receiving too much runoff. A typical inlet can accept about 4 cfs (0.1 m³/s). When inlets are placed along a curbline, they should not be spaced farther apart than about 250 linear feet (75 linear meters) to prevent excessive flow along the gutter. This spacing also allows access to the pipes for inspection and maintenance. Conversely, inlets should not be placed too close together because such spacing is needlessly expensive.

3. **Change of Direction.** Because storm sewer pipes must be straight, they must make sharp angles at every change of direction. To prevent clogging at the bend points and also to provide access to the pipes, special structures are provided at every change of direction. These structures typically are inlets or manholes.

4. **Change of Pipe Slope or Size.** For the same reasons as change of direction, inlets or manholes must be placed at each point where the slope or size of the pipe changes.

Figures 12-5 and 12-6 show two examples of storm sewer system layout. In Figure 12-5, several principles of street layout are illustrated. First, runoff is channeled to the inlets by flowing along the gutters, where it is intercepted by the inlets.

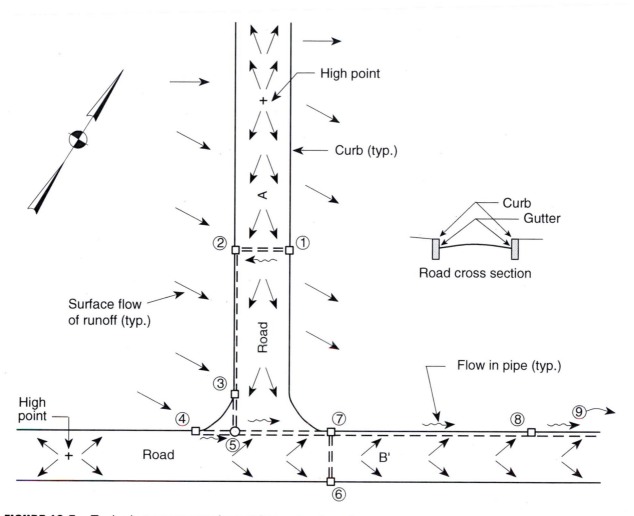

FIGURE 12-5   Typical storm sewer layout for a street system.

Inlet 2 intercepts runoff from the land west of Road A as well as runoff from the westerly half of the pavement of Road A. Inlet 1, however, intercepts runoff from the easterly half of Road A and nowhere else. Although Inlet 1 intercepts very little runoff compared to Inlet 2, it is included in the system to reduce the amount of gutter flow along the easterly side of Road A. Inlets 3 and 4 are placed at the uphill side of the intersection to prevent gutter flow from continuing across the intersection, where it would interfere with traffic movement. Manhole 5 is included to provide a junction for two branches coming together. The pipe segments crossing the roads, that is, between Inlets 1 and 2 and Inlets 6 and 7, are called cross drains and serve the purpose of conveying the gutter flow from one side of the road to the side where the main sewer line is running.

In Figure 12-6, inlets again are arranged to intercept runoff flowing along the curb, although in this case, the curb is part of the parking area for a building. Inlets must be placed at every low point in order to prevent puddling, and they must be numerous enough to prevent excessive buildup of runoff flow in the parking area. Notice the pipes leading from the two corners of the building conveying runoff from the roof. These pipes could also convey water from a footing drain if one had been installed.

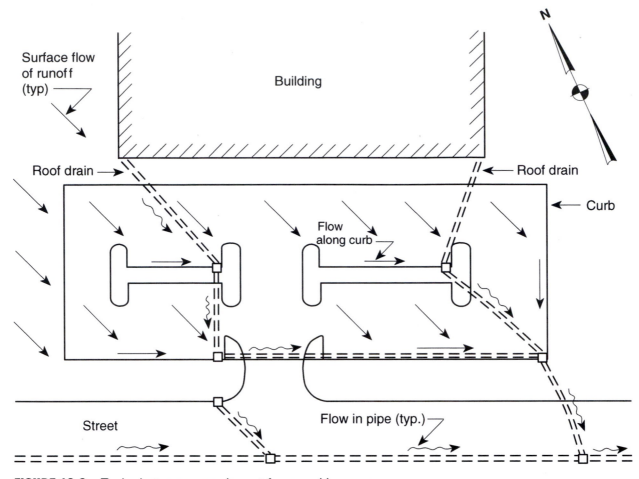

FIGURE 12-6 Typical storm sewer layout for a parking area.

12.4 HYDRAULIC DESIGN

After laying out the system in plan view, you can begin the hydraulic design. The principal goal of hydraulic design is to determine the pipe size, segment by segment, throughout the system. To accomplish this, peak discharge, Q_p, must be computed for each pipe segment using the Rational Method.

Figure 12-7 shows the same storm sewer system depicted in Figure 12-5 but with delineated drainage areas tributary to the individual inlets. These areas must be delineated by using topographic and site reconnaissance information. Also, hydraulic paths must be traced for each area in order to compute times of concentration.

Let us consider first the pipe segment from Inlet 1 to Inlet 2, which is the farthest upstream segment of the system. We will refer to this as Pipe Segment 1-2. All of the water flowing in this segment originates as runoff in its drainage area, referred to as Area 1. Computation of Q_p is done by using the procedure outlined in Section 11.1, including time of concentration and composite c-value. When Q_p is known, a size and slope are chosen for the pipe segment, and its corresponding capacity is determined. If the capacity is greater than Q_p, the pipe segment is considered adequate and is accepted in the design. If the capacity is less than Q_p, the pipe segment is not adequate, and a larger pipe size or steeper slope must be chosen.

In addition to checking pipe capacity, you must check inlet grate capacity. If Q_p exceeds 4 cfs (0.1 m³/s), you should either add another inlet at that location or shorten

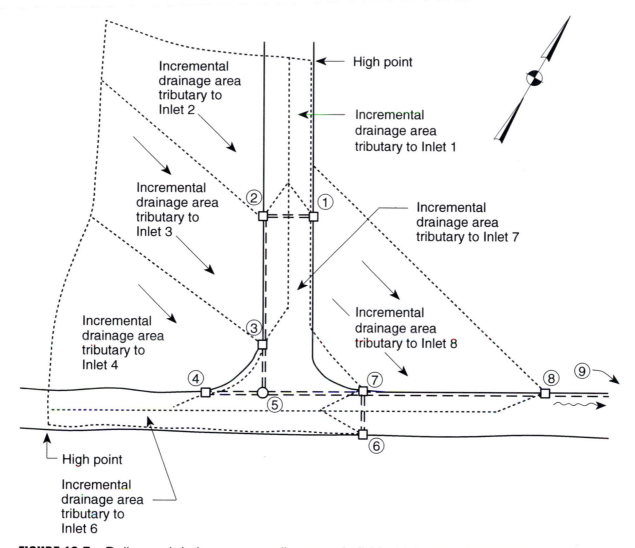

FIGURE 12-7   Delineated drainage areas tributary to individual inlets of a typical storm sewer system.

the distance between inlets, thus reducing the drainage area. In the case of Inlet 1, Q_p will be much less than 4 cfs (0.1 m³/s), since its tributary drainage basin consists of only a portion of road surface.

Because the drainage Area 1 is so small, you will find that time of concentration is also small. The remotest point in the basin is located in the center of the road at the high point, and most of the hydraulic path runs along the gutter. For very small basins like this, designers generally use a minimum value of time of concentration of 6 minutes. (Some designers use a higher value, such as 10 minutes.) So if a strict computation of t_c yields a value such as 2.8 minutes, use 6.0 minutes in your Rational Method calculations. This does not reduce the validity of the overall design.

Next, consider the pipe segment from Inlet 2 to Inlet 3. Water flowing in this pipe originates from two separate sources: some comes from Pipe Segment 1-2, while the remainder enters directly into Inlet 2. To compute Q_p for this pipe, you must use a tributary drainage area equal to the sum of the areas for Inlet 1 and Inlet 2.

Figure 12-8 shows how drainage areas are cumulative as you work your way down the system. Figure 12-8(b) shows the drainage area for Pipe Segment 2-3. To compute time of concentration for this area, follow the procedure outlined in

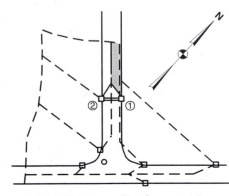

(a) Area Tributary to Pipe Segment 1-2

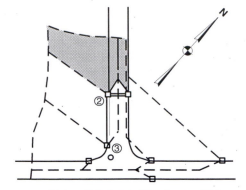

(b) Area Tributary to Pipe Segment 2-3

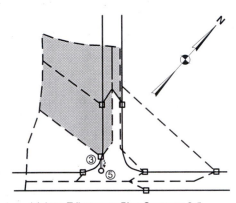

(c) Area Tributary to Pipe Segment 3-5

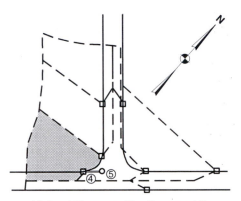

(d) Area Tributary to Pipe Segment 4-5

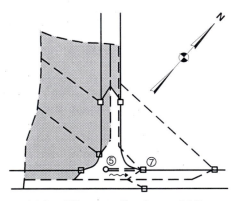

(e) Area Tributary to Pipe Segment 5-7

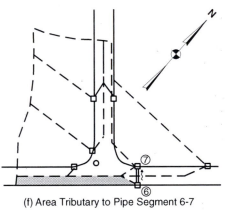

(f) Area Tributary to Pipe Segment 6-7

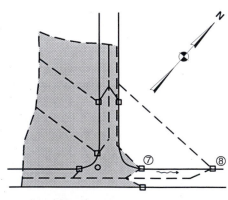

(g) Area Tributary to Pipe Segment 7-8

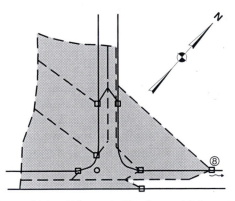

(h) Area Tributary to Pipe Segment 8-9

FIGURE 12-8 Drainage areas tributary to pipe segments through the storm sewer system.

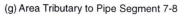
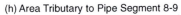

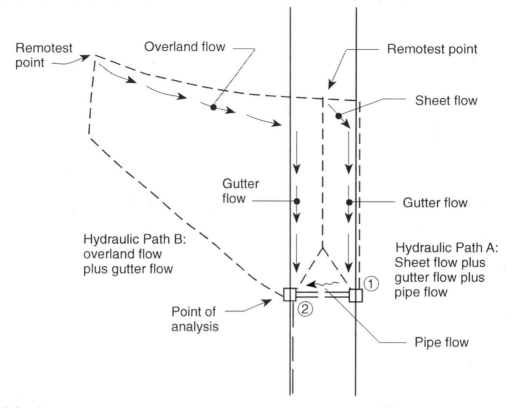

FIGURE 12-9   Two possible hydraulic paths for calculating Q_p for Pipe Segment 2-3.

Section 10.3 in which the longest hydraulic path is chosen. Figure 12-9 shows two possible hydraulic paths for calculation of t_c for Pipe Segment 2-3. Notice that both points terminate at Inlet 2, which is the point of analysis for Pipe Segment 2-3. Since Path B includes overland flow in addition to gutter flow, it will undoubtedly be longer in time than Path A. Therefore, Path B is chosen.

Next, we turn our attention to Pipe Segment 3-5. Figure 12-8(c) shows the drainage area tributary to this pipe, which includes the previous area plus the incremental area tributary to Inlet 3. To compute the time of concentration for this area, choose the longest hydraulic path of the three possible paths shown in Figure 12-10. Notice that all three paths terminate at Inlet 3, the point of analysis for Pipe Segment 3-5. Either Path B or Path C could have a longer travel time. This can be determined only by computing t_c for both paths and comparing values. Whichever path yields the higher value of t_c will be chosen, and that t_c will be used in calculating Q_p for Pipe Segment 3-5.

The next pipe segment is 4-5, but in this case, we do not add the previous drainage areas as we did with segment 3-5 above. Pipe segment 4-5 is a branch of the overall storm sewer system and therefore does not carry the discharge from the upstream areas. In Figure 12-8(d), we see that the drainage area for this segment is confined to the incremental area tributary to Inlet 4 referred to as Area 4. Time of concentration for this segment is simply the time of concentration for Area 4.

The next pipe segment is 5-7. Figure 12-8(c) shows that the drainage area tributary to this pipe includes the summation of all upstream incremental areas. No runoff is directly tributary to Pipe Segment 5-7 since Manhole 5 has no grate through which

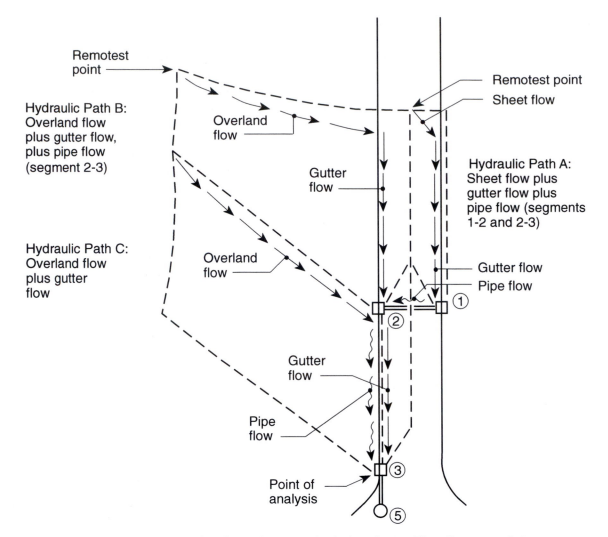

FIGURE 12-10 Three possible hydraulic paths for calculating Q_p for Pipe Segment 3-5.

water can enter. So all discharge flowing in Pipe Segment 5-7 comes from the two up-stream branches of the system. Manhole 5 represents the confluence of the two branches, as well as the point of analysis for calculating Q_p for Pipe Segment 5-7. Time of concentration for this calculation is based on the longest hydraulic path of the four possible paths originating in the four upstream incremental drainage areas.

The next pipe segment considered in the design is Segment 6-7. This is another branch segment (like Segment 4-5) and has a tributary drainage area as shown in Figure 12-8(f). Calculation of Q_p for this segment is similar to that for Segment 1-2, which has a comparable drainage area and time of concentration.

The next pipe segment is 7-8, which carries water from three different sources: Segment 6-7, accumulated flow in Segment 5-7, and runoff entering Inlet 7.

Figure 12-8 shows the tributary drainage area for this segment. Time of concentration is based on the longest hydraulic path, terminating at Inlet 7, of the six possible paths originating in the six upstream incremental drainage areas.

The last pipe segment in the system we are analyzing is Segment 8-9. Figure 12-7 shows Inlet 8 and a pipe extending eastward toward Inlet 9, although Inlet 9 is not actually shown. Figure 12-8(h) shows the tributary drainage area for this segment, which consists of the summation of all upstream incremental areas. Time of concentration for this segment is calculated in the same manner as the preceding segments, by selecting the hydraulic path that produces the longest travel time.

Example 12-1

Problem

Calculate the peak discharge in each pipe segment of the storm sewer system depicted in Figure 12-7 for a design storm frequency of 25 years. Assume that the project site is located in Pennsylvania, Region 1 and has the following parameters:

Inlet	Incremental Drainage Area (acres)	t_c* (min)	$c^\dagger$
1	0.07	6	0.95
2	0.46	10	0.45
3	0.52	10	0.48
4	0.65	9	0.41
5	——	——	——
6	0.10	6	0.95
7	0.15	6	0.95
8	0.70	14	0.38

*Time of concentration for each incremental drainage area.
†Composite runoff coefficient for each incremental drainage area.

Solution

Pipe Segment 1-2: Since area and runoff coefficient are already known, find rainfall intensity by use of the I-D-F curves for Pennsylvania (Region 1) in Appendix C-3. If we enter a duration of 6 minutes in the I-D-F graph, rainfall intensity for a 25-year storm is found to be

$$i = 5.5 \text{ in/h}$$

Peak runoff is then computed by using Equation 11-2:

$$\begin{aligned} Q_p &= Aci \\ &= (0.07)(0.95)(5.5) \\ &= 0.37 \text{ cfs} \quad \text{(Answer)} \end{aligned}$$

Pipe Segment 2-3: Drainage area is equal to the sum of the upstream incremental areas:

$$\begin{aligned} A &= 0.07 + 0.46 \\ &= 0.53 \text{ acre} \end{aligned}$$

Composite runoff coefficient is the weighted average of the runoff coefficients of the upstream incremental areas:

$$\begin{aligned} c &= \frac{(0.07)(0.95) + (0.46)(0.45)}{0.53} \\ &= 0.52 \end{aligned}$$

Time of concentration is based on the hydraulic path with the longest travel time. Total time to Inlet 2 along hydraulic path A as shown in Figure 12-10 is 6.0 minutes plus the travel time in Pipe Segment 1-2. For the purpose of this example, assume that this travel time is about 0.1 minute. Therefore, total time is 6.1 minutes. However, total time to Inlet 2 along hydraulic path B as shown in Figure 12-10 is 10 minutes (given). Thus, time of concentration is taken as

$$t_c = 10 \text{ min}$$

Rainfall intensity is found in Appendix C-3 by entering a duration of 10 minutes. Therefore,

$$i = 4.3 \text{ in/h}$$

Peak runoff is then computed by using Equation 11-2:

$$
\begin{aligned}
Q_p &= Aci \\
&= (0.53)(0.52)(4.3) \\
&= 1.2 \text{ cfs} \quad \text{(Answer)}
\end{aligned}
$$

Pipe Segment 3-5: Drainage area is equal to the sum of the upstream incremental areas:

$$
\begin{aligned}
A &= 0.07 + 0.46 + 0.52 \\
&= 1.05 \text{ acres}
\end{aligned}
$$

Composite runoff coefficient is the weighted average of the runoff coefficients of the upstream incremental areas:

$$
\begin{aligned}
c &= \frac{(0.07)(0.95) + (0.46)(0.45) + (0.52)(0.48)}{1.05} \\
&= 0.50
\end{aligned}
$$

Time of concentration is based on the hydraulic path with the longest travel time. Hydraulic Path A was eliminated in the analysis for Segment 2-3. Total time along Path B to Inlet 3 is 10 minutes plus the travel time in Pipe Segment 2-3, which we will assume for now to be 0.5 minutes. Therefore, total time is 10.5 minutes. Total time to Inlet 3 along Hydraulic Path C as shown in Figure 12-10 is 10 minutes (given). Thus, time of concentration is taken as

$$t_c = 10.5 \text{ min}$$

Rainfall intensity is found in Appendix C-3 by entering a duration of 10.5 minutes. Therefore,

$$i = 4.2 \text{ in/h}$$

Peak runoff is then computed by using Equation 11-2:

$$
\begin{aligned}
Q_p &= Aci \\
&= (1.05)(0.50)(4.2) \\
&= 2.2 \text{ cfs} \quad \text{(Answer)}
\end{aligned}
$$

Pipe Segment 4-5: This segment is a branch of the system and, as shown earlier, is treated as though it is the beginning of the system. Area and runoff coefficient are given. Rainfall intensity is found in Appendix C-3 by entering a duration of 9 minutes. Therefore,

$i = 4.5$ in/h

Peak runoff is then computed by using Equation 11-2:

$Q_p = Aci$
$= (0.65)(0.41)(4.5)$
$= 1.2$ cfs   (Answer)

Pipe Segment 5-7: Drainage area is equal to the sum of the upstream incremental areas:

$A = 0.07 + 0.46 + 0.52 + 0.65$
$= 1.70$ acres

Composite runoff coefficient is the weighted average of the runoff coefficients of the upstream incremental areas:

$$c = \frac{(0.07)(0.95)+(0.46)(0.45)+(0.52)(0.48)+(0.65)(0.41)}{1.70}$$
$$= 0.46$$

Time of concentration is based on Hydraulic Path B because it requires the greatest amount of time. We saw earlier that this path has a time of 10.5 minutes from its beginning to Inlet 3. However, for Pipe Segment 5-7, the point of analysis is Manhole 5. So the time of concentration is 10.5 minutes plus the travel time in Pipe Segment 3-5, which we will show later to be 0.1 minute. Therefore, total time is 10.6 minutes. Total time to Manhole 5 along any other path is less than 10.6 minutes. Thus, time of concentration is taken as

$t_c = 10.6$ min

Rainfall intensity is found in Appendix C-3 by entering a duration of 10.6 minutes. Therefore,

$i = 4.2$ in/h

Peak runoff is then computed by using Equation 11-2:

$Q_p = Aci$
$= (1.70)(0.46)(4.2)$
$= 3.3$ cfs   (Answer)

Pipe Segment 6-7: This segment is another branch of the system and therefore treated as though it is at the beginning. Area and runoff coefficients are given. Rainfall intensity for a duration of 6 minutes was already found to be

$i = 5.5$ in/h

Peak runoff is then computed by using Equation 11-2:

$Q_p = Aci$
$= (0.10)(0.95)(5.5)$
$= 0.52$ cfs   (Answer)

Pipe Segment 7-8: Drainage area is equal to the sum of the upstream incremental areas:

$$A = 1.70 + 0.10 + 0.15$$
$$= 1.95 \text{ acres}$$

Notice that in this computation, the first four incremental areas are summed in the first term: 1.70 acres. Composite runoff coefficient is a weighted average as computed previously:

$$c = \frac{(1.70)(0.46) + (0.10)(0.95) + (0.15)(0.95)}{1.95}$$
$$= 0.52$$

Notice that in this computation, the first four incremental areas were taken as one composite c value. This gives the same result as listing them separately. Time of concentration is once again based on Hydraulic Path B, which has a total time to Inlet 7 of 10.6 minutes plus the travel time in Pipe Segment 5-7, which we will show later to be 0.2 minute. Therefore, total time is 10.8 minutes. Total time to Inlet 7 along any other path is less than 10.8 minutes. Thus, time of concentration is taken as

$$t_c = 10.8 \text{ min}$$

Rainfall intensity is found in Appendix C-3 by entering a duration of 10.8 minutes. Therefore,

$$i = 4.1 \text{ in/h}$$

Peak runoff is then computed by using Equation 11-2:

$$Q_p = Aci$$
$$= (1.95)(0.52)(4.1)$$
$$= 4.2 \text{ cfs} \quad \text{(Answer)}$$

Pipe Segment 8-9: Drainage area is equal to the sum of the upstream incremental areas:

$$A = 1.95 + 0.70$$
$$= 2.65 \text{ acres}$$

Composite runoff coefficient is a weighted average as computed previously:

$$c = \frac{(1.95)(0.52) + (0.70)(0.38)}{2.65}$$
$$= 0.48$$

Time of concentration is, as always, based on the longest hydraulic path. Using Inlet 8 as point of analysis, Path B has a time of 10.8 minutes plus travel time in Pipe Segment 7-8, which we will show later to be 0.9 minutes. Therefore, total time for Path B is 11.7 minutes. However, total time for the hydraulic path within the incremental area tributary to Inlet 8 is 14 minutes. So this is now the longest hydraulic path to the point of analysis; therefore, time of concentration is taken as

$$t_c = 14 \text{ min}$$

Rainfall intensity is found in Appendix C-3 by entering a duration of 14 minutes. Therefore,

$$i = 3.75 \text{ in/h}$$

Peak runoff is then computed by using Equation 11-2:

$$\begin{aligned} Q_p &= Aci \\ &= (2.65)(0.48)(3.75) \\ &= 4.8 \text{ cfs} \quad \text{(Answer)} \end{aligned}$$

The calculations in this example can be conveniently arranged in tabulation form:

(1) Pipe Segment	(2) Incr. Area (acres)	(3) c	(4) Incr. Ac (acres)	(5) Cumm. Ac (acres)	(6) t_c (min)	(7) i (in/h)	(8) Q_p (cfs)
1-2	0.07	0.95	0.067	0.067	6	5.5	0.37
2-3	0.46	0.45	0.207	0.274	10	4.3	1.2
3-5	0.52	0.48	0.250	0.524	10.5	4.25	2.2
4-5	0.65	0.41	0.267	0.267	9	4.5	1.2
5-7	—	—	—	0.791	10.6	4.25	3.3
6-7	0.10	0.95	0.095	0.095	6	5.5	0.52
7-8	0.15	0.95	0.143	1.029	10.8	4.2	4.2
8-9	0.70	0.38	0.266	1.295	14	3.75	4.8

For a full understanding of the table in Example 12-1, you must study it carefully and in detail. First, look at column 4, labeled *Incremental Ac*. Each number in this column is the product of the corresponding numbers in columns 2 and 3. Column 5 then shows cumulative values from column 4, which accomplishes two computations at once: it computes cumulative area and composite c for the accumulated area. These operations were done separately earlier in the example.

The desired result, peak flow for each pipe segment, is shown in column 8. Each value in column 8 is computed by multiplying the corresponding values in columns 5 and 7. This multiplication is equivalent to using Equation 11-2, as we did throughout the example.

To understand better how the computations were done, analyze column 5 more closely. Each value represents the total area tributary to the particular pipe segment multiplied by the composite runoff coefficient of that area. The first three values are running totals of the incremental values in column 4. The fourth value, however, is not a running total because Pipe Segment 4-5 is a branch of the system and carries runoff solely from its incremental drainage area.

Now take a similar look at column 6. Notice that Pipe Segments 2-3, 3-5, 5-7, and 7-8 form a sequence of t_c's in which each t_c increases by an amount equal to the travel time in the previous pipe segment. Travel times are based on computations that will be explained in Example 12-2. Pipe Segments 4-5 and 6-7 are not in this sequence because they are branches and are not on the main stem of the system. Segment 8-9 is also not in the sequence, despite being part of the main stem, because a different hydraulic path was used to calculate time of concentration.

Each value in column 7 is a rainfall intensity found in Appendix C-3 corresponding to the time of concentration in column 6.

Peak runoff for Pipe Segment 8-9 represents the total peak runoff for the storm sewer system to that point (Inlet 8). If we had computed peak runoff for each incremental area and then added them together, the resulting total peak runoff would be greater than the 4.8 cfs computed. It would be incorrect to add the individual peak runoff values because such a procedure does not account for attenuation as the runoff travels from each incremental area to Inlet 8.

In performing these design calculations, you should be aware of peak runoff entering each individual inlet. In this case, it is evident that no single incremental area produces a peak runoff greater than 4 cfs. If we had suspected one area of exceeding its inlet capacity, we would have checked peak runoff for that area.

Pipe Size Computation

After computing peak discharge flow in each pipe segment, the next step in storm sewer design is to choose an appropriate size for the pipe. The slope of the pipe is chosen at this time as well, since both size and slope are needed to determine capacity. Also important to capacity is the type of pipe: for example, concrete, corrugated metal, or plastic. Usually, the pipe's material is selected first, since this decision is based primarily on cost and other factors.

Pipe slope is dictated to a great extent by surface grades, although some variation is available to the designer. So at this point in the design, a profile of the proposed sewer is very helpful, if not essential. Plotting a profile reveals not only the slope but also the pipe depth and any potential conflicts with other utilities.

Figure 12-11 shows a profile of the storm sewer system shown in Figure 12-7, which is the subject of Examples 12-1 and 12-2. Notice that the profile is drawn with an exaggerated vertical scale. That is, vertical distances are 10 times larger than horizontal distances. Profiles typically are drawn in this fashion to render very subtle slopes more obvious and easier to employ in design.

In performing the design, a profile like that in Figure 12-11 is drawn on a work sheet and the pipe segments added one at a time as their sizes are determined by the computations. It is a trial-and-error process in which a 12-inch pipe is chosen first and its capacity is compared to Q_p for that segment. If necessary, a larger size is then chosen. The following example illustrates the design process.

Example 12-2

Problem

Determine the pipe sizes for the storm sewer system depicted in Figure 12-7 for a design storm frequency of 25 years. Assume that the pipes are to be reinforced concrete pipes (RCP) with Manning's n-value of 0.015. Also, assume that the system has the following parameters:

Pipe Segment	Length (ft)	Slope (%)
1-2	30	2.0
2-3	200	3.25
3-5	25	2.5
4-5	25	2.0
5-7	50	0.5
6-7	30	2.0
7-8	220	0.5
8-9	——	0.5

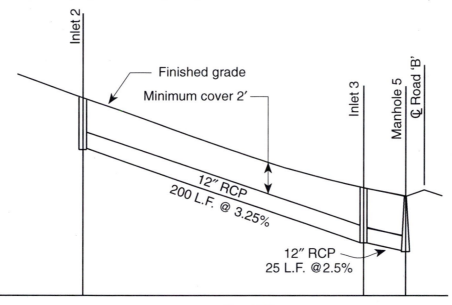

Road 'A'

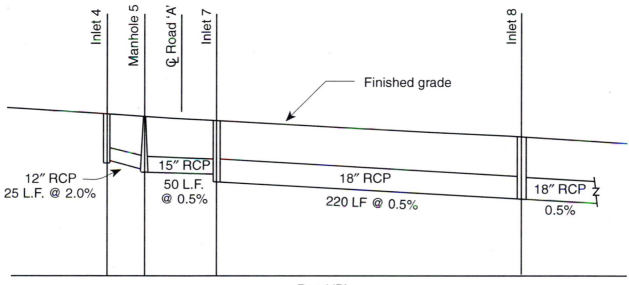

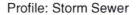

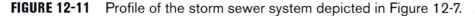

Road 'B'

Profile: Storm Sewer

FIGURE 12-11   Profile of the storm sewer system depicted in Figure 12-7.

Solution

Pipe Segment 1-2: Start by assuming a size of 12 inches, which we will take as the minimum size for this example. Now determine the capacity for a 12-inch diameter pipe with $n = 0.015$ and slope = 2.0 percent using Pipeflow Chart 35 in Appendix A-4. Locate the slope line (0.02 ft/ft) and find the upper end. From that point, trace straight down to the *Discharge* axis for $n = 0.015$, and read the answer: $Q = 4.4$ cfs.

Since this capacity is greater than the computed peak runoff of 0.37 cfs, the assumed pipe size is accepted.

Pipe Segment 2-3: Find the capacity for a 12-inch pipe at a slope of 3.25 percent using Chart 35. Interpolate between the slope lines for 0.03 ft/ft and 0.04 ft/ft, trace down to the discharge axis, and read the answer: $Q = 5.8$ cfs.

Since this capacity is greater than the computed peak runoff of 1.2 cfs, the assumed pipe size is accepted.

Pipe Segment 3-5: Find the capacity for a 12-inch pipe at a slope of 2.5 percent using Chart 35. Interpolate between the slope lines for 0.02 ft/ft and 0.03 ft/ft, and read the answer: $Q = 5.0$ cfs.

Since this capacity is greater than the computed peak runoff of 2.2 cfs, the assumed pipe size is accepted.

Pipe Segment 4-5: This segment uses the same pipe size and slope as Segment 1-2, so it has the same capacity: 4.4 cfs.

Since this capacity is greater than the computed peak runoff of 1.2 cfs, the assumed 12-inch pipe size is accepted.

Pipe Segment 5-7: Again, start by assuming a pipe size of 12 inches. The capacity for a 12-inch pipe with slope of 0.5 percent is found in Chart 35 to be $Q = 2.2$ cfs. Since this capacity is less than the computed peak runoff of 3.3 cfs, the assumed pipe size is not accepted.

Next, choose a pipe size of 15 inches. The capacity for a 15-inch pipe with slope of 0.5 percent is found in Chart 36 to be $Q = 4.0$ cfs. Since this capacity is greater than the computed peak runoff of 3.3 cfs, the 15-inch pipe is accepted.

Pipe Segment 6-7: This segment uses the same pipe size and slope as Segments 1-2 and 4-5, so it has the same capacity of 4.4 cfs. This capacity is greater than the computed peak runoff of 0.52 cfs, and so a 12-inch pipe is selected.

Pipe Segment 7-8: Start by assuming a pipe size of 15 inches, since pipe sizes must be equal to or greater than upstream pipes. The capacity for a 15-inch pipe with a 0.5 percent slope was determined previously to be 4.0 cfs.

Since this capacity is less than the computed peak runoff of 4.2 cfs, the assumed 15-inch pipe is not accepted and an 18-inch pipe is tried next. The capacity for an 18-inch pipe with a slope of 0.5 percent is found in Chart 37 to be $Q = 6.4$ cfs.

Since 6.4 cfs is greater than 4.2 cfs, the 18-inch pipe is accepted.

Pipe Segment 8-9: Start by assuming a pipe size of 18 inches, since pipe sizes must be equal to or greater than upstream pipes. The capacity of an 18-inch pipe with a slope of 0.5 percent was already determined to be 6.4 cfs.

Since 6.4 cfs is greater than 4.8 cfs, the 18-inch pipe is accepted. This hydraulic design can be presented in chart form as shown in Table 12-1. Charts of this type

TABLE 12-1   Drainage Calculation Chart for Example 12-2 (25-Year Storm, $n = 0.015$)

(1) Pipe Segment From	To	(2) A—Increm. Area (acre)	(3) C—Runoff Coefficient	(4) A·C—Increm.	(5) A·C—Cumul.	(6) t_c—Time of Conc. (min.)	(7) i—Rainfall Intensity (in/h)	(8) Q_p—Peak Runoff (cfs)	(9) Pipe Length (ft)	(10) Slope (%)	(11) Size (in)	(12) Capacity (full) (cfs)	(13) Velocity (fps) (Design Flow)	(14) Travel Time in Pipe (min)
1	2	0.07	0.95	0.067	0.067	6	5.5	0.37	30	2.0	12	4.4	3.4	0.15
2	3	0.46	0.45	0.207	0.274	10	4.3	1.2	200	3.25	12	5.8	5.6	0.6
3	5	0.52	0.48	0.250	0.524	10.6	4.25	2.2	25	2.5	12	5.0	6.0	0.1
4	5	0.65	0.41	0.267	0.267	9	4.5	1.2	25	2.0	12	4.4	4.8	0.1
5	7	—	—	—	0.791	10.7	4.25	3.3	50	0.50	15	4.0	3.6	0.2
6	7	0.10	0.95	0.095	0.095	6	5.5	0.52	30	2.0	12	4.4	3.7	0.1
7	8	0.15	0.95	0.143	1.029	10.9	4.2	4.2	220	0.50	18	6.4	3.9	0.9
8	9	0.70	0.38	0.266	1.295	14	3.75	4.8	—	0.50	18	6.4	4.0	—

typically are utilized as a format for storm sewer design calculations and can be prepared by using spreadsheet software.

A close and detailed scrutiny of Table 12-1 is important in understanding the storm sewer design process. This chart is an exact facsimile of those used universally by engineers for presentation of storm sewer design. Notice first that columns 1 through 8 are the same as the chart shown in Example 12-1. So let us now focus on columns 9 through 14.

These columns are arranged in the order in which the numbers are determined. First, pipe length is taken from the layout plan. Next, slope is determined by drawing a trial pipe on the profile worksheet. The size is also determined in the trial. Now that size and slope have been postulated, capacity is determined from the pipe flow charts, and the proposed size is accepted.

The remaining two columns are included to allow a computation of travel time in the pipe segment, which is needed to determine subsequent time of concentration. This is the computation referred to in Example 12-1.

Look first at column 13, Segment 1-2. The velocity of 3.4 ft/s was found in Chart 35 in Appendix A-4. This is the average velocity in Segment 1-2 for a discharge of 0.37 cfs. It is determined by entering the chart at a discharge of 0.37 cfs and tracing upward to the slope line of 0.02 ft/ft. From that point, trace to the left (keeping parallel to the velocity lines) to the velocity scale and interpolate between 3 ft/s and 4 ft/s.

Travel time in Pipe Segment 1-2 is then computed using the formula

$$\text{Time} = \frac{\text{Distance}}{\text{Velocity}}$$

where distance, in this case, is the pipe length of 30 ft. Therefore,

$$\begin{aligned}
\text{Time} &= \frac{30}{3.4} \\
&= 8.82 \text{ s} \\
&= 0.15 \text{ min}
\end{aligned}$$

The travel time is then entered in column 14. Each number in column 14 represents the travel time of the discharge in the corresponding pipe segment. These travel times are used to compute time of concentration as the design progresses down the system.

For instance, the time of concentration in column 6 for Segment 3-5 is 10.6 minutes, which is computed by adding 10 minutes (column 6, Segment 2-3) to 0.6 minute (column 14, Segment 2-3).

As another example, the time of concentration shown in column 6 for Segment 5-7 is 10.7 minutes, which is computed by adding 10.6 minutes (column 6, Segment 3-5) to 0.1 minute (column 14, Segment 3-5).

Of course, not all t_c values in column 6 are computed in this manner. Exceptions include segments with no upstream tributary pipes (Segments 1-2, 4-5, 6-7) and segments with hydraulic paths originating in their own incremental drainage area (Segments 2-3 and 8-9).

12.5 STORM SEWER OUTFALLS

Careful attention must be given to the design of the storm sewer outfall or point of discharge from the system. This is the point where collected stormwater is discharged from the system to the receiving body of water, and it is here that most soil erosion damage can occur.

One of the first considerations in outfall design is the outfall structure. A storm sewer pipe can simply emerge from the ground and terminate with no structure, or a headwall can be constructed at the discharge point. Figure 12-12 depicts in isometric views several outfall structures in general use today. In Figure 12-13, the structures are shown as they might appear on construction plans.

The purpose of a headwall or other outfall structure is to protect the soil around the discharge pipe from erosion and keep the slope in place. The outfall structure actually acts as a small retaining wall. Very few cases occur when a structure can be completely avoided.

In some cases, materials other than those shown in Figure 12-12 can be used to construct a headwall. Examples include gabions, grouted stone, and railroad ties.

Generally, storm sewer outfalls are configured in one of three ways (see Figure 12-14):

1. **Outfall at Stream Bank.** The storm sewer pipe extends all the way to the receiving stream, and the headwall is constructed in the bank.
2. **Channel Connecting Outfall with Stream.** The headwall or flared end section is located several feet from the stream and a channel is constructed to connect the two.
3. **Outfall Discharging onto Stream Overbank.** This arrangement is similar to item 2 except no channel is cut between the outfall and the stream. Discharge is allowed to flow overland across the overbank and eventually into the stream. This arrangement is selected often when the overbank area is environmentally sensitive, as in the case of wetlands, and excavating a channel is undesirable.

Discharge exiting from the outfall is in concentrated form and therefore potentially damaging to unprotected ground. Excessive velocity can damage the ground by dislodging soil particles and washing them away. Figure 12-15 shows an outfall with severely eroded ground immediately downstream.

An important part of the design process is the selection of a method for protecting the ground surface wherever velocities are destructive, such as at the outfall. Appendix A-2 shows a list of maximum allowable velocities for various types of ground cover. These velocities are a guide to use in designing an outfall.

Several methods are available for the control of erosion at a storm sewer outfall:

1. **Reduce Discharge Velocity.** This can be accomplished by reducing the slope of the last pipe segment before the outfall.
2. **Energy Dissipator.** In cases of very high velocity, specially designed obstruction blocks can be placed at the outlet to create a head loss and therefore reduction of velocity. Such a design is beyond the scope of this book.
3. **Stilling Basin.** A depression in the ground surface can be provided at the outlet to absorb excessive energy of the discharge. Such a basin is designed to trap water and therefore must have a provision for drainage between storms. This design is also beyond the scope of this book.

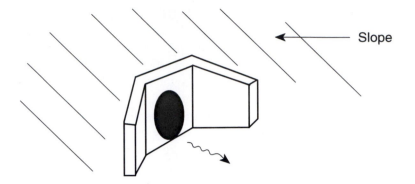

(a) Concrete Headwall with Wingwalls

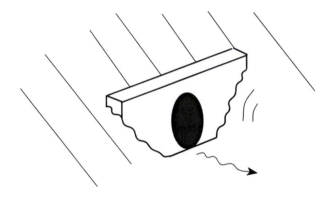

(b) Concrete Straight Headwall

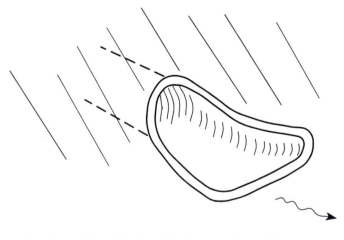

(c) Flared End Section (Preformed flared shape
connected to end of discharge pipe; materials
include concrete, corrugated metal, and plastic.)

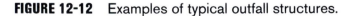

FIGURE 12-12   Examples of typical outfall structures.

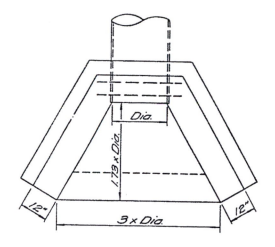

PLAN

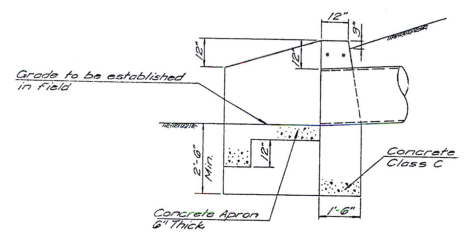

Grade to be established
in field

Concrete
Class C

Concrete Apron
6" Thick

OUTLET END

(a) Concrete Headwall and Apron

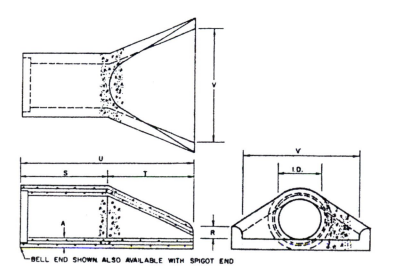

BELL END SHOWN ALSO AVAILABLE WITH SPIGOT END

(b) Concrete Flared End Section

FIGURE 12-13 Construction details of various outfall structures.

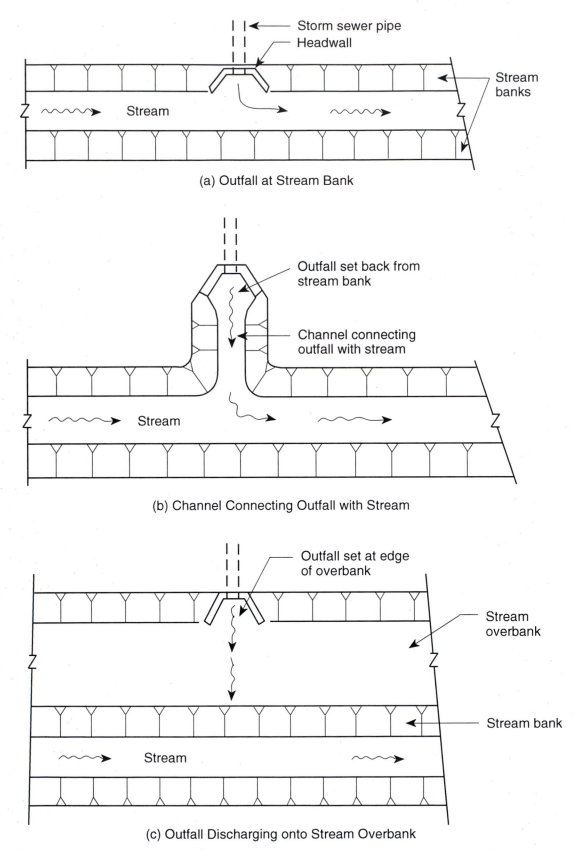

(a) Outfall at Stream Bank

(b) Channel Connecting Outfall with Stream

(c) Outfall Discharging onto Stream Overbank

FIGURE 12-14   Schematic representation of three conditions encountered for a storm sewer outfall at a stream.

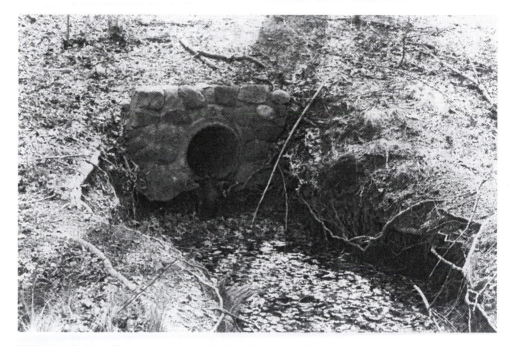

FIGURE 12-15 Storm sewer outfall with severely eroded ground immediately downstream.

4. **Riprap.** This is a lining of heavy rocks covering the vulnerable ground to protect the ground surface and slow the discharging velocity at the same time. Riprap design procedures can be found in many publications, especially agency design manuals.

5. **Erosion Control Mats.** A wide variety of commercially available products consist of mesh netting, which is placed on the ground to protect the surface and anchor a vegetative cover as it grows.

6. **Sod.** This is the application of sod strips to the vulnerable ground to provide a grass lining without the disadvantage of growing grass from seed. This protective lining is generally effective but expensive and labor intensive.

7. **Gabions.** Gabions are rectangular wire mesh baskets filled with rocks and placed on the ground as a protective lining similar to riprap.

Riprap

Riprap is a common erosion control lining used at storm sewer outfalls as well as culvert outlets, especially in areas where suitable rock materials are readily available. Figure 12-16 depicts a storm sewer outfall with riprap protection in place. A lining of the ground at a pipe outlet (using riprap or any other material) is generally referred to as an **apron**.

Design of riprap outfall protection includes many factors, the most basic of which are as follows:

1. Type of stone
2. Size of stone
3. Thickness of stone lining
4. Length of apron
5. Width of apron

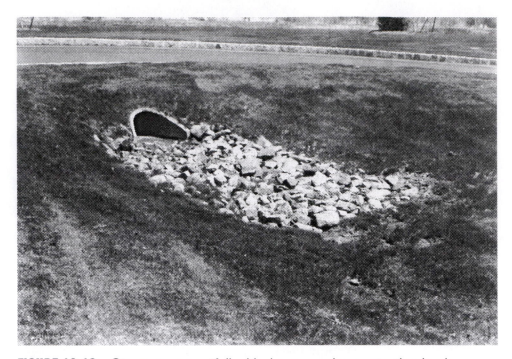

FIGURE 12-16 Storm sewer outfall with riprap erosion protection in place.

Procedures for determining these parameters are contained in many published design manuals in use today across the United States. When designing riprap, you should be aware of any design standard used by the agency reviewing your design and consider following it. However, a simple riprap design procedure is presented here for general use.

1. **Type of Stone.** The stones used for riprap should be hard, durable, and angular. Angularity, a feature of crushed stone from a quarry, helps to keep the stones locked together when subjected to the force of moving water.
2. **Size of Stone.** The stones should be well graded in a range of sizes referred to as gradation. Gradation is another factor promoting the interlocking of the stones. Size is defined as the median diameter, d_{50}, which is the diameter of stones of which 50 percent are finer by weight, and is selected using the following formulas:

$$d_{50} = \frac{0.02}{TW}\left(\frac{Q}{D_0}\right)^{4/3} \quad \text{(English units)} \tag{12-1}$$

where d_{50} = median stone size, ft
$\quad Q$ = design discharge, cfs
$\quad D_0$ = maximum pipe or culvert width, ft
$\quad TW$ = tailwater depth, ft

$$d_{50} = \frac{0.044}{TW}\left(\frac{Q}{D_0}\right)^{4/3} \quad \text{(SI units)} \tag{12-1a}$$

where d_{50} = median stone size, m
$\quad Q$ = design discharge, m³/s
$\quad D_0$ = maximum pipe or culvert width, m
$\quad TW$ = tailwater depth, m

Note: For this riprap design, tailwater is the flow depth in the pipe at the outlet.

3. **Thickness of Stone Lining.** The blanket of stones should be three times the median stone size if no filter fabric liner between the stones and the ground is used. If a filter fabric liner is used, the thickness should be twice the median stone size.

4. **Length of Apron.** The length, L_a, of the apron is computed using one of the formulas below.

If the design tailwater depth, TW, is greater than or equal to $\frac{1}{2}D_0$, then

$$L_a = \frac{3Q}{D_0^{3/2}} \quad \text{(English units)} \tag{12-2}$$

where L_a = apron length, ft
$\quad Q$ = design discharge, cfs
$\quad D_0$ = maximum pipe or culvert width, ft

$$L_a = \frac{5.4Q}{D_0^{3/2}} \quad \text{(SI units)} \tag{12-2a}$$

where L_a = apron length, m
$\quad Q$ = design discharge, m³/s
$\quad D_0$ = maximum pipe or culvert width, m

If TW (design) is less than $\frac{1}{2}D_0$, then

$$L_a = \frac{1.8Q}{D_0^{3/2}} + 7D_0 \quad \text{(English units)} \tag{12-3}$$

where L_a = apron length, ft
$\quad Q$ = design discharge, cfs
$\quad D_0$ = maximum pipe or culvert width, ft

$$L_a = \frac{3.26Q}{D_0^{3/2}} + 7D_0 \quad \text{(SI units)} \tag{12-3a}$$

where L_a = apron length, m
$\quad Q$ = design discharge, m³/s,
$\quad D_0$ = maximum pipe or culvert width, m

Figure 12-17 illustrates the dimensions involved with apron size.

5. **Width of Apron.** If a channel exists downstream of the outlet, the riprap width is dictated by the width of the channel. Riprap should line the bottom of the channel and part of the side slopes. The lining should extend

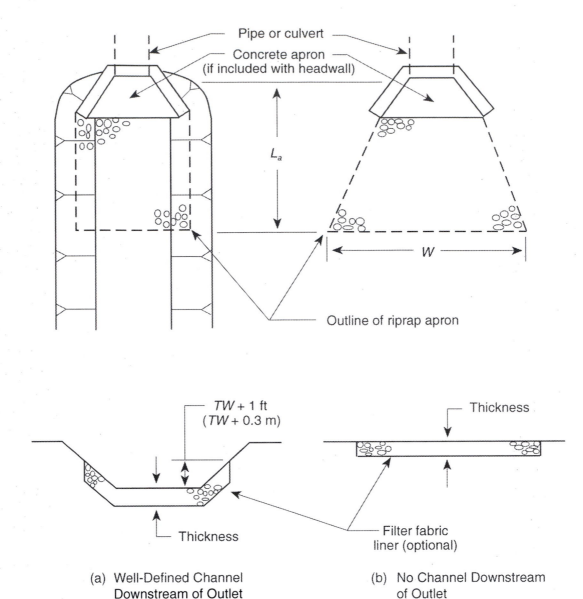

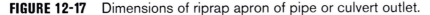

(a) Well-Defined Channel
Downstream of Outlet

(b) No Channel Downstream
of Outlet

FIGURE 12-17 Dimensions of riprap apron of pipe or culvert outlet.

1 foot (0.3 m) above the design tailwater depth. The extra 1-foot height is called **freeboard** and is employed as a safety measure.

If no channel exists downstream of the outlet, the width, W, of the apron is computed using one of the two formulas below.

If the design tailwater depth, TW is greater than or equal to $\frac{1}{2}D_0$, then

$$W = 3D_0 + 0.4L_a \tag{12-4}$$

where W = apron width, ft (m)
D_0 = max. pipe or culvert width, ft (m)
L_a = apron length, ft (m)

If TW (design) is less than $\frac{1}{2}D_0$, then

$$W = 3D_0 + L_a \tag{12-5}$$

where W = apron width, ft (m)
D_0 = max. pipe or culvert width, ft (m)
L_a = apron length, ft (m)

Example 12-3

Problem

A storm sewer outfall is to be designed for direct discharge to the ground (no channel). Design discharge is 70 cfs, and the last pipe segment is a 36-inch reinforced concrete pipe (RCP) with a 1.3 percent slope. The ground downstream of the outfall is predominantly silt loam.

Solution

First, determine the velocity of the design discharge at the outfall. Using Chart 43 of Appendix A-4, design velocity is found to be 10.5 fps. (The Manning's n-value is assumed to be 0.012.)

Next, compare the design velocity to the permissible velocity found in Appendix A-2. For silt loam, the permissible velocity is 3.0 fps.

Since design velocity exceeds permissible velocity, a protective lining will be required. Riprap is chosen based on cost and accessibility of the stone.

To design the riprap apron, first determine the size, d_{50}, using Equation 12-1. Before using Equation 12-1, TW is determined from Chart 43 to be 2.2 feet. Then, by using Equation 12-1,

$$d_{50} = \frac{0.02}{2.2}\left(\frac{70}{3}\right)^{4/3}$$
$$= 0.61 \text{ ft } \left(7\frac{1}{4} \text{ in}\right)$$

Specify 8-inch stone, since it is the next higher whole inch.

Next, determine the apron length, L_a. Since $TW = 2.2$ ft, which is greater than $\frac{1}{2}D_0$, use Equation 12-2:

$$L_a = \frac{(30)(70)}{(3)^{3/2}}$$
$$= 40.4 \text{ ft}$$

Specify 40 feet, since it is the rounded value of L_a.

Next, since there is no channel downstream of the outfall, determine the apron width, W. Since $TW > \frac{1}{2}D_0$, use Equation 12-4:

$$W = 3(3) + 0.4(40.4)$$
$$= 25.2 \text{ ft}$$

Specify 25 ft, since it is the rounded value of W.

The outfall design is summarized in the following drawing.

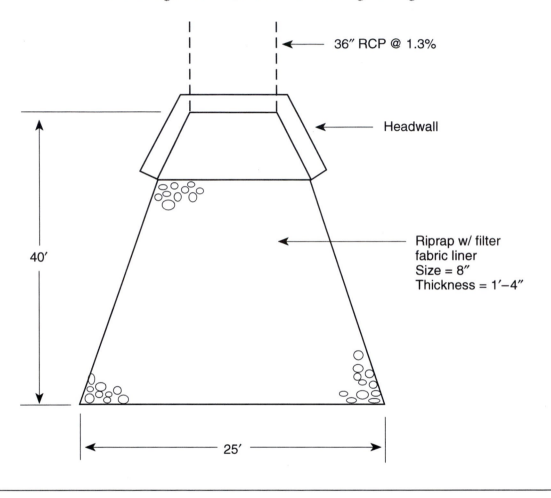

12.6 CASE STUDY

In this case, a residential subdivision is proposed for a 28.5-acre tract in suburban Atlanta, Georgia. The subdivision, named Tall Pines, consists of 25 building lots plus one additional lot at the northerly end for a detention basin. As shown in Figure 12-18, one principal road, Road A, traverses the tract from south to north, and two stub roads, Road B and Road C, intersect Road A and run to opposite property lines.

In this case study, we will analyze the storm sewer design for the subdivision, and in another case study in Chapter 15, we will analyze the detention design.

To analyze the storm sewer design, we will trace the following procedures normally included in such design:

1. Design investigation
2. System layout

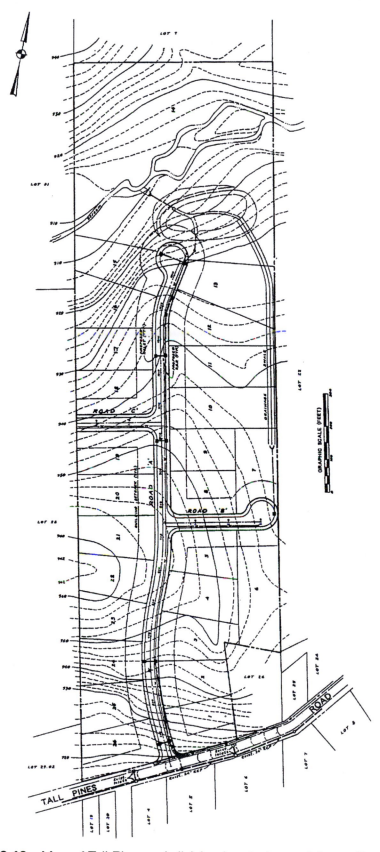

FIGURE 12-18   Map of Tall Pines subdivision located near Atlanta, Georgia.
(Courtesy of Jaman Engineering.)

3. Hydraulic design
4. Outfall design

The design investigation resulted in a topographic map used for the base map in Figure 12-18. Also, a site visit revealed that the tract is completely wooded in its existing condition. A meeting with the municipal engineer confirmed that the existing storm sewer in Tall Pines Road has sufficient capacity to accept additional discharge from the tract.

The subdivision was then designed in accordance with municipal zoning requirements. Roads A and B were proposed to extend to the property lines to provide access to adjoining tracts for future development.

Next, the storm sewer system was laid out in plan view to locate key drainage structures. Figures 12-19 and 12-20 show plans and profiles of the roads, including inlet and pipe segment locations. Since Road A has a high point at about Station 6 + 55, drainage must flow in two opposite directions. Some runoff flows southerly and is picked up by inlets at Station 0 + 75, while the remainder flows northerly toward the existing stream. Since Road B has a curbed cul-de-sac with a low point, an inlet was placed at its end to pick up all runoff flowing down the street.

No inlet is placed at the end of Road C even though it is pitched toward the adjoining property to the west. Any runoff flowing down Road C and onto adjoining property is kept to a minimum by placing an inlet at Station 9 + 93 to intercept discharge before it turns the corner. Normally, runoff in concentrated form should not be allowed to run on the ground onto another property because of the danger of erosion. But if the amount of flow can be reduced to a minor level, it might be allowed. Nonetheless, if the adjoining property owner objected, it would be necessary to design measures to eliminate the flow.

The pair of inlets at Station 9 + 93 are piped northerly down Road A to the cul-de-sac and then into the detention basin. The inlet at the end of Road B cannot be piped westerly toward Road A because Road B is pitched in the opposite direction, as shown in Figure 12-20. Therefore, the inlet is piped northerly to an outfall, and then a drainage ditch or swale runs northerly along the easterly property line to the detention basin. Figure 12-21 shows a profile of the drainage swale.

After completing the storm sewer layout, hydraulic design was initiated. Figure 12-22 shows the drainage area map for the subdivision, with incremental drainage basins delineated for each pipe segment. A close look at Figure 12-22 reveals that some of the basin divides do not follow the existing contours. This is because proposed grading will alter the contour lines, and it is the proposed contours that dictate basin divides. For example, in some lots, basin divides run along the rear sides of proposed houses because the lots will be graded to pitch toward the road. In other lots, such as Lots 15 through 18, it was impractical to place enough fill to pitch the lawns to the road, so these lots drain away from the road.

To start the hydraulic design process, key parameters were selected based on good design practice and local regulations:

Design storm frequency:	25-year
Pipe material:	reinforced concrete
Pipe Manning n-value:	0.015
Minimum pipe size	15 inches
Runoff coefficients:	Impervious: 0.90
	Lawn: 0.30
	Woods: 0.20

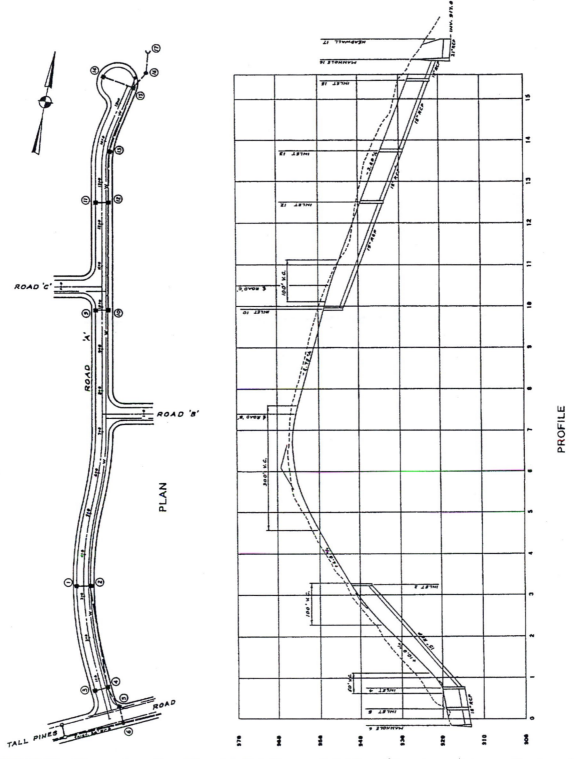

FIGURE 12-19   Plan and profile of Road A, Tall Pines subdivision. *(Courtesy of Jaman Engineering.)*

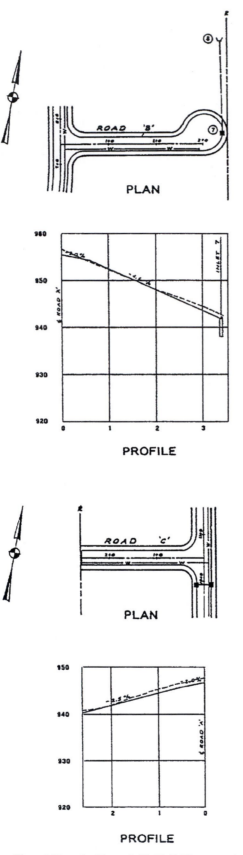

FIGURE 12-20   Plan and profile of Roads B and C, Tall Pines subdivision. *(Courtesy of Jaman Engineering.)*

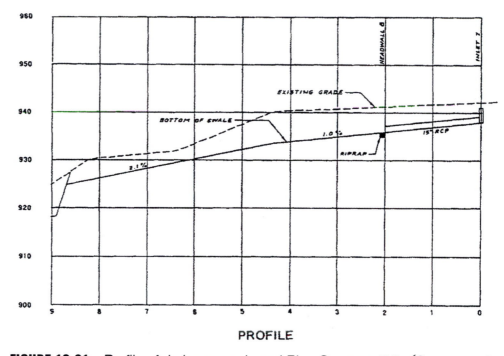

FIGURE 12-21   Profile of drainage swale and Pipe Segment 7-8. *(Courtesy of Jaman Engineering.)*

Next, drainage areas were measured, times of concentration computed, and a table of results prepared.

Times of concentration were determined by adding overland flow time and gutter flow time. Overland flow times were taken from Appendix C-2 using average grass surface, and gutter flow times were taken from Figure 10-9 using paved surface. Table 12-2 shows a summary of t_c computations, and Table 12-3 presents a summary of incremental areas, composite c-values, and times of concentration.

Storm sewers in this subdivision are divided into three separate systems, each corresponding to a different discharge or outfall point. Each system was designed separately starting with the southerly system, and results were recorded in the design table shown in Table 12-4.

Southerly System

Pipe Segment 1-2

Peak runoff tributary to this segment is computed in columns 2 through 8 in Table 12-4. The drainage area tributary to Segment 1-2 is called Incremental Area 1. The value Ac shown in column 5 is the product of incremental area, A, and runoff coefficient, c. Time of concentration of 11.9 minutes shown in column 6 is that computed previously for Incremental Area 1. Rainfall intensity of 6.9 in/h, shown in column 7, was determined from the rainfall intensity duration curves for Atlanta depicted in Appendix C-3. Peak runoff of 2.9 cfs shown in column 8 was computed by multiplying the values in columns 5 and 7.

Segment 1-2 is a cross drain and is assigned an arbitrary slope of 2.0 percent and minimum size of 15 inches. A 2.0 percent slope is used because it ensures

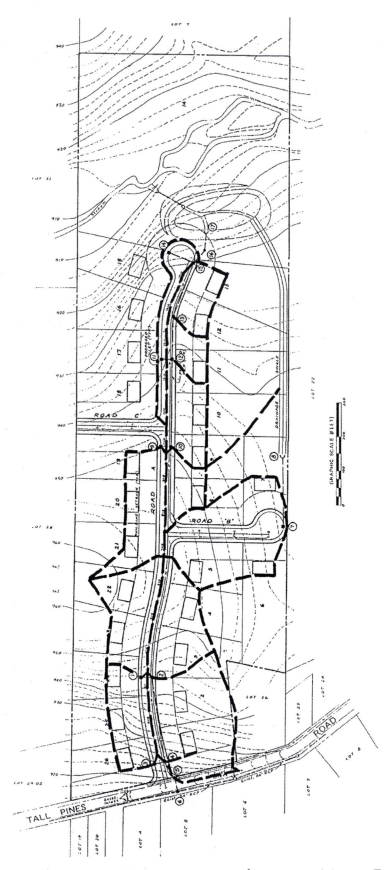

FIGURE 12-22 Drainage area map of Tall Pines subdivision. *(Courtesy of Jaman Engineering.)*

TABLE 12-2   Computation of t_c for Tall Pines Subdivision

Inlet		Time of Concentration	
1	Overland	100' @ 5.0%	$t_1 = 11.0$ min
	Shallow conc.	150' @ 6.0%	$t_2 = 0.6$ min
	Gutter	100' @ 6.0%	$t_3 = 0.3$ min
			$t_c = 11.9$ min
2	Overland	90' @ 2.0%	$t_1 = 12.0$ min
	Gutter	260' @ 4.7%	$t_3 = 1.0$ min
			$t_c = 13.0$ min
3	Overland	100' @ 7.0%	$t_1 = 10.0$ min
	Gutter	250' @ 8.0%	$t_3 = 0.7$ min
			$t_c = 10.7$ min
4	Overland	100' @ 6.0%	$t_1 = 10.5$ min
	Shallow conc.	150' @ 6.0%	$t_2 = 0.6$ min
	Gutter	130' @ 8.0%	$t_3 = 0.4$ min
			$t_c = 11.5$ min
5	Overland	100' @ 5.0%	$t_1 = 11.0$ min
	Shallow conc.	170' @ 9.0%	$t_2 = 0.6$ min
	Gutter	110' @ 3.0%	$t_3 = 0.5$ min
			$t_c = 12.1$ min
7	Overland	100' @ 5.0%	$t_1 = 11.0$ min
	Shallow conc.	150' @ 3.7%	$t_2 = 0.8$ min
	Gutter	80' @ 3.4%	$t_3 = 0.4$ min
			$t_c = 12.2$ min
9	Overland	100' @ 5.0%	$t_1 = 11.0$ min
	Shallow conc.	130' @ 2.3%	$t_2 = 0.9$ min
	Gutter	280' @ 2.7%	$t_3 = 1.4$ min
			$t_c = 13.3$ min
10	Overland	100' @ 2.0%	$t_1 = 12.5$ min
	Gutter	130' @ 2.7%	$t_3 = 0.6$ min
			$t_c = 13.1$ min

adequate capacity with sufficient vertical drop for ease of construction. Of course, the slope could be reduced if less drop is available, but in general, the flatter the slope of a storm sewer, the greater is the possibility of an error in construction.

The capacity of this segment was determined to be 8.0 cfs from Chart 36 in Appendix A-4 and then entered in Column 12 of Table 12-4. Since this capacity exceeds the design discharge of 2.9 cfs, the segment was accepted.

The design velocity was determined from Chart 36 to be 5.8 ft/s and entered in column 13 of Table 12-4. Time of flow in Segment 1-2 was then computed using velocity and distance to be 0.1 minute and entered in Column 14 of Table 12-4.

TABLE 12-3 Summary of Runoff Parameters for Tall Pines Subdivision

Inlet or Manhole	Incremental Drainage Area (acres)	Impervious Area (acres)	Lawn Area (acres)	Wooded Area (acres)	Composite c	t_c (min)
1	0.98	0.24	0.55	0.19	0.43	11.9
2	0.83	0.24	0.54	0.05	0.47	13.0
3	0.74	0.28	0.46	—	0.53	10.7
4	1.12	0.22	0.57	0.33	0.39	11.5
5	0.64	0.06	0.14	0.44	0.29	12.1
6	—	—	—	—	—	—
7	1.70	0.51	0.79	0.40	0.46	12.2
8	—	—	—	—	—	—
9	1.08	0.30	0.62	0.16	0.45	13.3
10	0.46	0.14	0.32	—	0.48	13.1
11	0.12	0.07	0.05	—	0.65	*
12	0.64	0.21	0.43	—	0.50	*
13	0.34	0.10	0.24	—	0.48	*
14	0.31	0.17	0.14	—	0.63	*
15	0.52	0.18	0.34	—	0.51	*
	9.04	2.66	5.04	1.34		

These times of concentration are, by inspection, less than any upstream time of concentration and therefore are not needed.

Pipe Segment 2-4

Column 5 of Table 12-4 shows cumulative Ac to be 0.81, the sum of the first two incremental Ac values. Time of concentration is 13.0 minutes, which is based on the hydraulic path for the incremental drainage area tributary to Inlet 2. The value 13.0 minutes was chosen because it is larger than the time of concentration obtained by using the hydraulic path starting in Incremental Area 1 and continuing through Pipe Segment 1-2. That t_c is $11.9 + 0.1 = 12.0$ minutes, which is smaller than 13.0 minutes. Rainfall intensity, based on a duration of 13.0 minutes, was found in Appendix C-3 to be 6.5 in/h. Therefore, Q_p was computed to be 5.3 cfs and recorded in Column 8 of Table 12-4.

Pipe Segment 2-4 is shown on the profile in Figure 12-19 to be a 15-inch pipe with a length of 250 feet and a slope of 8.8 percent. Inlet 4 is located at station 0 + 75, which is a shift from the first trial location at station 0 + 50 in order to fit the pipe under the vertical curve and maintain sufficient cover. The capacity was determined to be 17.0 cfs using Chart 36 in Appendix A-4. Since the capacity is greater than Q_p, the pipe segment was accepted.

The design velocity was determined from Chart 36 to be 12 fps. Although this velocity is near the high end of acceptable values, it was not considered problematic, since the horizontal deflection between Segment 2-4 and Segment 4-5 is relatively small, thus presenting little probability of surcharging Inlet 4.

Pipe Segment 3-4

This segment is a branch of the system and a cross drain. Peak discharge is computed in columns 2 through 8 to be 2.7 cfs. The size and slope were chosen, as with

TABLE 12-4   Drainage Calculation Chart for Tall Pines Subdivision (25-Year Storm, $n = 0.015$)

(1) Pipe Segment		(2) A—Increm. Area (acre)	(3) C—Runoff Coefficient	(4) A·C—Increm.	(5) A·C—Cumul.	(6) t_c—Time of Conc. (min)	(7) i—Rainfall Intensity (in/h)	(8) Q_p—Peak Runoff (cfs)	(9) Pipe Length (ft)	(10) Slope (%)	(11) Size (in)	(12) Capacity (full) (cfs)	(13) Velocity (fps) (Design Flow)	(14) Travel Time in Pipe (min)
From	To													
Southerly system														
1	2	0.98	0.43	0.42	0.42	11.9	6.9	2.9	30	2.0	15	8.0	5.8	0.1
2	4	0.83	0.47	0.39	0.81	13.0	6.5	5.3	250	8.8	15	17.0	12.0	0.3
3	4	0.74	0.53	0.39	0.39	10.7	7.0	2.7	30	2.0	15	8.0	5.8	0.1
4	5	1.12	0.39	0.44	1.64	13.3	6.3	10.3	50	1.6	18	11.5	7.3	0.1
5	6	0.64	0.29	0.19	1.83	13.4	6.3	11.5	40	1.6	18	11.5	7.4	—
Road B														
7	8	1.70	0.46	0.78	0.78	12.2	6.7	5.2	200	1.0	15	5.5	5.0	0.3
Northerly system														
9	10	1.08	0.45	0.49	0.49	13.3	6.3	3.1	30	2.0	15	8.0	6.0	0.1
10	12	0.46	0.48	0.22	0.71	13.4	6.3	4.5	260	3.8	15	11.0	8.2	0.5
11	12	0.12	0.65	0.08	0.08	6.0	8.5	0.7	30	2.0	15	8.0	4.0	—
12	13	0.64	0.50	0.32	1.11	13.9	6.2	6.9	125	3.8	15	11.0	9.1	0.2
13	15	0.34	0.48	0.16	1.27	14.1	6.2	7.9	170	3.8	15	11.0	9.5	0.3
14	15	0.31	0.63	0.20	0.20	6.0	8.5	1.7	80	2.0	15	8.0	5.0	—
15	16	0.52	0.51	0.27	1.74	14.4	6.1	10.6	40	3.8	15	11.0	10.0	0.1
16	17	—	—	—	1.74	14.5	6.1	10.6	50	1.0	21	14.0	6.3	—

Segment 1-2, to be 15-inch and 2.0 percent, respectively. The resulting capacity of 8.0 cfs is greater than Q_p, and therefore the segment was accepted.

Pipe Segment 4-5

Discharge in this segment consists of all upstream pipes plus runoff directly entering Inlet 4. Therefore, cumulative Ac shown in column 5 of Table 12-4 is 1.64, which represents the sum of the first four incremental Ac values. Time of concentration is 13.3 minutes based on the hydraulic path starting in Incremental Area 1 and continuing through Pipe Segments 1-2 and 2-4. All other hydraulic paths yield smaller times of concentration. In Table 12-4, the value 13.3 minutes is obtained by adding the travel time of 0.3 minute in column 14 to the time of concentration of 13.0 minutes in column 6 for Segment 2-4. Rainfall intensity of 6.3 in/h was found in Appendix C-3 for a duration of 13.3 minutes. Therefore, Q_p was computed to be 10.3 cfs and entered in column 8.

Pipe Segment 4-5 is shown on the profile to have a length of 50 feet and a slope of 1.6 percent. The capacity first was determined for a 15-inch pipe to be 7.1 cfs using Chart 36 in Appendix A-4. Since this capacity is less than Q_p, the next higher pipe size of 18 inches was considered. The capacity of an 18-inch pipe was determined to be 11.5 cfs using Chart 37 in Appendix A-4. Since this capacity is greater than Q_p, the segment was accepted as an 18-inch pipe.

Pipe Segment 5-6

Like Segment 4-5 before it, this segment carries discharge from all upstream incremental areas plus runoff entering Inlet 5. Therefore, the cumulative Ac of 1.83 represents the sum of the five incremental Ac values in the southerly system. Time of concentration is 13.4 minutes, which was computed by adding the 0.1 minute travel time in Segment 4-5 to the previous t_c of 13.3 minutes. All other hydraulic paths yield smaller times of concentration. Rainfall intensity of 6.3 in/h was found in Appendix C-3 for a duration of 13.4 minutes. Therefore, Q_p was computed to be 11.5 cfs and entered in column 8.

Pipe Segment 5-6 is shown on the profile to be an 18-inch pipe with a length of 40 feet and a slope of 1.6 percent. The capacity was determined to be 11.5 cfs using Chart 37 in Appendix A-4. Since this capacity is equal to Q_p, the segment was accepted.

At Manhole 6, the southerly system connects to the existing 24-inch storm sewer in Tall Pines Road. The proposed 18-inch pipe should connect at an elevation in which the crowns of the two pipes match. This then became a vertical constraint on the southerly system and helped determine the 1.6 percent grade of the last two segments.

Road B

Pipe Segment 7-8

Peak runoff tributary to this segment was computed to be 5.2 cfs, as is shown in columns 2 through 8 in Table 12-4. The inlet grate was considered adequate to pass 4.5 cfs discharge because it is located at a low point where a few inches of head can build up above the grate, thus increasing its capacity.

The profile in Figure 12-20 shows a 15-inch pipe with a length of 100 feet and a slope of 1.0 percent. The 100-foot length was needed to get past the proposed house before beginning the swale, and the slope of 1.0 percent was dictated by the existing grade as shown on the profile. The capacity was found to be 5.5 cfs by using Chart 36 in Appendix A-4. Since the capacity is greater than design discharge, the pipe segment was accepted.

Drainage Swale

Pipe Segment 7-8 discharges into a swale that runs to the detention basin. As is shown on the profile in Figure 12-21, the swale starts with a slope of 1.0 percent, which then increases to 2.1 percent before reaching the detention basin.

To design the swale, first the peak discharge, Q_p, was computed. To compute Q_p, the tributary drainage area was delineated as shown in Figure 12-22. Normally, in designing a drainage swale, the point of analysis is taken as the downstream end of the swale because this gives the most conservative result. However, in this case, as shown in Figure 12-22, because of the peculiar slope of the land, the tributary drainage area extends only about 150 feet downstream of the pipe outfall. So this was taken as the point of analysis for computation of Q_p.

Tributary drainage area, A, was measured to be 2.36 acres, which includes the 1.70 acres tributary to Pipe Segment 7-8. Composite runoff coefficient was computed to be 0.40 on the basis of the following quantities:

Impervious area: 0.51 acre
Lawn area: 1.17 acres
Wooded area: 0.68 acre

Time of concentration was computed based on the hydraulic path to Inlet 7 plus Pipe Segment 7-8 plus 150 feet of the swale:

t_c to inlet 7: 12.2 min
Travel time in Segment 7-8: 0.3 min
Travel time in first 150 ft of swale: 1.6 min
   (based on Figure 10-9, unpaved)

Total t_c = 12.2 + 0.3 + 1.6 = 14.1 min

Rainfall intensity was taken from Appendix C-3 for a duration 14.1 minutes:

$i = 6.2$ in/h

Therefore, Q_p was computed by using Equation 11-2:

$$Q_p = Aci$$
$$= (2.36)(0.40)(6.2)$$
$$= 5.9 \text{ cfs}$$

When Q_p was known, the next step was to select a trial cross section and test it for depth and velocity. For trial 1, a trapezoidal channel with a 4-foot bottom width was chosen but was found to be larger than necessary. For trial 2, a triangular channel with side slopes of 2.5 horizontal to 1 vertical was selected.

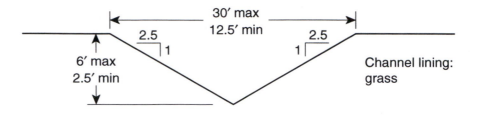

To determine normal depth and velocity, the trial-and-error procedure outlined in Section 6.4 was used. An *n*-value of 0.10 was taken from Appendix A-1 based on highway channels and swales with maintained vegetation, fair stand any grass, length 12 inches, depth 0.7 foot–1.5 feet, 2 fps.

This *n*-value was determined only after a trial-and-error process to determine approximate depth of flow and velocity.

The resulting depth of flow was 1.4 feet, and velocity was 1.1 fps, as shown in Table 12-5.

Normal depth and velocity were also checked for the steeper portion of the swale where the slope is 2.1 percent. The resulting depth of flow was 1.2 feet and velocity was 1.5 fps, as shown in Table 12-6.

Because the maximum design depth of 1.4 feet remains within the swale with adequate freeboard and the maximum design velocity of 1.5 fps is noneroding, the proposed triangular swale was accepted.

Outfall Erosion Protection

To determine whether a riprap outfall apron is needed, the design velocity in Pipe Segment 7-8 was compared to the values in Appendix A-2. As is shown in column 13 in Table 12-4, the velocity is 5.0 fps.

In Appendix A-2, the allowable velocity for silt loam is 3.0 fps. The choice of silt loam is based on observations made during site reconnaissance.

Therefore, since the pipe velocity exceeds the allowable velocity, a protective lining is needed. Riprap was chosen as the lining material.

TABLE 12-5 Computation of Normal Depth in First Section of Drainage Swale in Tall Pines Subdivision

$$\frac{1.49}{n}s^{1/2} = 1.49$$

D (ft)	a (ft²)	p (ft)	R (ft)	R²/³ —	v (fps)	Q (cfs)
1.0	2.5	5.4	0.463	0.598	0.64	1.6
2.0	10.0	10.8	0.93	0.95	1.0	10.0
1.5	5.63	8.1	0.69	0.78	1.2	6.6
1.4	4.9	7.54	0.65	0.75	1.1	5.5

Note: Normal depth and velocity were also checked for the steeper portion of the swale, where the slope is 2.1%. The resulting depth of flow was 1.2 feet and velocity was 1.5 fps, as shown in Table 12-6.

TABLE 12-6 Computation of Normal Depth in Steeper Section of Drainage Swale in Tall Pines Subdivision

$$\frac{1.49}{n}s^{1/2} = 2.16$$

D (ft)	a (ft²)	p (ft)	R (ft)	R²/³ —	v (fps)	Q (cfs)
1.4	4.9	7.54	0.65	0.75	1.6	7.9
1.0	2.5	5.4	0.463	0.598	1.3	3.2
1.2	3.6	6.5	0.557	0.677	1.5	5.3

First, stone size was determined by using Equation 12-1. Tailwater depth was found in Chart 36, Appendix A-4, for a 15-inch pipe with slope 1.0 percent, n-value 0.015, and discharge 5.2 cfs to be 0.95 feet:

$$
\begin{aligned}
d_{50} &= \frac{0.02}{TW}\left(\frac{Q}{D_0}\right)^{4/3} \\
&= \frac{0.02}{0.95}\left(\frac{5.2}{1.25}\right)^{4/3} \\
&= 0.14 \text{ ft} = 1.7 \text{ in}
\end{aligned}
$$

Although the computed size was 1.7 inches, 4-inch stone was chosen because it is more stable and has little cost difference.

Next, the apron length was computed by using Equation 12-2, since TW is greater than $\tfrac{1}{2}D_0$:

$$
\begin{aligned}
L_a &= \frac{3Q}{D_0{}^{3/2}} \\
&= \frac{(3)(5.2)}{1.25^{3/2}} \\
&= 11.2 \text{ ft}
\end{aligned}
$$

Therefore, an apron length of 12.0 feet was chosen as a rounding up of the computed length. The height of the riprap was set 1.0 foot above the tailwater depth, or 0.95 + 1.0 = 1.95 feet. Figure 12-23 shows the riprap design.

Northerly System

Pipe Segment 9-10

This segment is a cross drain and is designed much like Segment 1-2. Peak discharge was computed to be 3.1 cfs, as is shown in columns 2 through 8 of Table 12-4. The size and slope were chosen to be 15-inch and 2.0 percent, respectively, which result in a capacity of 8.0 cfs.

Pipe Segment 10-12

Peak discharge was computed in a manner similar to that for Segment 2-4. Cumulative Ac is the sum of the first two incremental Ac values, and t_c is the sum of t_c for

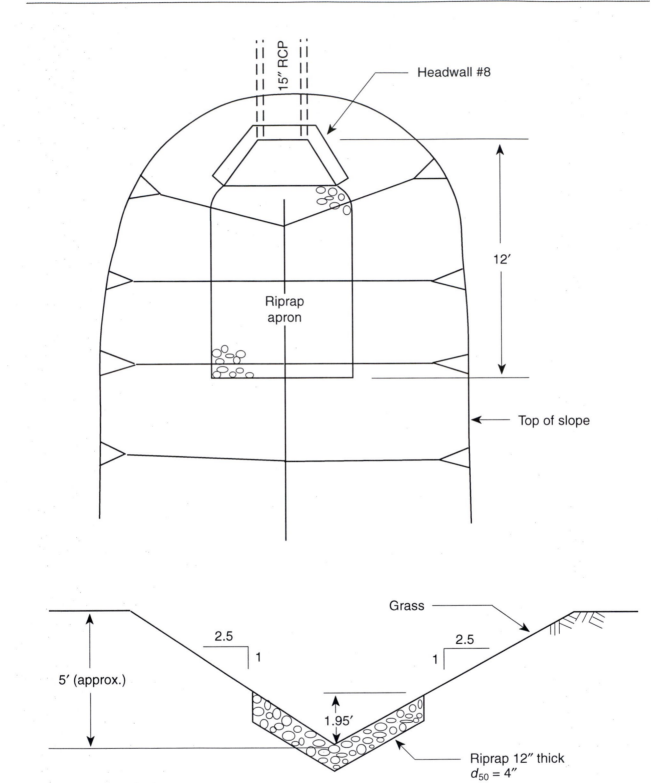

FIGURE 12-23 Riprap outfall protection at Headwall 8.

incremental area 9 plus travel time in Segment 9-10. Therefore, Q_p was computed to be 4.5 cfs.

Pipe Segment 10-12 is shown on the profile in Figure 12-19 to be a 15-inch pipe with a slope of 3.8 percent. From Chart 36 in Appendix A-4, the capacity was found to be 11.0 cfs, which is greater than the computed design discharge.

Pipe Segment 11-12

Like Segment 3-4, this is a branch of the system and a cross drain and therefore is determined to be a 15-inch pipe with a slope of 2.0 percent.

Pipe Segment 12-13

Discharge in this segment consists of flow from all upstream pipes plus runoff directly entering Inlet 12. Therefore, cumulative Ac shown in column 5 of Table 12-4 is 1.11, which represents the sum of the first four incremental Ac values. Time of concentration is 13.9 minutes, which was computed by adding the travel time (column 14) in Segment 10-12 to the time of concentration to Inlet 10. (13.4 min + 0.5 min = 13.9 min.) All other hydraulic paths yield smaller times of concentration. Rainfall intensity of 6.2 in/h was found in Appendix C-3 for a duration of 13.9 minutes. Therefore, Q_p was computed to be 6.9 cfs.

Pipe Segment 12-13 is shown on the profile to have a length of 125 feet and a slope of 3.8 percent. Capacity for a 15-inch pipe was determined to be 11.0 cfs using Chart 36. Since this capacity is greater than Q_p, the segment was accepted.

Pipe Segment 13-15

This segment continues the discharge from the previous segment with the addition of runoff directly entering Inlet 13. Therefore, cumulative Ac shown in column 5 to be 1.27 is the sum of the previous value of 1.11 and the incremental Ac value of 0.16. Similarly, time of concentration shown in column 6 to be 14.1 minutes is the sum of the previous value of 13.9 minutes and the travel time of 0.2 minute shown in column 14. Rainfall intensity of 6.2 in/h was found in Appendix C-3 just as in the previous segment. Therefore, Q_p was computed to be 7.9 cfs.

The profile shows Segment 13-15 to have a slope of 3.8 percent, thus giving it the same capacity as the previous segment: 11.0 cfs. Since this capacity is greater than 7.5 cfs, the segment was accepted.

Pipe Segment 14-15

Inlet 14 was placed at the low point of the cul-de-sac to prevent puddling. The resulting Pipe Segment 14-15 is a branch of the system and is designed much like Segment 11-12.

Pipe Segment 15-16

This segment conveys discharge from all upstream segments plus runoff directly entering Inlet 15. Cumulative Ac, shown in column 5 to be 1.74, is the sum of cumulative Ac values for Segments 13-15 and 14-15 and incremental Ac for inlet 15. (1.27 + 0.20 + 0.27 = 1.74.) This value also represents the sum of all incremental values shown in column 4. Time of concentration, shown as 14.4 minutes, is computed by adding the travel time in Segment 13-15 of 0.3 minute to the time of concentration to Inlet 13 of 16.2 minutes. (14.1 min + 0.3 min = 14.4 min.) Rainfall intensity of 6.1 in/h was found in Appendix C-3 using a duration of 14.4 minutes. Therefore, Q_p was computed to be 10.6 cfs.

The slope of Segment 15-16 is shown on the profile to be 3.8 percent, thus giving it a capacity of 11.0 cfs; the segment was accepted.

Manhole 16 was included in the layout to reduce the slope of the last pipe segment so that the velocity at the outfall to the detention basin could be kept under control. The profile in Figure 12-19 shows that a drop occurs at Manhole 16, allowing Pipe Segment 16-17 to have a 1.0 percent slope. If the manhole were not included, the pipe would have a slope of approximately 6 percent, resulting in a velocity of about 13 fps, which would be excessive at the outfall.

Pipe Segment 16-17

Since no runoff can enter through the top of the manhole, it has no tributary drainage area; consequently, columns 2, 3, and 4 of Table 12-4 are blank. However, the value 1.74 was entered in column 5 because all upstream incremental areas are tributary to Manhole 16, just as they are to Inlet 15. Time of concentration is shown in column 6 to be 14.5 minutes, which is the sum of the time of concentration to Inlet 15 and the travel time in Pipe Segment 15-16. Rainfall intensity of 6.1 in/h was found in Appendix C-3 by using a duration of 14.5 minutes. Therefore, Q_p was computed to be 10.6 cfs.

As was stated above, the slope of Segment 16-17 was set at 1.0 percent. At this slope, a 15-inch pipe has a capacity of 5.5 cfs, which is less than the design discharge. Therefore, capacity was checked for an 18-inch pipe using Chart 37 in Appendix A-4 and found to be 9.2 cfs, which is still less than the design discharge. Next, a 21-inch pipe was considered and capacity found in Chart 38 to be 14.0 cfs. Also using Chart 38, design velocity for 10.1 cfs was found to be 6.3 fps. Therefore, since its capacity is greater than design discharge and its velocity is reasonably low, the segment was accepted.

It should be noted that a 21-inch RCP is an uncommon size and might not be readily available. Therefore, a 24-inch RCP, which is a more common size, could have been specified in this case, since it would perform as well and vertical clearance is not a factor.

The structure chosen for Outfall 17 is a flared-end section because the gentle slope of the detention basin fits well against the slope of the flared-end section and therefore no wingwalls are needed. Figure 12-13 shows a detail of a flared-end section. The apron lining for Outfall 17 was designed as part of the detention basin.

PROBLEMS

1. A 24-inch RCP outfall discharges directly onto the ground. The pipe has a slope of 1.75 percent and *n*-value of 0.015 and carries a design discharge of 20. cfs. Design a riprap apron for the outfall.

2. A 60-inch RCP outfall discharges into an earth channel with a bottom width of 5.0 feet and side slopes of 2 horizontal to 1 vertical. The pipe has a slope of 0.8 percent and *n*-value of 0.012 and carries a design discharge of 85 cfs. Design a riprap apron for the outfall.

3. A concrete box storm sewer 4 feet high by 8 feet wide discharges into an earth channel with a bottom width of 10 feet and side slopes of 3 horizontal to 1 vertical. The storm sewer has a slope of 0.5 percent and an *n*-value of 0.015 and carries a design discharge of 215 cfs. Design a riprap apron for the outfall.

4. A 48-inch RCP outfall discharges directly onto the ground. The pipe has a slope of 2.0 percent and an *n*-value of 0.012 and carries a design discharge of 75 cfs. Design a riprap apron for the outfall.

5. Following is a plan view of a small storm sewer system:

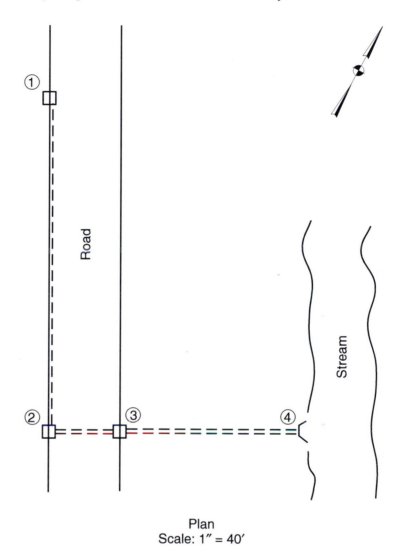

Plan
Scale: 1″ = 40′

The site is located in Atlanta, Georgia. Using a design chart like that in Table 12-4, complete the hydraulic design. Key parameters are as follows:

    Design storm: 25-year
    Pipe material: reinforced concrete
    Manning's *n*: 0.012
    Minimum pipe size: 12 inches

Segment	Incremental Area (acres)	*c*	t_c (min)	Pipe Slope (%)
1-2	1.24	0.46	18	1.8
2-3	0.86	0.62	16	0.9
3-4	0.52	0.80	6	0.5

6. A site plan for a proposed warehouse located near Pittsburgh, Pennsylvania (Region 1), is shown in Figure 12-24. Inlet locations and incremental drainage areas have already been determined. The on-site storm sewer system connects through an easement to the existing system in Brickel Avenue. Using a design chart like that in Table 12-4, complete the hydraulic design for this storm sewer system. Key parameters are as follows:

Design storm: 15-year
Pipe material: reinforced concrete
Manning's n: 0.012
Minimum pipe size: 12 inches

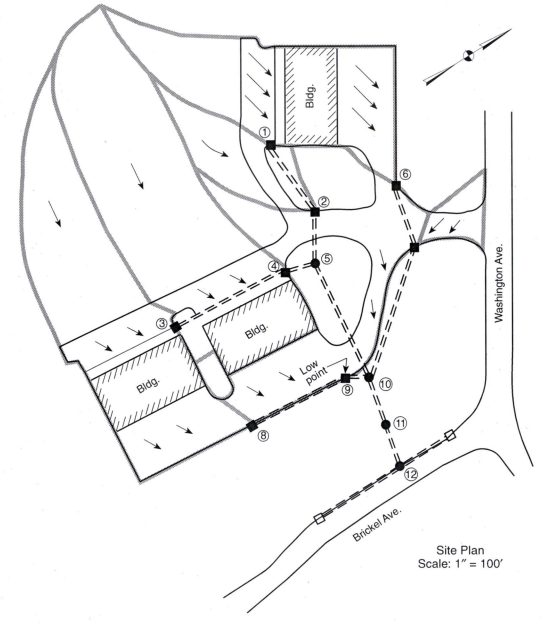

FIGURE 12-24   Site plan showing drainage areas tributary to the inlets.

Segment	Incremental Area (acres)	c	t_c (min)	Pipe Slope %
1-2	0.65	0.62	16	2.5
2-5	0.34	0.34	15	2.1
3-4	1.16	0.28	18.5	1.1
4-5	1.79	0.26	19.0	2.4
5-10	—	—	—	1.0
6-7	0.31	0.89	6	2.8
7-10	0.15	0.65	12	3.5
8-9	0.29	0.90	6	1.0
9-10	1.10	0.66	10	2.2
10-11	—	—	—	3.0
11-12	—	—	—	1.0

Note: *All paved areas are curbed. Roof drains connect to inlets 1, 3, and 4.*

7. Design a storm sewer system for Whitebirch Court and Warren Place, located in northern New Jersey, which are shown in Figure 12-25. The storm sewer connects to the existing sewer in McDonald Drive at the manhole shown at the intersection. Your design should include drainage area delineation and hydraulic design using a chart like the one in Table 12-4. System layout is shown in the figure. Assume all roads are curbed and crowned. Also, assume that no runoff enters Warren Place from the road to its south. Wooded areas are delineated with a symbol for wood lines. Suggested design parameters and pipe slopes are shown below:

   Design storm: 25-year
   Pipe material: reinforced concrete
   Manning's *n*: 0.012
   Minimum pipe size: 12 inches
   Runoff coefficients: paved, 0.90; grass, 0.35; wooded, 0.25

Pipe Segment	Slope (%)
1-3	1.5
2-3	2.5
3-5	1.0
4-5	1.0
5-6	6.0
6-7	1.2

8. Design a storm sewer system for the site development located near Atlanta, Georgia, and shown in Figure 12-26. The system should outfall at the headwall shown in the southeast corner of the tract. Your design should include system layout, drainage area delineation, hydraulic design, and outfall apron design. Assume that all paved areas are curbed. Wooded areas are delineated with

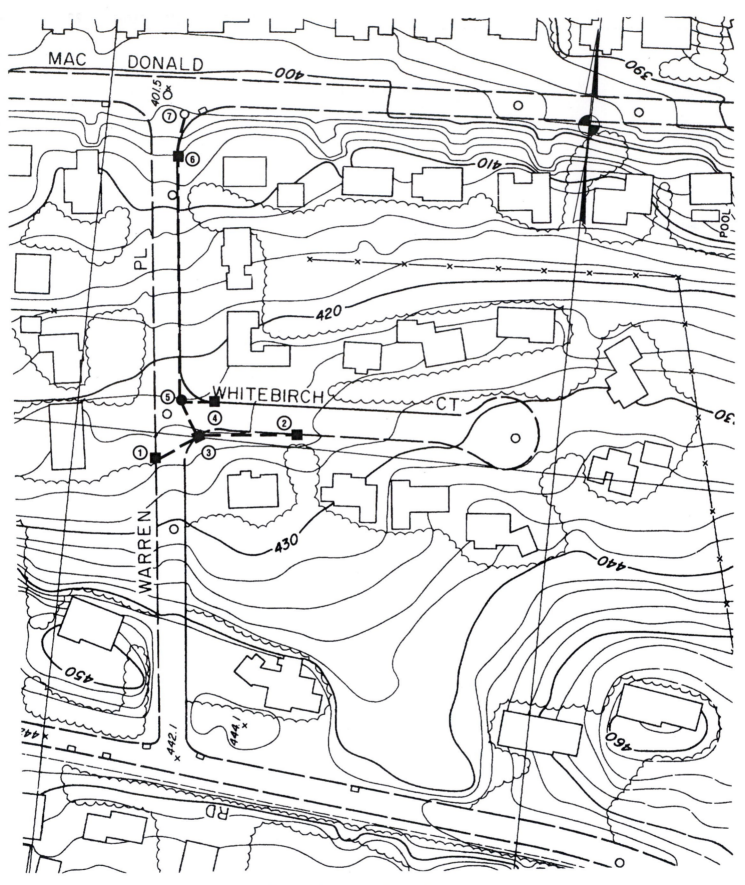

Plan of Proposed Storm Sewer
Scale: 1″ = 100′
Contour Interval 2′

FIGURE 12-25 Plan of proposed storm sewer for problem 7.

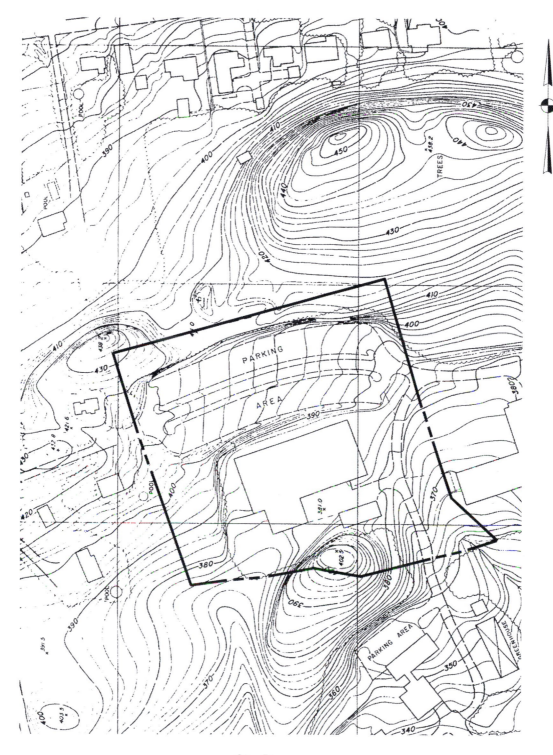

Site Plan
Scale: 1″ = 200′
Contour Interval 2′

FIGURE 12-26   Topographic map of developed site near Atlanta, Georgia. *(Map adapted from Aero Service.)*

wood lines. Suggested design parameters are listed below.

Design storm: 25-year
Pipe material: reinforced concrete
Manning's n: 0.012
Minimum pipe size: 12 inches
Runoff coefficients: Impervious: 0.95
                      Grass: 0.32
                      Wooded: 0.25

FURTHER READING

Debo, T., and Reese, A. (1995). *Municipal Storm Water Management*. Boca Raton, FL: Lewis Publishers.

Joint Committee of ASCE and Water Pollution Control Federation (2000). *Design and Construction of Sanitary and Storm Sewers*. New York: ASCE and WPCF.

Mays, L. W., ed. (2001). *Stormwater Collection Systems Design Handbook*. New York: McGraw-Hill.

Urban Water Resources Research Council of ASCE and the Water Environment Federation (1992). *Design and Construction of Urban Stormwater Management Systems*. New York and Alexandria, VA: ASCE.

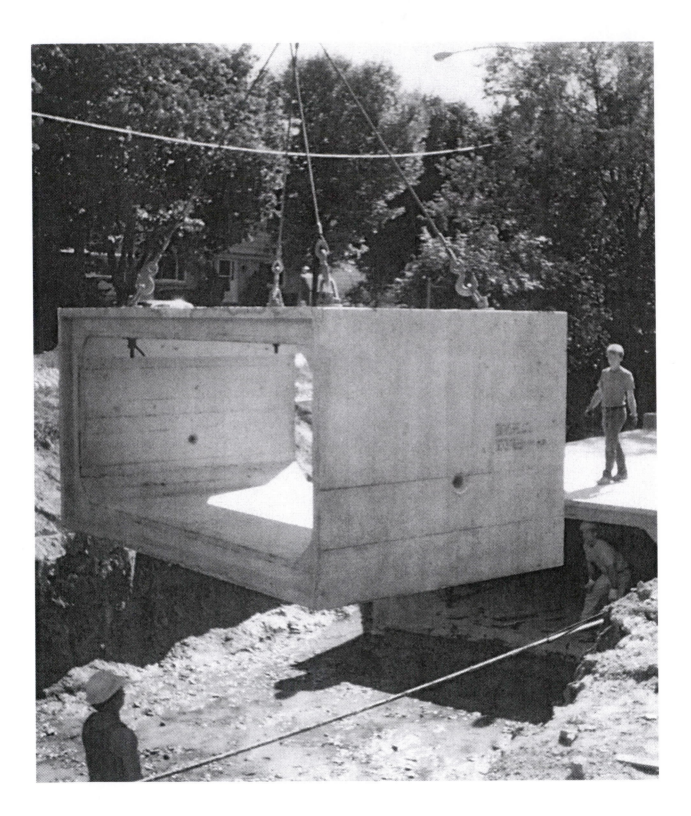

CULVERT DESIGN

Methods for calculating flow through a culvert were presented in Chapter 9. In this chapter, we will see how to apply those calculations to the design of actual culverts in typical field applications.

Many factors must be considered in performing any engineering design, and the design principles outlined here for culverts illustrate that assertion. However, it should be remembered that the principal emphasis is on hydraulic design. There are other factors, such as structural stability, cost, and traffic control, which will not be treated with as much detail.

OBJECTIVES

After completing this chapter, the reader should be able to:

- Assess an existing culvert for hydraulic adequacy
- Interpret plans showing a culvert profile
- Choose an appropriate layout for a new culvert
- Choose an appropriate layout for a culvert replacement
- Design a culvert size for a new embankment or a culvert replacement
- Design riprap protection for a culvert inlet and outlet
- Relate culvert design to an actual case study

13.1 FUNDAMENTAL CONCEPTS

Design considerations focus on two general concepts: *outcome* and *construction*. Outcome includes all factors that determine the finished product while construction involves factors that control the actual building process. The principal goal of outcome design for a culvert is determination of the size and alignment of the culvert and provisions for erosion control. The term *size* refers to the dimensions of the barrel, also called the *opening* of the culvert, while alignment is concerned with orientation, primarily horizontal.

Additional goals of outcome design include structural stability, durability, cost, ease of maintenance, and safety. Thus, the designer visualizes the culvert in its completed, functioning state and seeks to ensure that the completed structure will have sufficient hydraulic capacity, sufficient strength, ability to be maintained, and all the other desired attributes at an affordable cost.

Principal design goals for the construction phase of the project include erosion control of disturbed soil, control of traffic, safety of workers, control of flooding that may occur during construction, and the routing of heavy trucks through residential areas.

Each culvert design project is unique, but two general categories of project can be identified from the range of individual cases:

- *New embankment*, which involves the design of a new culvert to convey a stream through a new embankment.
- *Culvert replacement*, which involves the design of a culvert to replace an existing culvert (usually undersized) in an existing embankment.

Each of these design categories is described individually later in this chapter.

The general procedure for hydraulic design is similar for both project categories and is shown in flow chart form in Figure 13-1.

First, the design storm and method of computation must be selected. These are usually specified by the governmental agency that has jurisdiction over the culvert. Typically, the design storm is a 100-year storm computed by the NRCS Method. However, for minor culverts, a lesser-frequency storm may be acceptable.

Allowable headwater elevation (A.H.E.) is a key design parameter and constitutes the maximum height of headwater that will be allowed for the design storm. This height or elevation usually is prescribed by agency regulations and may be the upstream crown of the culvert, the lowest point of the top of the embankment, or some other specific height. If no regulation applies, the designer must determine the maximum height that the headwater will be allowed to rise during the design storm. The higher the allowable headwater elevation, the smaller the culvert and therefore the more economical the design. Consideration must be given to potential damage caused by the upstream pool of water.

The next preliminary design step is the computation of design discharge. To do this, the watershed must be delineated on a suitable topographic map using the culvert location as the point of analysis. In choosing runoff parameters, the designer must choose between existing watershed ground conditions and conditions of future development.

The more conservative design allows for future development in the watershed and is therefore preferable. Future development usually means more impervious area and shorter time of concentration and therefore greater peak runoff. However, with the proliferation of detention basins that are designed to reduce peak runoff, future runoff might not be greater than that occurring at present.

Finally, the water level in the existing stream, which will become the tailwater for the culvert, is determined. If no significant obstructions are present downstream and therefore no backwater effect exists at the culvert location, water level is assumed to be normal depth and is computed by using Manning's equation. However, if backwater is suspected, then water level must be computed by using a special method such as standard step calculations. Since this method is beyond the scope of this text, cases involving backwater will not be included. In most cases involving

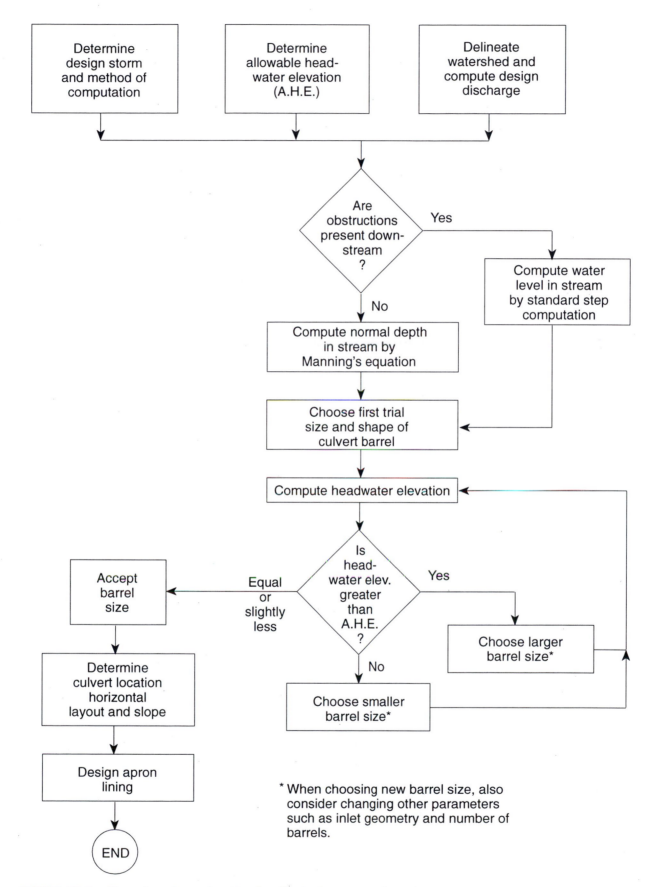

FIGURE 13-1   Flowchart for culvert hydraulic design procedure.

backwater computations, appropriate computer software such as HEC-RAS is employed. A list of applicable software currently available is included in Appendix E.

After all the preliminary computations and plottings are complete, the essential hydraulic design may begin. The first step is to choose an initial trial size and shape of the culvert. This includes barrel dimensions, type of wingwalls, and entrance geometry. Then compute the headwater elevation using the procedures outlined in Chapter 9. If the resulting headwater elevation is greater than the allowable headwater elevation, another trial must be made that uses a larger cross section. If the size of the culvert becomes too large to fit under the road, multiple barrels may be used. However, the number of barrels should be kept to a minimum. It is desirable that the opening size of each barrel be as large as possible because small culvert openings are more easily clogged by debris. To find the headwater depth for two culvert barrels, for example, divide design discharge by 2 and proceed as if for one barrel. Figure 13-2 shows a typical multiple-barrel culvert.

If the resulting headwater elevation is less than the allowable elevation, the chosen culvert is larger than necessary, and consideration should be given to trying a smaller size.

After the barrel opening has been determined, the position or alignment of the culvert can be fixed. In the case of a culvert replacement, the location usually coincides with that of the existing culvert, although there are exceptions. For new culverts, the location is chosen on the basis of a variety of factors, both horizontal and vertical. Figure 13-3 shows some typical culvert alignments. To assist in vertical alignment, profiles of the streambed and the top of embankment are plotted.

Generally, the culvert should follow the streambed in both horizontal and vertical alignment. However, the shortest culvert results from placement perpendicular to the embankment. This may require relocation of a portion of the existing stream, as shown in Figure 13-3(a).

Once the culvert size has been established, an apron lining both upstream and downstream of the culvert should be considered. To design an outlet apron lining,

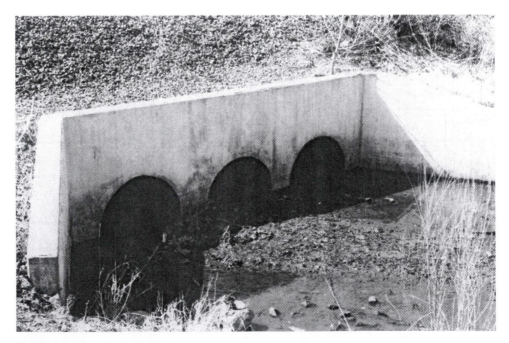

FIGURE 13-2 Typical three-barrel pipe culvert.

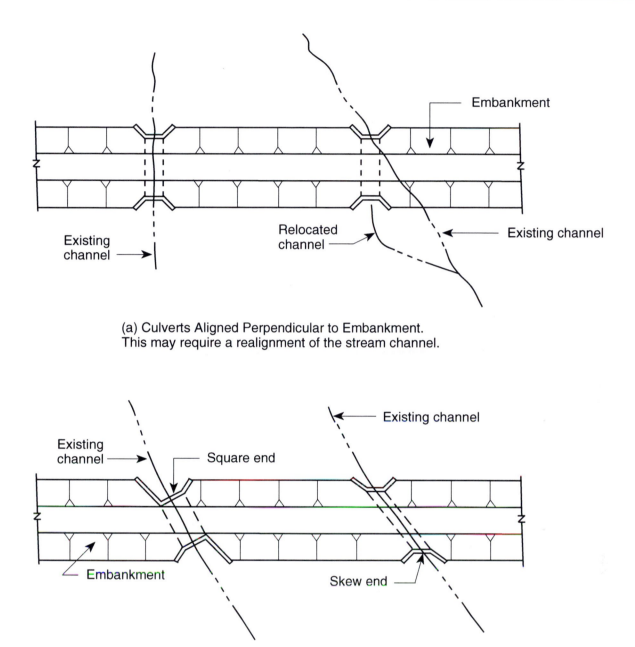

(a) Culverts Aligned Perpendicular to Embankment.
This may require a realignment of the stream channel.

(b) Culverts Aligned at a Skew to the Embankment.
The face of the barrel end may be square or skewed.

FIGURE 13-3   Some examples of horizontal alignments of culverts.

compute velocity at the outlet of the culvert by using the continuity equation, $Q = va$.
Cross-sectional area is computed by one of three methods:

1. If tailwater depth, TW, is less than critical depth, use critical depth together
   with barrel dimensions to compute cross-sectional area.
2. If tailwater depth is greater than critical depth, use tailwater depth together
   with barrel dimensions to compute cross-sectional area.
3. If tailwater level is above the crown of the outlet, use the cross-sectional
   area of the entire barrel opening.

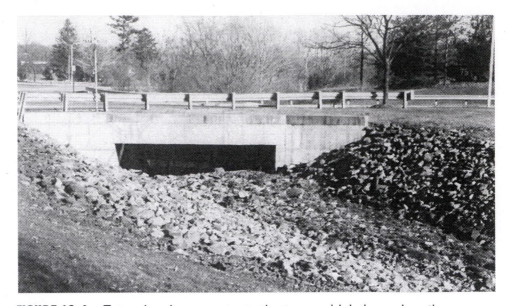

FIGURE 13-4 Extensive riprap protects the trapezoidal channel on the downstream side of this new concrete box culvert.

Using this velocity, design an apron lining in accordance with the procedure outlined in Section 12.5 or any other accepted procedure. Figure 13-4 shows typical riprap lining on the downstream side of a new culvert.

To design an inlet apron lining, compute velocity at the inlet of the culvert by using the continuity equation. Cross-sectional area is computed by using the head-water depth, *HW*, together with barrel dimensions. If the headwater is above the crown, use the cross-sectional area of the entire barrel opening.

After computing velocity, design the apron lining in accordance with any accepted procedure. For instance, if riprap is to be the lining, stone size may be computed by using Equation 12-1 or 12-1a, and apron length may be determined at the discretion of the designer.

When computing the cross-sectional area of a culvert, if the face of the culvert is skewed, as shown in the right-hand sketch in Figure 13-3(b), do not use the actual skew dimensions. Use the dimensions perpendicular to the long axis of the barrel.

Example 13-1

Problem

Find the outlet velocity for a 4 foot by 8 foot box culvert with a discharge of 200 cfs and tailwater depth of 3.2 feet.

Solution

First, find critical depth by using Chart 7 in Appendix A-3. Critical depth is 2.7 feet.

Since tailwater depth is greater than critical depth, compute cross-sectional area, using tailwater depth:

$$a = (8)(3.2) = 25.6 \text{ ft}^2$$

Finally, compute velocity, using the continuity equation:

$$v = \frac{Q}{a} = \frac{200}{25.6} = 7.8 \text{ ft/s} \quad \text{(Answer)}$$

Other environmental considerations are important in culvert design and should be discussed at preliminary meetings with the reviewing agencies. One of these is fish habitat. If the stream is important to fish habitat or production, it might be necessary to design the culvert to protect such conditions. Figure 13-5 depicts

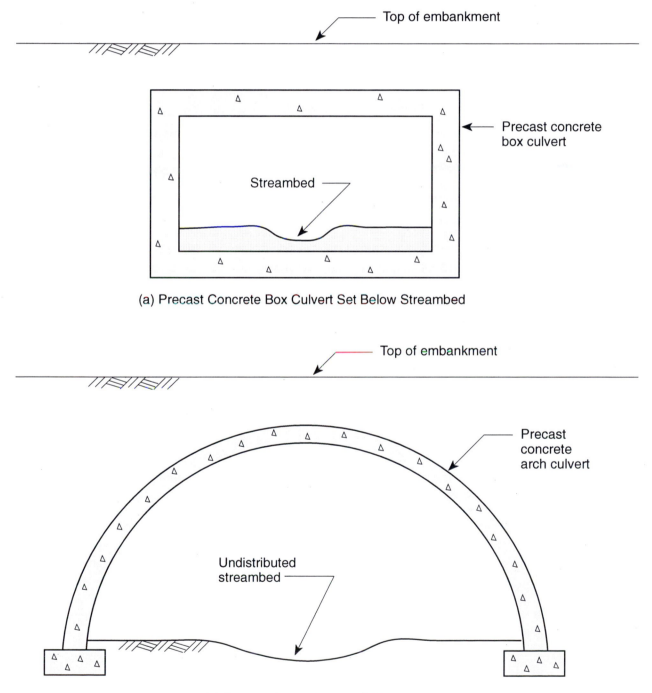

(a) Precast Concrete Box Culvert Set Below Streambed

(b) Precast Concrete Arch Culvert

FIGURE 13-5   Examples of methods to preserve existing stream conditions in culverts.

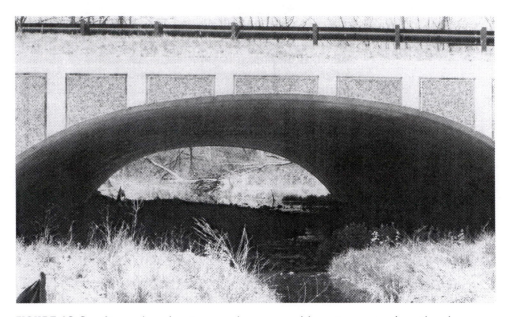

FIGURE 13-6 An arch culvert spanning a sensitive stream and wetland area.

two measures designed to protect the fish community. In Figure 13-5(a), a precast concrete culvert is placed lower than the stream invert so that the bed will consist of an unbroken natural channel as it goes through the culvert. In Figure 13-5(b), an arch culvert is placed over a stream to leave the bed and overbank completely undisturbed. Figure 13-6 shows an example of an arch culvert constructed in a new embankment for a road leading to a residential development. The culvert was constructed without touching the streambed and adjacent wetlands.

These environmental considerations have virtually no effect on hydraulic calculations. The only possible effect is the change in roughness due to the presence of streambed instead of a concrete surface. However, this difference is minor and results in very little discernible difference in headwater elevation.

Another environmental consideration is the potential for flooding downstream from the culvert. In cases of culvert replacement, if the existing culvert is severely undersized, it might have been causing significant upstream pooling during severe storms, thus reducing the downstream flow rate. In effect, the culvert and embankment act in such cases as a detention basin, which attenuates or lessens the flow rate downstream. This effect is analyzed in Chapter 14. Therefore, to replace the undersized culvert with an adequately sized culvert would remove the attenuation and increase the flow downstream, possibly creating flooding problems. If this detrimental effect of increasing the size of a culvert is suspected, a routing analysis should be conducted to assess the downstream flooding problem. The resulting decision to increase the culvert size or to maintain the existing size would typically be a public agency policy decision.

13.2 DESIGN INVESTIGATION

Before a culvert design is begun, a project meeting should be conducted, and then certain essential data must be acquired, much as in the case of storm sewer design. These are summarized as follows:

1. Relevant maps
2. Site reconnaissance
3. Applicable regulations and engineering design or reports for completed projects relating to the design

Project Meeting

The project meeting that defines the scope of the design is similar to that described for storm sewer design. It might also be necessary, however, to hold a meeting at the agency that exercises jurisdiction over the proposed culvert.

Culverts generally are considered major hydraulic structures and are directly or indirectly regulated by counties, states, or both. In many cases, a special permit or approval is required before construction of a culvert, and the application process can be complex. Therefore, a *preapplication* meeting often is needed to clarify how the regulations apply to the project in question and to coordinate between designer and reviewer what design information will be presented with the application.

Relevant Maps

Relevant maps required for design purposes usually consist of a boundary survey and two topographic maps. The boundary survey is needed to be sure that the culvert will be laid out on the owner's property, which usually consists of a road or railroad right-of-way. Certain details of the culvert design, namely, the wingwalls and riprap apron, cannot be determined without the use of topography of the culvert area. Also dependent on this information are certain key vertical relationships, such as the distance from the streambed to the top of the embankment. These applications of the topographical data require a high degree of precision; therefore, contour lines of 1-foot (0.3 m) or 2-foot (0.6 m) intervals are preferred. In addition, certain spot elevations might be necessary. All existing utilities must also be accurately depicted. Therefore, supplementary field topography might be required.

Topography is also required to delineate the watershed tributary to the culvert. Since the watershed is often quite large in comparison to the construction site, it might be impractical to use 2-foot (0.6 m) contours, and a smaller-scale, less precise topographic map might suffice for runoff calculations. USGS quadrangle sheets drawn to a scale of 1:24,000 typically are used for this purpose.

Site Reconnaissance

A site visit must be conducted to verify the topography and make note of any features that are not clearly depicted on the maps. Also, the stream and overbank must be observed to determine Manning n-values and whether obstructions are present downstream.

Regulations and Design Reports

Finally, any applicable regulations must be obtained and reviewed, and if any reports of previous engineering design relating to the project exist, they should also be reviewed.

After all the engineering data have been obtained, the design process may begin.

13.3 DESIGN OF NEW CULVERT

Consider the case of a new road embankment proposed in an alignment that intersects an existing stream. This type of design has some advantages over replacing an existing culvert because there are usually fewer existing constraints, thus allowing more flexibility to the designer. For instance, since the road profile has not yet been established, the height of the proposed culvert could possibly be increased and the proposed road raised to compensate. This is not often an option for an existing road.

Another example of increased flexibility is the lack of existing underground utilities such as water, gas, and sanitary sewer mains. Also, the absence of improved building lots adjacent to the stream allows increased latitude in horizontal layout of the proposed culvert.

These factors that affect the design of a new culvert in a new road embankment are illustrated by the following example.

Example 13-2

Problem

A new road is proposed to connect from Shawn Court to Oakwood Avenue, as shown in Figure 13-7. Design a culvert to convey the existing stream through the proposed embankment.

Solution

The hydraulic design process follows the outline presented in Figure 13-1. Design storm is determined by local regulation to be the 100-year, 24-hour storm as computed by the NRCS Method. This computation is then performed and yields a design discharge of 480 cfs.

Allowable headwater elevation (A.H.E.) is determined by local regulation to be the upstream culvert crown.

From the topographic information obtained for the culvert vicinity, a profile of the proposed road centerline is prepared as depicted in Figure 13-8. (At first, the trial culvert openings and road grades are not included; they will be added later.)

Now we may begin hydraulic calculations. The first step is to determine tailwater depth. Since no obstructions are present downstream, flow depth in the stream is computed using Manning's equation. For a design discharge of 480 cfs, tailwater depth is found to be 3.7 feet.

Next, we choose a culvert size as a first trial. Choose a 4-foot by 8-foot concrete box culvert with 45-degree wingwalls and a square edge entrance. To check headwater depth, first assume inlet control. Using Chart 1 of Appendix B-1, we find that $Q/B = 61$ cfs/ft, which leads to a value of HW/D in scale (1) of the headwater depth

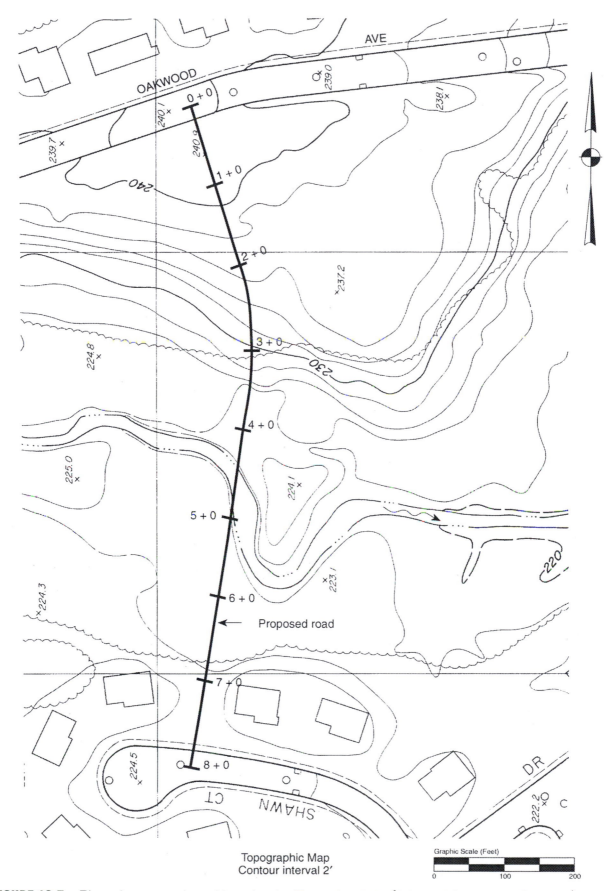

Topographic Map
Contour interval 2'

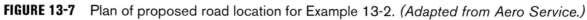

Graphic Scale (Feet)

0   100   200

FIGURE 13-7 Plan of proposed road location for Example 13-2. *(Adapted from Aero Service.)*

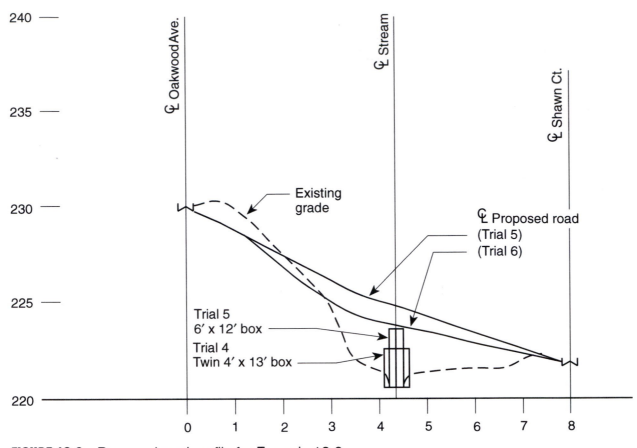

FIGURE 13-8   Proposed road profile for Example 13-2.

scale of 2.9. Therefore, $HW = 11.6$ feet. This obviously exceeds the A.H.E., which requires a depth of 4 feet at the culvert crown. Therefore, 4 feet by 8 feet is too small, and a larger opening must be tried. Note that it is not necessary to compute HW for outlet control. Why?

For Trial 2, choose a 4-foot by 16-foot culvert. From Chart 1, HW/D is found to be 1.25, so $HW = 5.0$ feet, which still exceeds the A.H.E. Therefore, this culvert size is rejected.

For Trial 3, choose a two-barrel culvert with 4-foot by 12-foot openings. To find HW for inlet control, use a design discharge of 240 cfs conveyed by a single 4-foot by 12-foot culvert. From Chart 1, HW/D is found to be 0.91, which yields a value of HW of 3.64 ft, below the A.H.E. Now, check outlet control.

To find HW assuming outlet control, first find critical depth. From Chart 10 in Appendix A-3, critical depth for 240 cfs is found to be 2.3 feet. Then

$$TW' = \frac{2.3 + 4.0}{2} = 3.15 \text{ ft}$$

Since TW is greater than TW', use TW for tailwater. By using Chart 8 in Appendix B-2 for $k_e = 0.4$, and $L = 50$ ft, H is found to be 0.63 foot. Then,

$$HW = TW + H - Ls$$
$$= 3.7 + 0.63 - 0.25$$
$$= 4.1 \text{ feet}$$

Therefore, the culvert operates under outlet control, and the headwater is above the crown. Consequently, this size is rejected.

For Trial 4, choose a two-barrel culvert with 4-foot by 13-foot openings. After computing HW as in the previous trial, the culvert is found to be operating under outlet control with $HW = 4.0$ feet. Therefore, a twin 4-foot by 13-foot box culvert is hydraulically adequate.

However, other shapes and sizes could be adequate as well, provided that the resulting headwater is below the crown. For instance, suppose we chose a box culvert with a height of 6 feet. Then for Trial 5, you could choose a single 6-foot by 12-foot box culvert. Assuming inlet control, HW is found from Chart 1 to be 5.82 feet. Assuming outlet control, HW is found from Chart 8 to be 4.55 feet. Therefore, this culvert operates under inlet control, and $HW = 5.82$ feet, which is below the A.H.E. So by the applicable headwater criterion, this culvert also is adequate.

Which culvert is the better choice: twin 4-foot by 13-foot box or single 6-foot by 12-foot box? The latter size would be much less expensive, but it would have two disadvantages. First, it would result in a headwater elevation of 227.32, which is 2.12 feet higher than the 100-year flood level occurring without a culvert. For the homes located at the westerly end of Shawn Court, this could be very damaging. Second, the higher culvert would require a higher grade for the proposed road and therefore much more fill to construct the embankment. Figure 13-8 shows the alternative culvert openings and resulting road profiles.

Therefore, the twin 4-foot by 13-foot box culvert is the better choice because it results in a headwater elevation only 0.3 foot higher than existing and requires a significantly smaller roadway embankment than would the higher culvert. Figure 13-9 shows a profile of the accepted culvert design.

If the A.H.E. was determined by allowing no rise in upstream water surface over existing conditions, as is required in some locations, the twin 4-foot by 13-foot box culvert would be nearly adequate. In such a case, the smallest adequate culvert would be a twin 4-foot by 14-foot box.

Next, the horizontal layout is determined. Figure 13-10 shows three alternative layouts to fit site conditions. The first alternative, shown in Figure 13-10(a), is the simplest and least expensive. It is perpendicular to the proposed road and has a length of 50 feet. Due to the meandering of the stream, a 160-linear foot channel realignment must be constructed downstream to blend into the existing channel. However, such a modification of the stream might not be allowed by the regulating agency for environmental reasons.

> *Note:* A linear foot is a unit of horizontal measure that may follow a curved as well as straight line.

The next alternative, shown in Figure 13-10(b), is an attempt to follow the path of the stream to avoid extensive channel realignment. However, even with this layout,

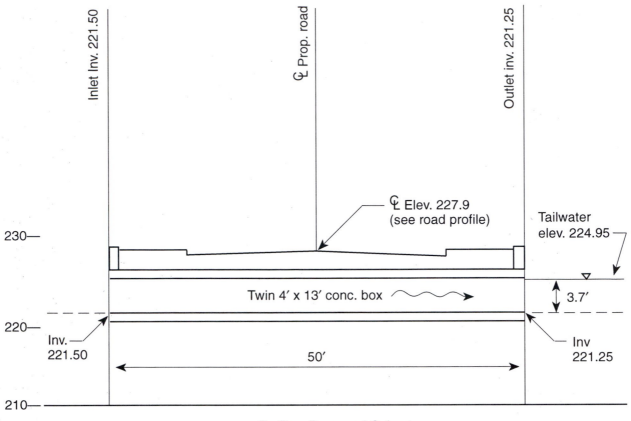

Profile—Proposed Culvert

FIGURE 13-9 Stream profile for Example 13-2.

a small realignment of 60 linear feet is necessary. The amount of skew of the culvert is kept to a minimum because the greater the skew, the longer is the culvert. (The skew angle is defined as the angle made by the long axis of the culvert and a line perpendicular to the road.) In this case, the culvert is 95 feet long, which is nearly double the length of alternative (a) and increases the cost precipitously. The culvert ends are square because a 45-degree skew at the end of a culvert is very severe, creating structural problems and adding more cost to the project.

The third alternative, (c), also attempts to follow the stream path but employs only a 25-degree skew. In this case, a channel realignment of 50 linear feet is needed at the upstream end to blend with the existing stream. A significant problem with this layout is the orientation of the culvert with the downstream channel. Discharge water is forced to make a sharp left turn as it flows from the culvert into the stream. This could create an erosion problem and also could result in higher tailwater, which could necessitate the increase of the size of the culvert opening.

Another alternative could be to realign the proposed road in a westerly direction to intercept the stream at a straighter section. This would probably require changing the point of intersection on Oakwood Avenue, which might not be possible because of other constraints, such as land ownership.

The choice of layout can affect the culvert opening in two ways. First, as we mentioned above, different downstream channel conditions lead to different tailwater

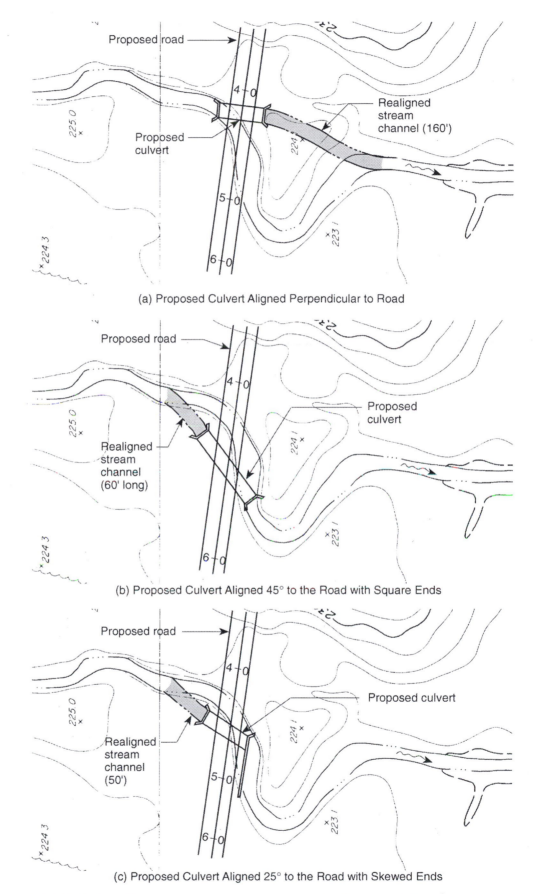

(a) Proposed Culvert Aligned Perpendicular to Road

(b) Proposed Culvert Aligned 45° to the Road with Square Ends

(c) Proposed Culvert Aligned 25° to the Road with Skewed Ends

FIGURE 13-10   Three alternative culvert layouts for Example 13-2. *(Map adapted from Aero Service.)*

depths, and second, different barrel lengths can affect headwater depth. Both of these effects apply to culverts operating under outlet control; if the culvert operates under inlet control, layout has little effect on opening size.

For the purpose of this example, we choose layout alternative (a).

Finally, design velocity is computed, and the need for any aprons, upstream and downstream, is assessed. Velocity at the outlet is found by using the continuity equation, $Q = va$. Cross-sectional area, a, is the area of a rectangle in which the width is 13.0 feet and the height is 3.7 feet. TW is used for the height instead of D_c because TW is the greater of these values:

$$a = (13.0)(3.7) = 48.1 \text{ ft}^2$$

$$v = \frac{Q}{a} = \frac{240}{48.1} = 5.0 \text{ ft/s}$$

Referring to Appendix A-2 for earth channels, we find that the permissible velocity for graded loam to gravel is 5.0 ft/s. Since the downstream channel will be constructed for a length of 160 linear feet as part of the project, the soil material can be specified as graded soil, silt to cobbles, and then no additional apron is required.

Velocity at the inlet of the culvert is found in the same manner, except using HW as the height. Thus,

$$a = (4.0)(13.0) = 52.0 \text{ ft}^2$$

$$v = \frac{Q}{a} = \frac{240}{52} = 4.6 \text{ ft/s}$$

Therefore, no apron is required at the upstream end of the culvert as well.

13.4 CULVERT REPLACEMENT

Now consider the case of an existing road with an existing culvert that is proposed to be replaced. In many culvert replacements, the existing culvert is hydraulically inadequate because of various factors. The culvert could have been constructed when design standards were not as conservative as current standards, development in the watershed could have caused an increase in peak runoff, or rerouting of pipes and channels upstream of the culvert could have increased the tributary drainage area.

The engineer's job in designing a culvert replacement often is made difficult by the physical constraints within which the design must be accomplished. For example, there might be very little vertical clearance from the stream invert to the top of the existing road. This means that the culvert cannot be made higher, just wider. In some cases, the road can be raised, but this adds considerable cost to the project.

Another typical constraint is the presence of established improvements and utilities adjacent to the existing culvert and stream. This eliminates the option of changing culvert layout.

In performing design of a culvert replacement, the existing culvert is normally analyzed first for its hydraulic adequacy to determine whether the existing opening must be enlarged. Then determination should be made as to whether the road is scheduled for future widening so that the new culvert could be designed longer if necessary.

These design considerations for a culvert replacement project are illustrated in the following example.

Example 13-3

Problem

The existing 36-inch RCP culvert under Washington Road as depicted in Figure 13-11 is proposed to be replaced. Design a replacement culvert.

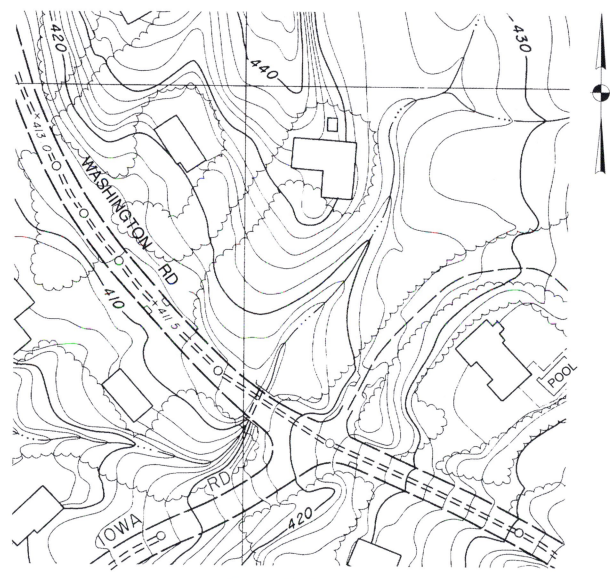

Topographic Map
Scale: 1" = 100'
Contour interval 2'

FIGURE 13-11   Topographic map used in Example 13-3. *(Map adapted from Aero Service.)*

Solution

First, the existing culvert is assessed for hydraulic adequacy. If it is found to be inadequate, a new culvert is designed following the outline presented in Figure 13-1.

Design storm is determined by local regulation to be the 100-year, 24-hour storm as computed by the NRCS Method. This computation is then performed and yields a design discharge of 131 cfs.

Allowable headwater elevation (A.H.E.) is determined by local regulation to be the inundation of the road or the elevation at which floodwater will start to run over the road. This elevation is determined from the topography to be 415.0. (Note: Even though the low-point elevation of the road profile is 411.50, the controlling elevation of 415.0 occurs just west of the culvert on the north side of the road at a low point in the stream bank.)

Existing road and culvert profiles are depicted in Figures 13-12(a) and 13-13(a), respectively.

As is shown in Figure 13-13(a), the existing culvert consists of a 36-inch RCP at the upstream end with a 48-inch CMP finishing at the downstream end. The upstream end has no wingwall, and the downstream end is set in an elaborate concrete apron and wingwall structure. Evidence of considerable erosion at the downstream end is manifest by the drop in stream invert at the end of the apron.

Apparently, the original 36-inch RCP culvert was previously extended for road widening by slipping a 48-inch CMP over the concrete pipe.

To assess the hydraulic adequacy of the existing culvert, first check inlet control. Using Chart 2 in Appendix B-1 for a 36-inch-diameter pipe and design discharge of 131 cfs, *HW/D* is found on scale (3) to be 4.7. Therefore,

$$HW = (4.7)(4.0) = 18.8 \text{ ft}$$

and the headwater elevation is equal to the upstream invert plus *HW*, or

$$411.7 + 18.8 = 430.5$$

which clearly exceeds the A.H.E. of 415.0. Therefore, the existing culvert is inadequate.

Normally, the first step in designing a replacement culvert would be determination of opening size. However, in this case, since vertical alignment can affect capacity, layout will be analyzed first. The horizontal layout will follow the existing culvert because of property constraints. However, as we can see in the profile, Figure 13-13(a), considerable vertical variation is available. Currently, the downstream invert is about 4.5 feet above the stream invert, so the entire culvert could be lowered to match the stream invert. However, this would create a conflict with the existing sanitary sewer main that crosses under the culvert, although the main could be lowered, as shown in Figure 13-12(b).

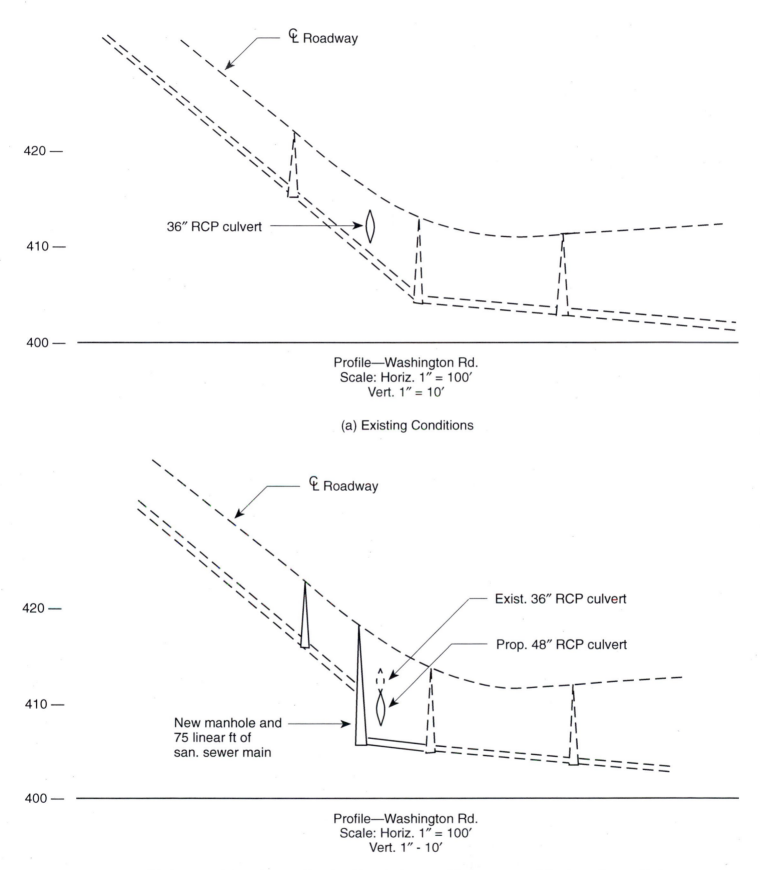

Profile—Washington Rd.
Scale: Horiz. 1″ = 100′
Vert. 1″ = 10′

(a) Existing Conditions

Profile—Washington Rd.
Scale: Horiz. 1″ = 100′
Vert. 1″ - 10′

(b) Proposed Conditions, Showing New Culvert and Reconstructed Sanitary Sewer Main

FIGURE 13-12 Profiles of Washington Road for existing and proposed conditions.

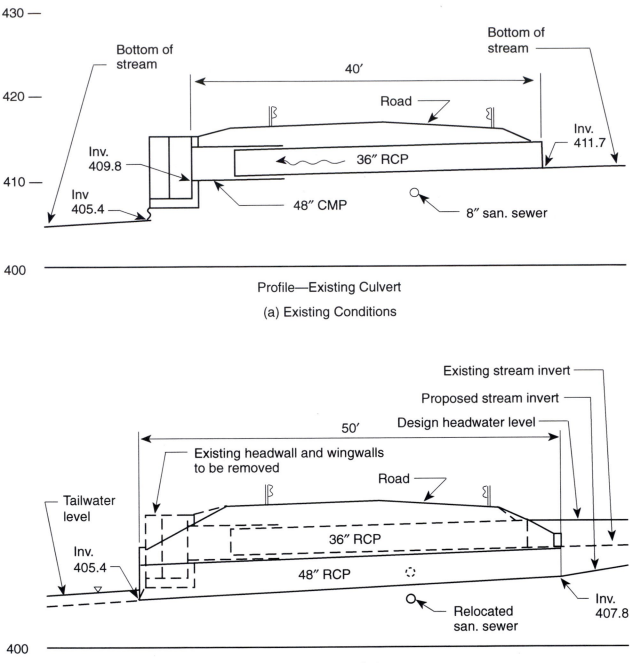

Profile—Existing Culvert

(a) Existing Conditions

Profile—Proposed Culvert

(b) Proposed Conditions Showing New Culvert and Lowered Stream Channel at Upstream End

FIGURE 13-13 Profiles of existing and proposed culverts for Example 13-3.

If the new culvert is lowered at the outlet end, it could also be lowered at the inlet end, as shown in Figure 13-13(b). This would create the advantage of allowing a headwater pool to develop during the design storm, which would increase the capacity of the culvert. However, this is true only if the culvert operates under inlet control. If outlet control prevails, then lowering the inlet end would have no effect on capacity.

Following this reasoning, choose a 36-inch RCP at the lower profile shown in Figure 13-13(b) for Trial 1. Let the new culvert have wingwalls and a square edge. To check inlet control use Chart 2 in Appendix B-1. For a 36-inch pipe, with entrance type (1),

$$\frac{HW}{D} = 5.6$$
$$HW = (5.6)(3.0) = 16.8 \text{ ft}$$

and headwater elevation is

$$407.8 + 16.8 = 424.6$$

Since this elevation exceeds the A.H.E., Trial 1 is rejected.

For Trial 2, choose a 48-inch RCP at the lower profile used in Trial 1. To check inlet control, use Chart 2 in Appendix B-1. For a 48-inch pipe with entrance type (1),

$$\frac{HW}{D} = 1.8$$
$$HW = (1.8)(4) = 7.2 \text{ ft}$$

and headwater elevation is

$$407.8 + 7.2 = 415.0$$

Since this elevation equals the A.H.E., check outlet control.

To check outlet control, first compute tailwater depth, TW. Since the stream has no downstream obstructions, Manning's equation is used. From the topographic map, the gradient of the stream is computed to be 5.0 percent, and a field observation is used to determine an n-value of 0.04 (mountain stream, no vegetation in channel, steep banks, cobbles on bottom). The channel cross section (looking downstream) is shown in Figure 13-14. Using Manning's equation, normal depth is found to be 1.25 feet. This depth is taken as TW. Note that this very shallow depth is due to the steep slope of the stream.

Next, compute critical depth. From Chart 45 in Appendix A-4,

$$D_c = 3.4 \text{ ft}$$

Therefore, TW' is computed as

$$TW' = \frac{(D_c + D)}{2}$$
$$= \frac{3.4 + 4}{2} = 3.7 \text{ ft}$$

Since $TW' > TW$, use TW' to compute headwater elevation. Next, determine H, using Chart 9 in Appendix B-2. For $Q = 131$ cfs, $k_e = 0.5$,

$$H = 2.9 \text{ ft}$$

Therefore, headwater elevation is

$$405.4 + 3.7 + 2.9 = 412.0$$

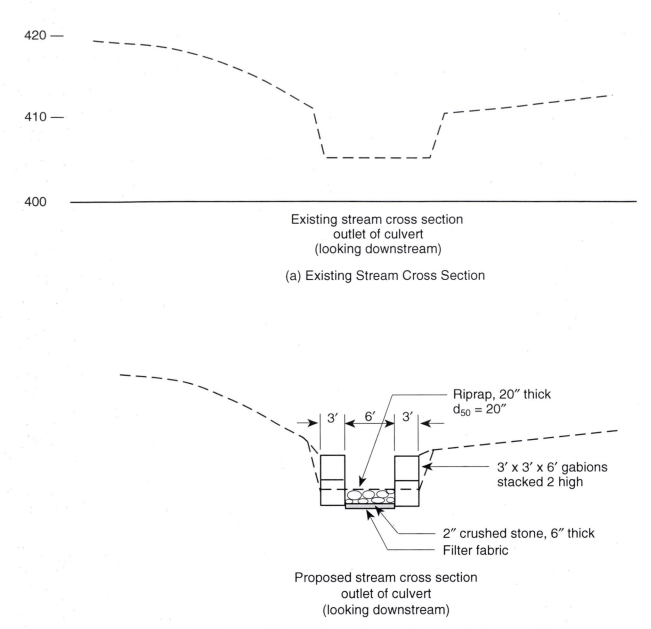

FIGURE 13-14 Cross section of the stream at the downstream end of the culvert for existing and proposed conditions for Example 13-3.

Since a higher headwater elevation is computed for inlet control, the culvert operates under inlet control, and headwater elevation is 415.0.

Therefore, the culvert defined in Trial 2 is adequate.

As we saw in Example 13-2, other culvert arrangements might also be hydraulically adequate. So consider some other trials. The fact that the existing culvert already consists of a 48-inch CMP at the outlet end suggests the possibility of simply replacing the 36-inch RCP and extending the 48-inch CMP up to the inlet end. This alternative would be far less expensive than Trial 2, since the existing wingwalls could be preserved and the sanitary sewer could be left in place. So Trial 3 is a 48-inch CMP at the existing elevation. Unfortunately, we can see immediately that if the inlet end is at a higher elevation than Trial 2, the headwater level will exceed the A.H.E., and the trial must be rejected.

Another problem with Trial 3 is that preserving the downstream wingwall would not make allowance for future road widening, which would be accomplished by Trial 2.

For Trial 4, let's consider a 4-foot by 4-foot concrete box culvert at the lower elevation used in Trial 2. To check inlet control, use Chart 1 in Appendix B-1:

$$\frac{Q}{B} = \frac{131}{4} = 32.75 \text{ cfs/ft}$$

Thus,

$$\frac{HW}{D} = 1.33$$
$$HW = (1.33)(4.0) = 5.3 \text{ ft}$$

Therefore, headwater elevation is

$$407.8 + 5.3 = 413.1$$

To check outlet control, first determine critical depth from Chart 3 in Appendix A-3 or from Equation 6-3:

$$D_c = 3.2 \text{ ft}$$

Therefore, TW' is computed as

$$TW' = \frac{(D_c + D)}{2}$$
$$= \frac{3.2 + 4}{2} = 3.6 \text{ ft}$$

Since $TW' > TW$, use TW' to compute headwater elevation. Next, determine H, using Chart 8 in Appendix B-2:

$$H = 1.7 \text{ ft}$$

Therefore, headwater elevation is

$$405.4 + 3.6 + 1.7 = 410.7$$

Since a higher headwater elevation is computed for inlet control, the culvert operates under inlet control, and headwater elevation is 413.1.

Therefore, the culvert defined in Trial 4 is adequate.

In fact, since the headwater elevation for Trial 4 is 1.9 feet lower than the A.H.E., the inlet end of the culvert could be raised by that amount, thus decreasing the amount of excavation required for installation. However, raising the culvert 1.9 feet to elevation 409.7 would not eliminate the need to reconstruct the sanitary sewer main as in Trial 2.

With all cost factors considered, Trial 4 is significantly more expensive than Trial 2. Therefore, Trial 2 is accepted as the hydraulic design for the culvert replacement project.

Finally, design velocity is computed, and the need for any aprons, upstream and downstream, is assessed. Velocity at the outlet is found by using the continuity equation. Cross-sectional area, a, is the area of a segment of a circle with diameter 4.0 feet. Depth of flow is critical depth, 3.4 feet, since $D_c > TW$. By using Figure 7-3, 3.4 feet is entered as a percent of the diameter, or

$$\frac{3.4}{4.0} = 100\% = 85\%$$

and the corresponding area is read as a percentage—or 90 percent of total area. Therefore,

$$a = (.90)(12.57) = 11.3 \text{ ft}^2$$

and velocity is

$$v = \frac{Q}{A} = \frac{131}{11.3} = 11.6 \text{ ft/s}$$

Referring to Appendix A-2, all permissible velocities for earth channels are exceeded. Therefore, a riprap lining is designed as an outlet apron. From Equation 12-1,

$$d_{50} = \frac{0.02}{1.25}\left(\frac{131}{4}\right)^{4/3}$$
$$= 1.67 \text{ ft} = 20 \text{ in}$$

From Equation 12-2,

$$L_a = \frac{(3)(131)}{4^{3/2}}$$
$$= 49 \text{ ft} \quad (\text{use } 50 \text{ ft})$$

Since a channel exists downstream of the culvert, the riprap will line the channel cross section to a height of 1.0 foot above the tailwater depth. However, a close look at Figure 13-14(a) reveals very steep side slopes. Riprap should not be placed on a slope steeper than two horizontal to one vertical. Therefore, to accommodate riprap, the downstream channel banks should be regraded with two horizontal to one vertical slopes. Unfortunately, not enough room is available in the channel for such grades without severely cutting into adjacent properties. Therefore, we will propose a combination of riprap on the channel bottom and gabions on the sides running for 50 feet along the channel, as shown in Figure 13-14(b).

The riprap thickness is only 20 inches because the relatively large stone size should be stable and a blanket of crushed stone with a filter fabric is provided below the riprap. Next, design velocity is computed at the inlet end of the culvert. Since the culvert operates in a submerged condition, the cross-sectional area is that of the entire opening: 12.57 ft². Therefore,

$$v = \frac{131}{12.57} = 10.4 \text{ ft/s}$$

Referring to Appendix A-2, we find that all permissible velocities for earth channels are again exceeded. Therefore, a protective lining is needed for the channel approaching the culvert. Part of the overall culvert design involves a reconstructed stream channel for a distance of 25 linear feet to drop the stream invert to the new lower invert of the culvert. This results in a channel slope over 10 percent, which will cause excessive velocities under low-flow conditions. That is, the most erosive conditions are not during the 100-year storm but during lesser storms that do not cause ponding at the culvert inlet. Riprap design for this condition is beyond the scope of this text.

The best design solution for erosion protection at the upstream side of this culvert is the use of gabions, grouted riprap, or a concrete slab lining.

13.5   CASE STUDY

In this case, a road is proposed to be reconstructed along a 2200-linear-foot length, including wider pavement, new curbs, storm sewers, and two culvert replacements. The road, named Southern Boulevard, is located in eastern Massachusetts.

This case study focuses on one of the culvert replacements, Culvert No. 1, located at Station 182 + 70. The existing culvert is a 4-foot by 4-foot box culvert conveying a tributary to Black Brook, as shown in Figure 13-15. Because the road will be widened from 22 feet to 36 feet and because the existing culvert construction is substandard, the decision was made to replace the culvert completely.

The first step in the design process was to determine the design storm and method of computation. These are based on the requirements of the regulating and reviewing agency. In this case, the culvert is owned by the county in which it is located and therefore must be reviewed and approved by the county engineering department. County regulations required a 100-year design storm to be computed by the NRCS Method.

Allowable headwater elevation was set by county regulations to be no higher than the lowest point of the road profile. That is, the road could not be overtopped by the headwater pool.

Design Discharge

The next step was to calculate design discharge. The watershed tributary to the culvert was delineated using the USGS Quad sheet covering the project area, together with information from a site reconnaissance.

Drainage area was measured by planimeter to be 231 acres. Therefore,

$A_m = 234$ acres $= 0.361$ s.m.

The curve number, CN, was computed to be 68 on the basis of soils delineated on the county soil survey map, cover conditions shown on the Quad sheet, and observations made during a site visit.

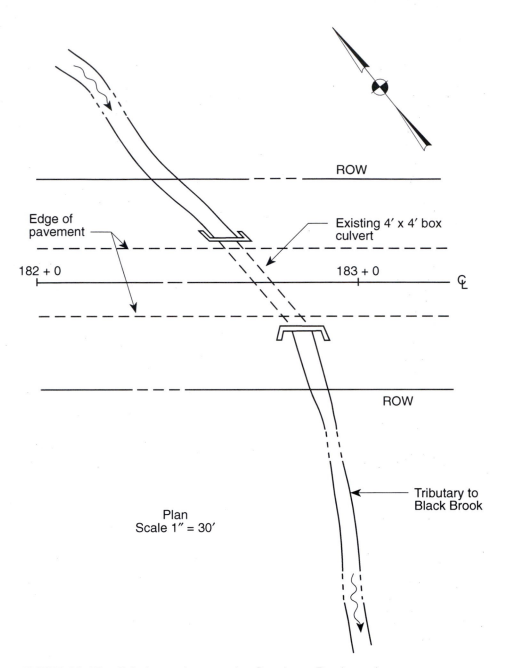

FIGURE 13-15 Existing culvert under Southern Boulevard.

Precipitation for the 100-year, 24-hour storm in eastern Massachusetts was found in Appendix D-3:

$P = 6.7$ in

Next, runoff depth, Q, was determined by using Figure 11-11:

$Q = 3.2$ in

Time of concentration was determined to be 1.10 hours.

Rainfall distribution was found in Appendix D-4 to be

Type III

Next, unit peak discharge, q_u, was determined for a type III rainfall distribution:

$$I_a = 0.941 \quad \text{(from Table 11-2)}$$

$$\frac{I_a}{P} = \frac{0.941}{6.7} = 0.14$$

Using Appendix D-5 (type III rainfall), we have

$$q_u = 270 \text{ csm/in}$$

Finally, peak runoff, q_p, was computed by using Equation 11-6:

$$
\begin{aligned}
q_p &= q_u A_m Q \\
&= (270)(0.361)(3.2) \\
&= 312 \text{ cfs}
\end{aligned}
$$

Existing Culvert Adequacy

Now that design discharge was determined, the existing culvert could be checked for hydraulic adequacy. First, inlet control was assumed. Using Chart 1 in Appendix B-1, we have

$$\frac{Q}{B} = \frac{312}{4} = 78.0 \text{ cfs/ft}$$

and

$$\frac{HW}{D} = 4.2$$

$$HW = (4.2)(4.0) = 16.8 \text{ ft}$$

Therefore, headwater elevation was computed to be equal to the invert elevation at the inlet plus HW, or

$$244.0 + 16.8 = 260.8$$

which was far above the low point of the road centerline, which had elevation 249.72, as shown in Figure 13-16. The actual headwater elevation would be much less than the computed 260.8 but greater than 249.72, because as headwater rises above the road, the backwater pool begins to flow over the road as though it is a large weir. Therefore, actual discharge would be a combination of culvert flow and weir flow, resulting in a headwater elevation about 8 inches above the road, or approximately 250.4.

This computation established the fact that the existing culvert was hydraulically inadequate because the road would be overtopped. Since the road cannot be overtopped, the allowable headwater elevation (A.H.E.) became that of the proposed road low point, or 249.42.

Hydraulic Design

With the allowable headwater elevation established, hydraulic design of the proposed culvert could begin. First, tailwater elevation was computed by using Manning's equation, since the downstream channel contained no significant

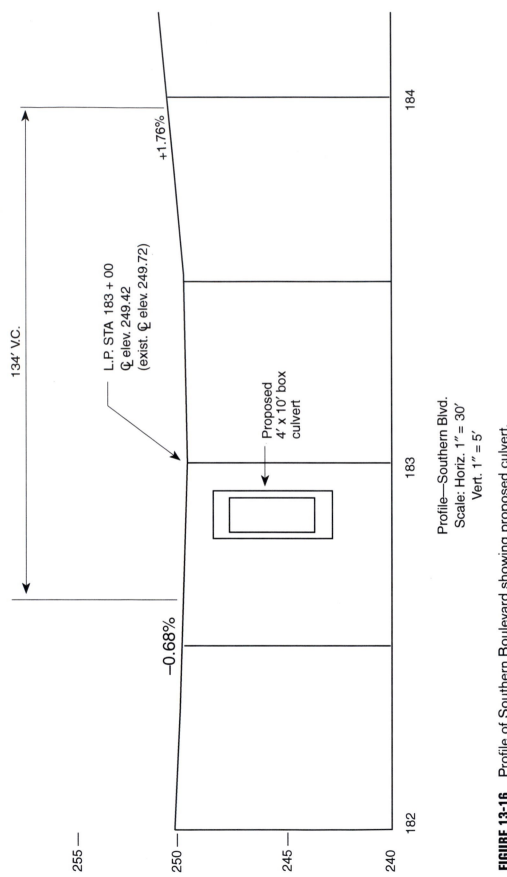

FIGURE 13-16   Profile of Southern Boulevard showing proposed culvert.

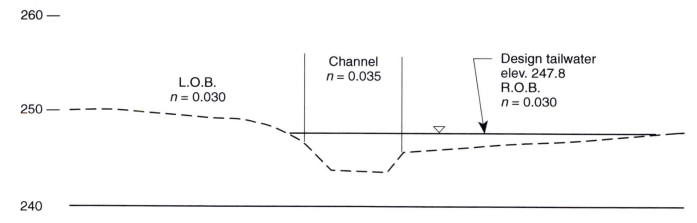

Stream Cross-Section at Outlet of Culvert (looking downstream)
Scale: 1″ = 10′

FIGURE 13-17   Cross section of stream at outlet end of culvert.

obstructions creating a backwater condition. A cross section of the stream at the culvert outlet is shown in Figure 13-17. Normal depth was determined to be 4.13 feet, giving a tailwater elevation of 247.80, which was above the culvert crown. What does this tell you about inlet control?

For a first trial in selecting culvert size, a box culvert with height 4 feet was assumed, since the proposed road elevation would not allow a culvert with greater height. So trial 1 was taken as a 4-foot by 8-foot box culvert.

Since tailwater was above the crown, outlet control was assumed. Entrance coefficient, k_e, was found in Appendix B-3 to be 0.4 for flared wingwalls and square edge. Then, using Chart 8 of Appendix B-2, we have

$$H = 2.3 \text{ ft}$$

Therefore, headwater elevation was equal to tailwater elevation plus H, or

$$247.8 + 2.3 = 250.1$$

This elevation exceeds the A.H.E. of 249.42, so Trial 1 was rejected.

For Trial 2, a 4-foot by 10-foot box culvert was assumed. Again using Chart 8 in Appendix B-2, we have

$$H = 1.5 \text{ ft}$$

Therefore, headwater elevation was equal to tailwater elevation plus H, or

$$247.8 + 1.5 = 249.3$$

This elevation is less than the A.H.E., so Trial 2 was accepted, and the culvert size was set at 4 feet by 10 feet.

Layout

The next step was the culvert layout. Because the land outside the road right-of-way was not owned by the county, any redirection of the stream was precluded and the only culvert layout option was a skew similar to the orientation of the existing culvert. Figure 13-18 illustrates the process used to determine the layout.

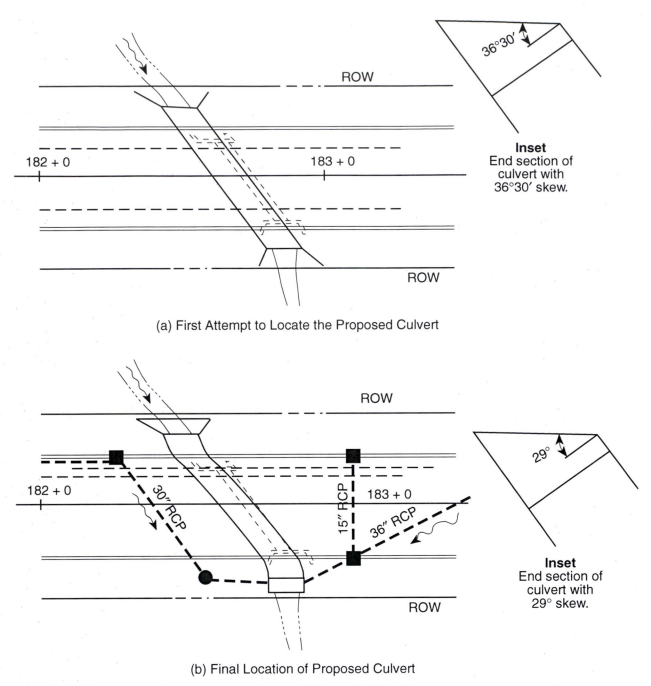

FIGURE 13-18 Location of proposed culvert within road right-of-way.

In Figure 13-18(a), a precast concrete box culvert was laid out with sufficient length to clear the proposed road with extra room for sidewalks on both sides. This resulted in a skew angle of 36°30′, which created difficulties in manufacturing the two end sections. A solution was conceived by adding bend sections near the two ends, as shown in Figure 13-18(b). Slightly bending the culvert resulted in end sections with 29° skews, which was within acceptable manufacturing limits. The bend sections are illustrated more clearly in Figure 13-19, which shows the final culvert design. The slight bending of the culvert would not significantly alter its hydraulic functioning.

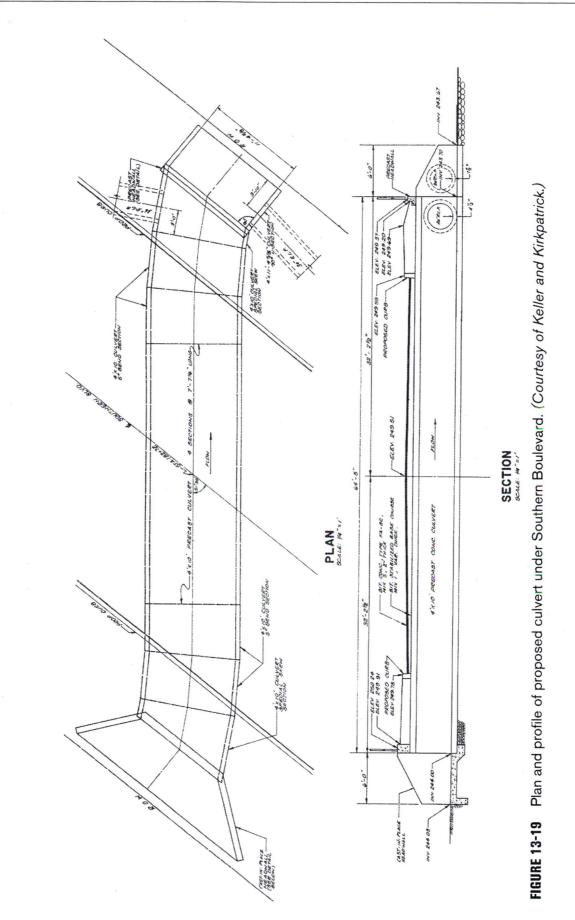

FIGURE 13-19 Plan and profile of proposed culvert under Southern Boulevard. (*Courtesy of Keller and Kirkpatrick.*)

Apron Design

Finally, a riprap lining for the stream was designed. The outlet velocity was computed by using the continuity equation, taking the full culvert opening for cross-sectional area because tailwater was above the crown. Therefore,

$$v = \frac{Q}{a}$$
$$= \frac{312}{40}$$
$$= 7.8 \text{ ft/s}$$

This velocity exceeds all permissible velocities included in Appendix A-2, so riprap was chosen as a suitable channel lining. Stone size was computed by using Equation 12-1:

$$d_{50} = \frac{0.02}{TW}\left(\frac{Q}{D_0}\right)^{4/3}$$
$$= \frac{0.2}{4.13}\left(\frac{312}{10}\right)^{4/3}$$
$$= 0.48 \text{ ft} = 5.7 \text{ in} \quad (\text{use } d_{50} = 6 \text{ in})$$

The riprap lining length was computed by using Equation 12-2:

$$L_a = \frac{3Q}{D_0^{3/2}}$$
$$= \frac{(3)(315)}{10^{3/2}}$$
$$= 29.9 \text{ ft} \quad (\text{use } L_a = 30.0 \text{ ft})$$

Therefore, riprap was proposed for a length of 30 feet downstream from the culvert using a median stone size of 6 inches and thickness of 12 inches with filter fabric on the bottom. The riprap was proposed to extend to the top of the right bank, which is only 2 feet high, and to the top of the left bank, which is about 3 feet high.

The downstream riprap would be contained within an existing stream easement. On the upstream end of the culvert, no riprap was proposed, since no easement existed or could be obtained outside the extent of the road right-of-way. However, as is shown in Figure 13-19, an upstream concrete apron was provided.

PROBLEMS

1. A 30-foot-wide road is proposed to be constructed over an existing stream as shown in Figure 13-20. Determine the best layout for a proposed 10-foot-wide box culvert to fit the following constraints:

    a. The culvert must extend 10 feet beyond each edge of the proposed road.

    b. The cost of the proposed culvert is $2000 per linear foot.

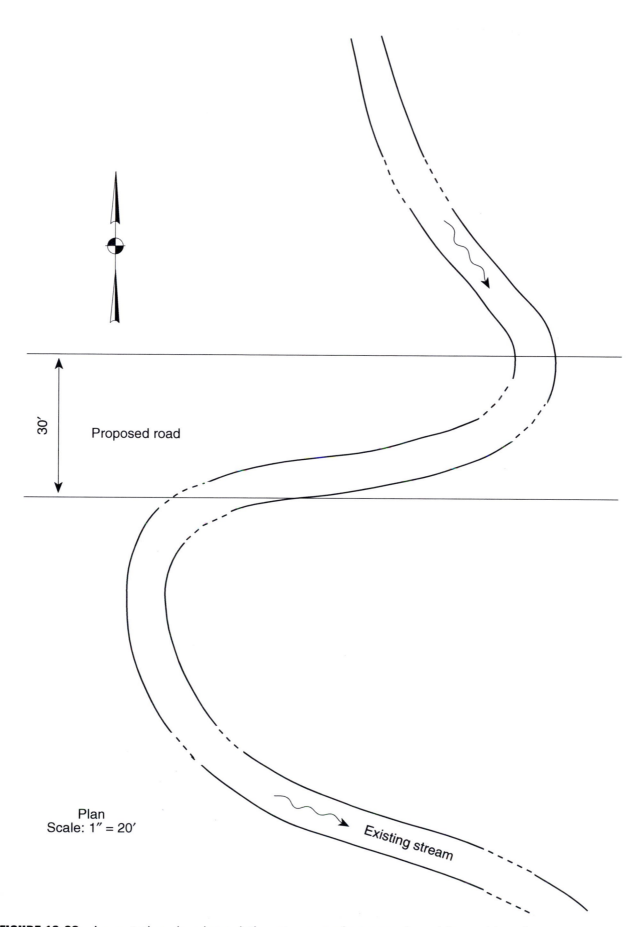

30′

Proposed road

Plan
Scale: 1″ = 20′

Existing stream

FIGURE 13-20 Layout plan showing existing stream and proposed road for problem 1.

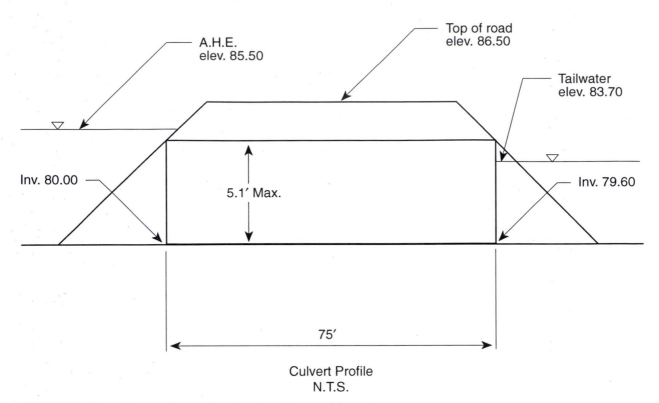

FIGURE 13-21   Schematic profile of culvert for problem 2.

   c. The cost of stream relocation is $250 per linear foot.

   d. The maximum culvert skew is 24°.

To analyze this problem, place a piece of transparent vellum over Figure 13-20 and trace the plan, then sketch the proposed culvert on the vellum.

2. The opening size of a proposed culvert under a new road is to be determined. The culvert, shown schematically in Figure 13-21, will have a height no greater than 5.1 feet. Design discharge has been computed to be 420 cfs. Find the culvert opening dimensions for the following shapes:

   a. Circular concrete pipe

   b. Concrete box

   Note: Multiple barrels are allowed, and each culvert has 45-degree wingwalls and a square edge entrance. Which shape would you choose?

3. Figure 13-22 shows an existing road and existing culvert. Evaluate the hydraulic adequacy of the culvert for a design discharge of 860 cfs and A.H.E. equal to the top of road, or elevation 184.5. Computed tailwater depth is 3.9 feet, giving a tailwater elevation of 181.3.

   If the culvert is inadequate, design a replacement culvert using flared wingwalls and a square edge entrance. Also, design riprap outlet protection if needed. Figure 13-23 shows the existing stream profile.

4. Figure 13-24 shows an existing road and existing culvert consisting of three 30-inch concrete pipes. Evaluate the hydraulic adequacy of the culvert for a design discharge of 152 cfs and A.H.E. equal to the top of road, or elevation

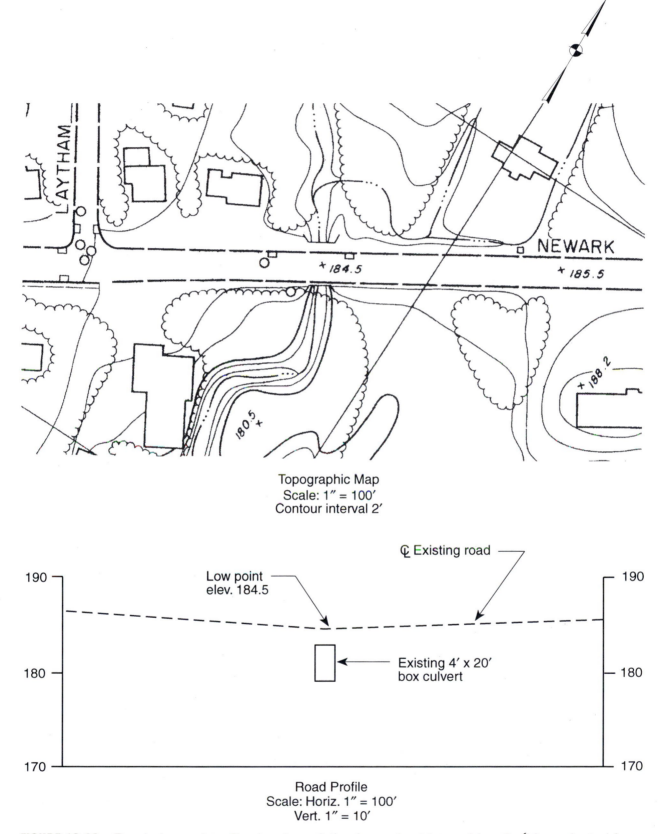

Topographic Map
Scale: 1″ = 100′
Contour interval 2′

Road Profile
Scale: Horiz. 1″ = 100′
Vert. 1″ = 10′

FIGURE 13-22 Road plan and profile showing existing box culvert for problem 3. *(Map adapted from Aero Service.)*

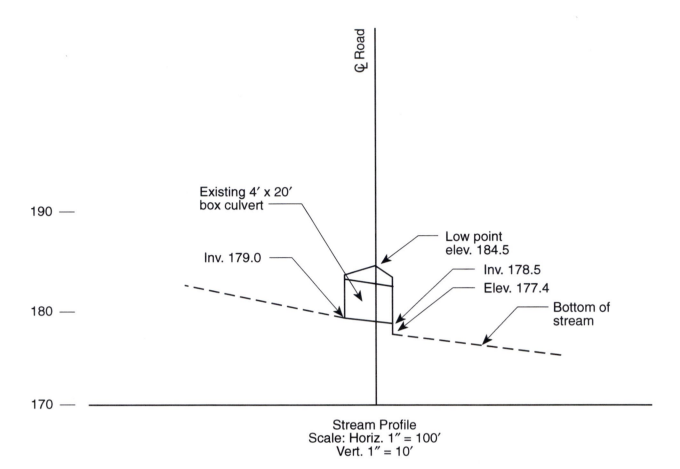

FIGURE 13-23 Stream profile showing existing culvert for problem 3.

320.9. Computed tailwater depth is 3.25 feet, giving a tailwater elevation of 320.00.

If the culvert is inadequate, design a replacement culvert using flared wing-walls and a square edge entrance. Also design riprap outlet protection if needed. Keep in mind that the culvert crown cannot be made much higher because of the existing road. Figures 13-25 and 13-26 show profiles of Brickel Avenue and the stream, respectively.

5. Figure 13-27 shows the location of a proposed road to connect Carol Place to Dwight Street. Design a culvert to convey the existing stream under the proposed road. Design discharge has been computed to be 340 cfs. Figures 13-28 and 13-29 show profiles of the proposed road and existing stream, respectively.

Notice the water surface profile shown in Figure 13-29. The profile shows a flow depth of 3.25 feet upstream of the proposed culvert and 3.0 feet downstream. The upstream depth is needed to evaluate the A.H.E., which is defined as being no higher than 0.2 foot above existing water level.

Also, design riprap outlet protection, if needed.

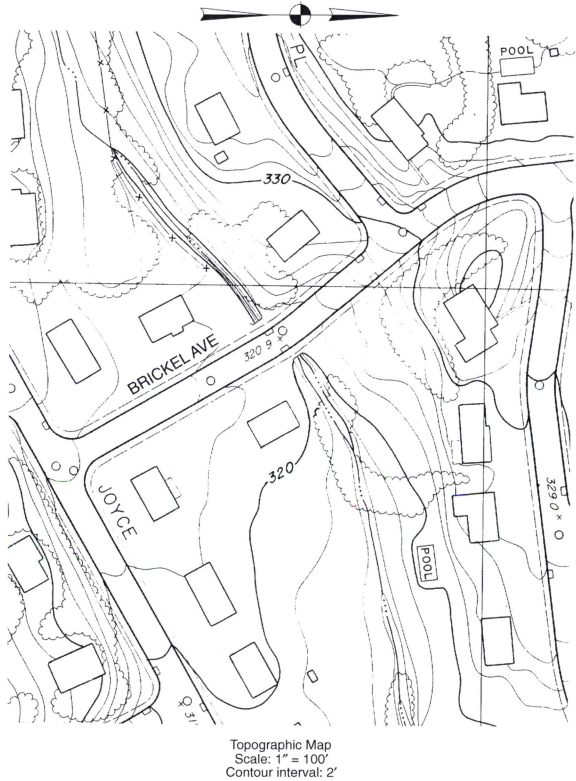

Topographic Map
Scale: 1″ = 100′
Contour interval: 2′

FIGURE 13-24   Plan of existing culvert for problem 4. *(Map adapted from Aero Service.)*

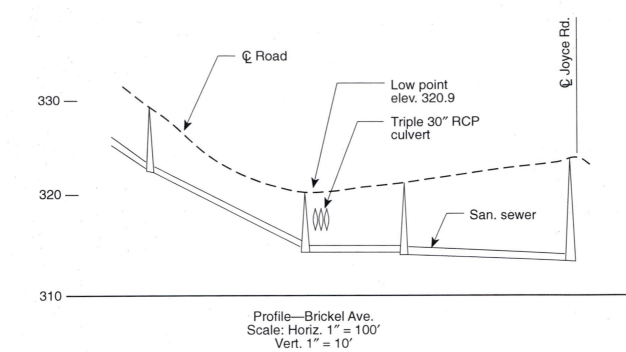

Profile—Brickel Ave.
Scale: Horiz. 1″ = 100′
Vert. 1″ = 10′

FIGURE 13-25 Profile of road showing existing culvert for problem 4.

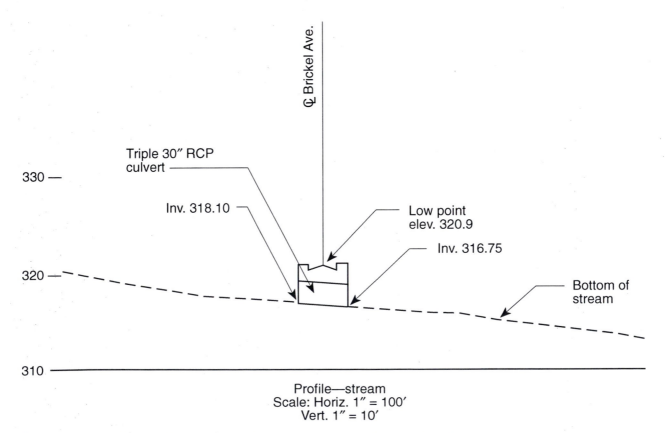

Profile—stream
Scale: Horiz. 1″ = 100′
Vert. 1″ = 10′

FIGURE 13-26 Profile of stream showing existing culvert for problem 4.

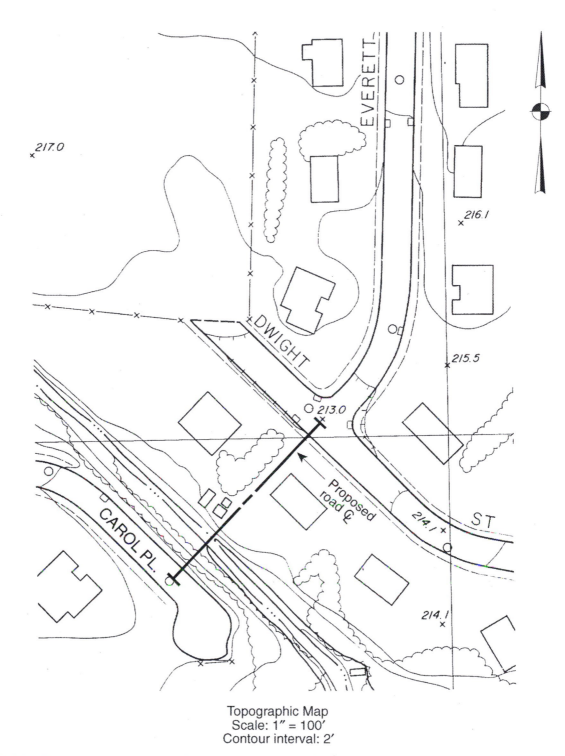

Topographic Map
Scale: 1" = 100'
Contour interval: 2'

FIGURE 13-27   Plan of proposed road location for problem 5. *(Map adapted from Aero Service.)*

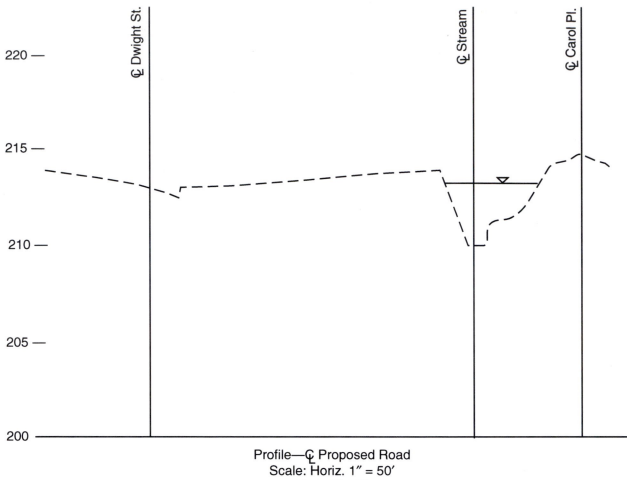

Profile—℄ Proposed Road
Scale: Horiz. 1″ = 50′
Vert. 1″ = 5′

FIGURE 13-28 Profile of proposed road for problem 5.

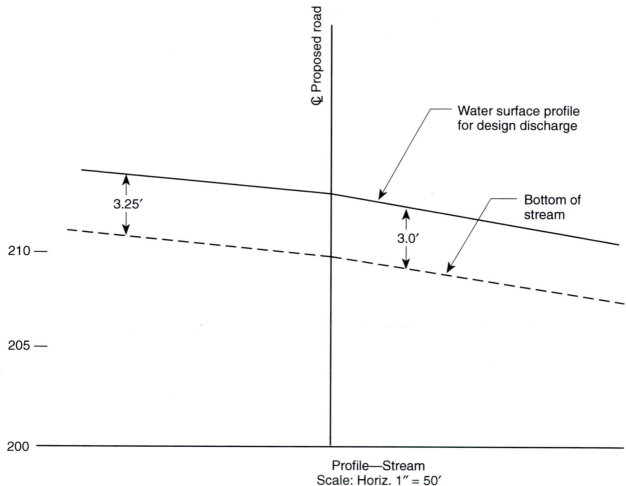

FIGURE 13-29 Profile of existing stream for problem 5.

FURTHER READING

Herr, L. (1965 revision). *Hydraulic Charts for the Selection of Highway Culverts,* Hydraulic Engineering Circular No. 5. Washington, DC: U.S. Department of Commerce, Bureau of Public Roads.

U.S. Department of Transportation, Federal Highway Administration (1967). *Use of Riprap for Bank Protection,* Hydraulic Engineering Circular No. 11. Washington, DC: Department of Transportation.

U.S. Department of Transportation, Federal Highway Administration (1975). *Design of Stable Channels with Flexible Linings,* Hydraulic Engineering Circular No. 15. Washington, DC: Department of Transportation.

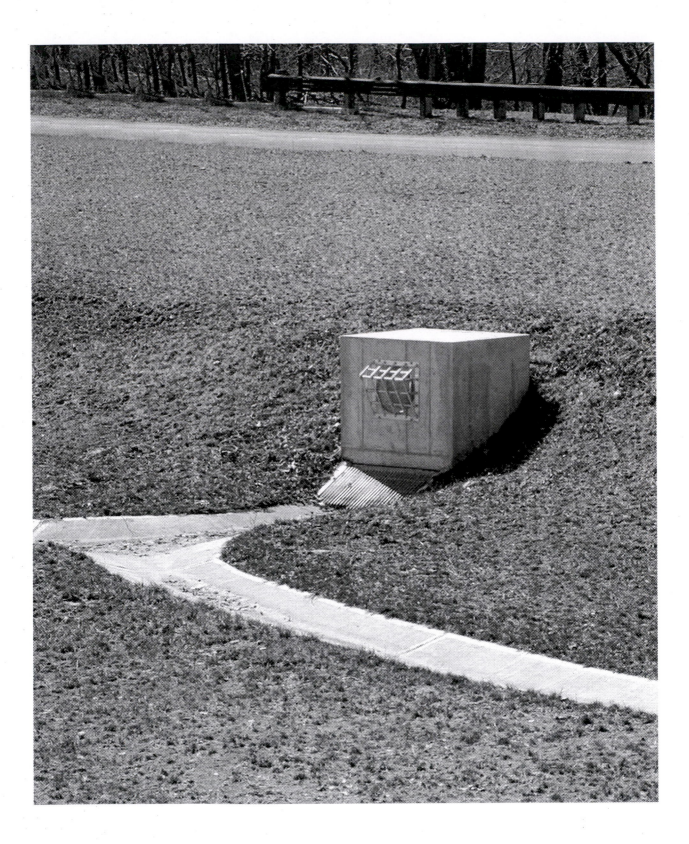

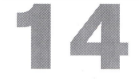

STORMWATER DETENTION

Detention of stormwater is based on the concept of storing runoff temporarily and then releasing it in a controlled manner to limit the rate of runoff leaving a site of development and mitigate the destructive effects of increased runoff. Other purposes of stormwater detention include water quality control and recharge.

In this chapter, we will learn the fundamental principles governing the detention process and the methods used to calculate the results. The storage and controlled release of stormwater are described mathematically as the routing of a runoff hydrograph. The concept of routing was introduced in Section 10.6 as it applies to streams. In this case, it will be applied to stormwater impoundments or reservoirs. Also discussed are the key components of detention basins, including the outlet structure and the emergency spillway.

OBJECTIVES

After completing this chapter, the reader should be able to:

- Compute impoundment volume by the elevation-area method
- Compute impoundment outflow using orifice and weir
- Compute a reservoir routing by hand

14.1 STORMWATER IMPOUNDMENT

The **impoundment** is the volume of water temporarily stored in a detention basin during a rainfall event. In the case of a wet basin, it is the volume of water stored above the permanent water level, that is, not including the permanent pool. The usual impoundment is provided by excavating an open cut in the ground and allowing stormwater to accumulate in the open cut. In some cases, an earth **berm** must be constructed at one end of the detention basin to provide sufficient storage volume. Figure 14-1 shows two cases of open-cut impoundments, one requiring an earth berm and one not needing a berm.

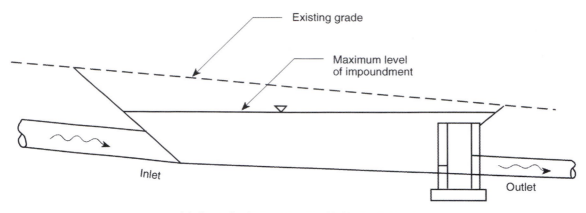

(a) Open-Cut Impoundment with No Berm Needed

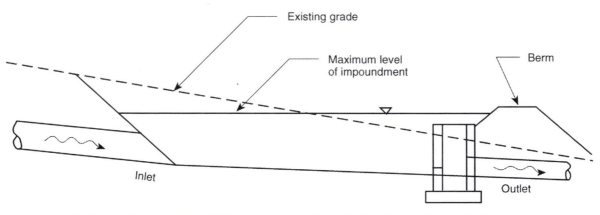

(b) Open-Cut Impoundment with Berm Required at Low End to Contain Stormwater Storage

FIGURE 14-1 Cross section views of two examples of open-cut impoundments.

The usual method for computing storage volume is the elevation-area method. In this method, contour lines are traced around the proposed basin, and the area contained within each contour is measured. A table of elevations and corresponding areas is then made. The volume contained between any two adjacent contours is estimated as the average of the two areas multiplied by the vertical distance between them. Each volume thus computed is an incremental volume, and the total volume is the sum of the incremental volumes.

The elevation-area method is illustrated in the following example.

Example 14-1

Problem

Find the volume contained in the open-cut detention basin shown in Figure 14-2 up to the elevation 236. Areas contained within the contours were measured by planimeter as follows:

Elevation (ft)	Area (ft^2)
230	0
231	250
232	840
233	1350
234	2280
235	3680
236	5040

Solution

Prepare a chart with four columns as shown below, the first two columns being a copy of the data shown above.

(1) Elevation (ft)	(2) Area (ft^2)	(3) Incremental Volume (ft^3)	(4) Cumulative Volume (ft^3)
230	0	0	0
231	250	125	125
232	840	545	670
233	1350	1095	1765
234	2280	1815	3580
235	3680	2980	6560
236	5040	4360	10,920

Each value in column 3 represents the volume contained between that elevation and the next lower elevation. The first value is zero because elevation 230 is the lowest elevation and there is no volume contained beneath it. The second value in column 3 is found by averaging the first two values in column 2 and multiplying by the difference between the first two elevations in column 1:

$$\frac{250+0}{2} \times 1 = 125 \text{ ft}^3$$

The third value in column 3 is computed by averaging the second and third values in column 2 and multiplying by the difference between the second and third elevations in column 1:

$$\frac{840+250}{2} \times 1 = 545 \text{ ft}^3$$

The rest of the values in column 3 are computed in like manner.

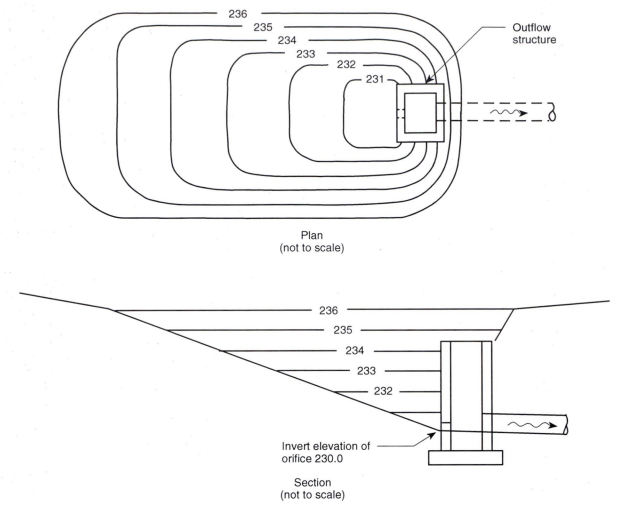

FIGURE 14-2 Schematic illustration of a proposed open-cut detention basin showing 1-foot contour intervals.

Each value in column 4 represents the sum of all values in column 3 up to and including that elevation. The first value is zero because the first value in column 2 is zero. The second value is computed by adding the first two values in column 3:

$$0 + 125 = 125 \text{ ft}^3$$

The third value is computed by adding the first three values in column 3:

$$0 + 125 + 545 = 670 \text{ ft}^3$$

The remaining values in column 4 are computed in like manner.

The total volume up to elevation 236 is the value in column 4 opposite elevation 236, or 10,920 ft^3. (Answer)

For underground detention basins using pipes for storage, the elevation-area method for computing volume is not convenient, so another method must be used. The easiest computation is by the average end-area method that is illustrated by the following example.

Example 14-2

Problem

Find the volume contained in the pipe detention basin shown in Figure 14-3.

Solution

Prepare a chart with four columns, as shown below:

(1)	(2)	(3)	(4)
	Downstream	Upstream	
Elevation	Area	Area	Volume
(ft)	(ft^2)	(ft^2)	(ft^3)
520	0	0	0
521	2.39	0	239
522	6.29	2.39	868
523	10.1	6.29	1639
524	12.6	10.1	2270
525	12.6	12.6	2520

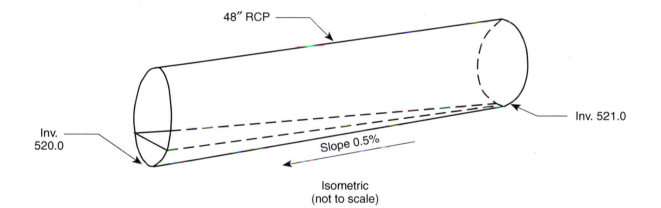

Isometric
(not to scale)

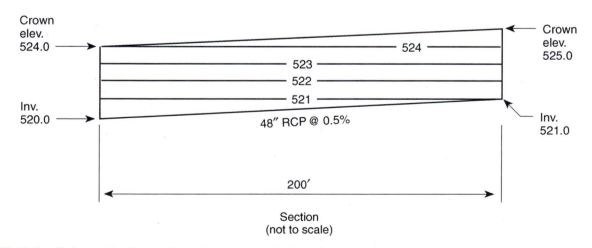

Section
(not to scale)

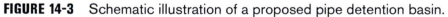

FIGURE 14-3   Schematic illustration of a proposed pipe detention basin.

Each value in column 2 represents the area of the segment of a circle related to the depth of water at the downstream end of the pipe. (The pipe is designed with a slight gradient so that it will completely drain after each storm.)

The first value is zero because elevation 520 is at the invert of the pipe. To find the second value in column 2, use Figure 7-3. Elevation 521 represents a depth of 1.0 foot, which is 25 percent of the pipe diameter. Therefore, enter Figure 7-3 at 25 percent depth of flow, and extend a line to the right until it intersects the area line. From this intersection, drop a line straight down and read the percentage on the Hydraulic Elements scale. The resulting area is 19 percent of the full cross-sectional area, which is 12.57 ft^2. Therefore, the area is

$$(12.57)(0.19) = 2.39 \text{ ft}^2$$

The third value in column 2 corresponds to elevation 522, which represents a depth of 2.0 feet, 50 percent of the pipe diameter. Therefore, enter Figure 7-3 at 50 percent and read 50 percent on the Hydraulic Elements scale. The area is thus

$$(12.57)(0.50) = 6.29 \text{ ft}^2$$

The fourth value corresponds to elevation 523, which represents a depth of 3.0 feet, 75 percent of the pipe diameter. Enter Figure 7-3 at 75 percent, and the Hydraulic Elements scale reads 80 percent. Therefore, the area is

$$(12.57)(0.80) = 10.1 \text{ ft}^2$$

The fifth value corresponds to elevation 524, which represents full depth at the downstream end of the pipe. Therefore, the area is 12.6 ft^2.

The sixth value corresponds to elevation 525, which also represents full depth at the downstream end of the pipe. Therefore, the area again is 12.6 ft^2.

Each value in column 3 represents the area of the segment of a circle related to the depth of water at the upstream end of the pipe. The first value is zero because there is no water in the pipe. The second value also is zero because when the water level reaches elevation 521, it just reaches the invert at the upstream end, which represents a depth of zero foot at that end.

The third value in column 3 corresponds to elevation 522, which represents a depth of 1.0 foot. By using Figure 7-3, the area is 19 percent of full area, or 2.39 ft^2.

The remaining values in column 3 are determined in the same manner as those in column 2.

Each value in column 4 is found by computing the average of the two corresponding end areas in columns 2 and 3 and then multiplying by the distance between the ends. The first value is

$$\frac{0+0}{2} \times 200 = 0 \text{ ft}^3$$

The second value is

$$\frac{2.39+0}{2} \times 200 = 239 \text{ ft}^3$$

The third value is

$$\frac{6.29 + 2.39}{2} \times 200 = 868 \text{ ft}^3$$

The remaining values are determined by using the same method. The total volume is the value in column 4 corresponding to the highest elevation of the pipe, or 2520 ft³.   (Answer)

> *Note:* It would be much faster to compute total volume as you would a cylinder: end area multiplied by length. However, the full tabular format is needed for subsequent detention basin design calculations.

14.2   OUTLET STRUCTURE

Impounded water in a detention basin is released slowly through the outlet structure, which usually consists of an orifice or combination orifice and weir. The simplest outlet structure consists of a single pipe with invert set at the lowest elevation of the basin. This is called a *single-stage outlet* because water is allowed to flow out through only one opening. However, another higher outlet generally is provided as an emergency relief to be used only if the outlet structure cannot handle the entire storm runoff. Emergency spillways are analyzed separately in the next section.

Figure 14-4 shows a single-stage outlet in the form of a single pipe installed in the berm of a detention basin. Although an open-cut basin is depicted, single-stage outlets can be used with underground detention as well.

The sketch in Figure 14-4 suggests that this single-stage outlet resembles a culvert, and indeed, it does act hydraulically as a culvert, usually with inlet control. However, such a single-stage arrangement is usually modeled as an orifice because the orifice model yields discharges very similar to a culvert acting with inlet control, especially for impoundment depths above the pipe crown. In these cases, the pipe experiences Type B flow, as shown in Figure 9-6.

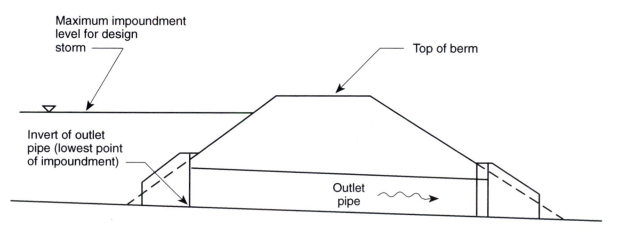

FIGURE 14-4   Typical single stage outlet.

As part of the detention basin calculations, a **discharge rating** of the outlet is computed. That is, for a series of hypothetical water levels in the impoundment, corresponding discharge through the orifice is determined. The following example illustrates this computation.

Example 14-3

Problem

An outlet consisting of a 12-inch pipe is proposed for the detention basin shown in Figure 14-4. The invert of the pipe is 322.0, and the top of berm is set at elevation 327.0. Compute the discharge rating for the outlet.

Solution

Assume that the pipe opening is a 12-inch orifice and that discharge is computed by using Equation 5-3. Then compute discharge for water level elevations of 322, 323, 324, 325, 326, and 327.

For water level elevation 322, head is equal to zero because water level is at the invert of the orifice. Discharge therefore also is zero.

For water level elevation 323, head is determined to be 0.5 foot, as shown in the figure below.

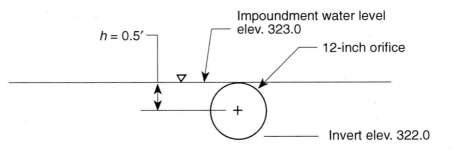

The area of the orifice is

$$a = \frac{\pi(1.0)^2}{4} = 0.785 \text{ ft}^2$$

and the discharge, Q, is

$$Q = ca\sqrt{2gh}$$
$$= (0.62)(0.785)\sqrt{2(32.2)(0.5)}$$
$$= 2.76 \text{ cfs} \quad \text{(Answer)}$$

For water level elevation 324, head is determined to be 1.5 feet, as shown in the figure below.

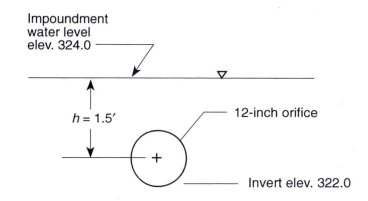

Therefore, discharge is

$$Q = ca\sqrt{2gh}$$
$$= (0.62)(0.785)\sqrt{2(32.2)(1.5)}$$
$$= 4.78 \text{ cfs} \quad \text{(Answer)}$$

For water level elevation 325, head is determined to be 2.5 feet. Therefore, discharge is

$$Q = (0.62)(0.785)\sqrt{2(32.2)(2.5)}$$
$$= 6.18 \text{ cfs} \quad \text{(Answer)}$$

For water level elevation 326, head is determined to be 3.5 feet. Therefore, discharge is

$$Q = (0.62)(0.785)\sqrt{2(32.2)(3.5)}$$
$$= 7.31 \text{ cfs} \quad \text{(Answer)}$$

Finally, for water level elevation 327, head is determined to be 4.5 feet, and discharge is computed as

$$Q = (0.62)(0.785)\sqrt{2(32.2)(4.5)}$$
$$= 8.29 \text{ cfs} \quad \text{(Answer)}$$

These results are then summarized in the following table:

W.L. Elev. (ft)	12″ Orifice	
	h (ft)	Q (cfs)
322	0	0
323	0.5	2.76
324	1.5	4.78
325	2.5	6.18
326	3.5	7.31
327	4.5	8.29

Multistage Outlet

Often, a detention basin design requires a two-stage outlet, or multiple stages beyond two, to create a special distribution of discharges to meet particular design conditions. Figures 14-5 and 14-6 show typical two-stage and three-stage outlet structures, respectively.

To compute a discharge rating for this type of outlet structure, each stage is considered separately, and then all discharges are added to give the total discharge.

The following example illustrates typical computations for a multiple stage outlet structure.

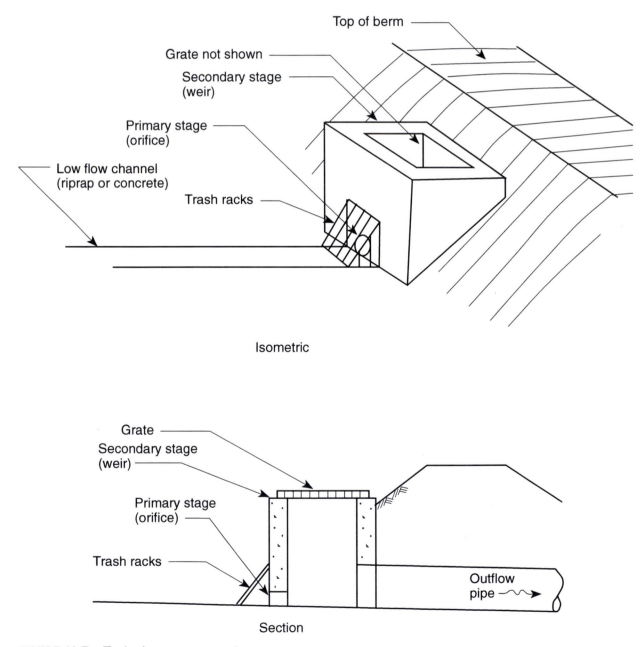

Isometric

Section

FIGURE 14-5 Typical two-stage outlet structure.

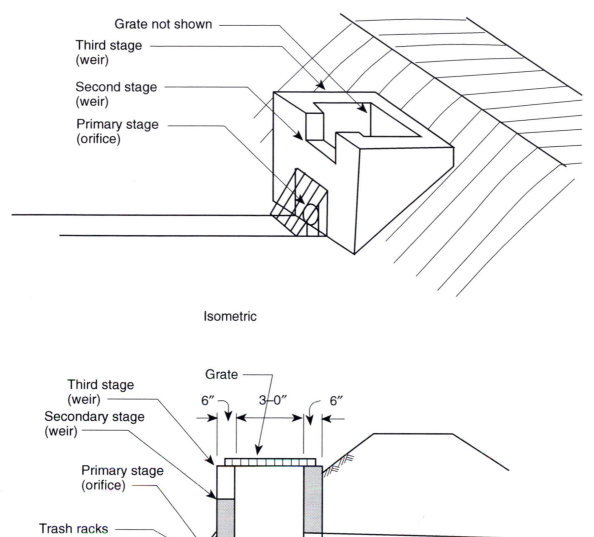

Isometric

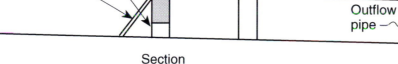

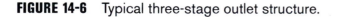

Section

FIGURE 14-6   Typical three-stage outlet structure.

Example 14-4

Problem

A three-stage outlet structure similar to that shown in Figure 14-6 is proposed for a detention basin design. Key elevations are as follows:

1. Primary stage (4-inch orifice): Invert elevation 560.0
2. Second stage (1.5-foot weir): Crest elevation 562.67
3. Third stage (12.5-foot weir): Crest elevation 563.67
4. Top of berm: elevation 565.0
5. Outflow pipe: (48-inch diameter)—Invert elevation 558.0

Note: For this example, assume no emergency spillway.

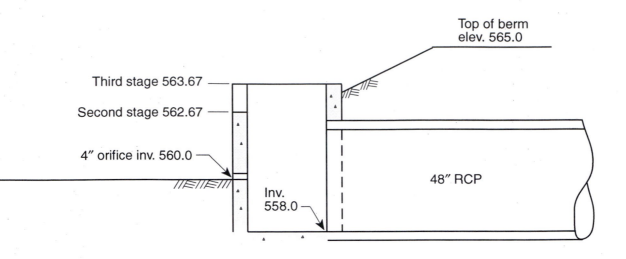

Compute the discharge rating for the outlet structure.

Solution

To create a discharge rating, compute discharge for a series of elevations ranging from the bottom of the basin (elevation 560.0) to the top of the berm (elevation 565.0). The elevations can be every whole foot but should include each stage along the way. Thus, the water level elevations to be considered are 560, 561, 562, 562.67, 563.67, 564, and 565.

For water level elevation 560, head for the orifice is equal to zero because water level is at the invert of the orifice. Discharge therefore also is zero.

For water level elevation 561, head is determined to be 0.83 foot, as shown below.

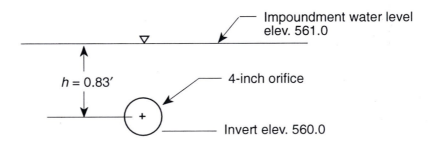

The area of the orifice is

$$a = \frac{\pi(0.333)^2}{4}$$
$$= 0.087 \text{ ft}^2$$

and the discharge, Q, is

$$Q = ca\sqrt{2gh}$$
$$= (0.62)(0.087)\sqrt{2(32.2)(0.83)}$$
$$= 0.39 \text{ cfs}$$

For water level elevation 562, head is determined to be 1.83 feet because it is 1.0 foot higher than the previous value of head. Therefore, discharge is

$$Q = (0.62)(0.087)\sqrt{2(32.2)(1.83)}$$
$$= 0.59 \text{ cfs}$$

For water level elevation 562.67, head is determined to be 2.5 feet. Therefore, discharge is

$$Q = (0.62)(0.087)\sqrt{2(32.2)(2.5)}$$
$$= 0.68 \text{ cfs}$$

For water level elevation 563.67, head is determined to be 3.5 feet. Therefore, discharge is

$$Q = (0.62)(0.087)\sqrt{2(32.2)(3.5)}$$
$$= 0.81 \text{ cfs}$$

For water level elevation 564, head is determined to be 3.83 feet. Therefore, discharge is

$$Q = (0.62)(0.087)\sqrt{2(32.2)(3.83)}$$
$$= 0.85 \text{ cfs}$$

For water level elevation 565, head is determined to be 4.83 feet. Therefore, discharge is

$$Q = (0.62)(0.087)\sqrt{2(32.2)(4.83)}$$
$$= 0.95 \text{ cfs}$$

Next, discharge over the second-stage weir is computed by using Equation 5-4. For water level elevations 560, 561, and 562, discharge is zero because the water is below the weir crest. At elevation 562.67, water level is just at the crest, so head is equal to zero, and once again discharge is zero.

For water level elevation 563.67, head is determined to be 1.0 foot. Since the outlet structure wall thickness is 0.5 foot, discharge coefficient, c, is found in Appendix A-5 to be 3.32 for all values of head equal to and greater than 1.0 foot. Therefore, discharge is

$$Q = cLH^{3/2}$$
$$= (3.32)(1.5)(1.0)^{3/2}$$
$$= 4.98 \text{ cfs}$$

For water level elevation 564, head is determined to be 1.33 feet. Therefore, discharge is

$$Q = (3.32)(1.5)(1.33)^{3/2}$$
$$= 7.64 \text{ cfs}$$

For water level elevation 565, head is determined to be 2.33 feet. Therefore, discharge is

$$Q = (3.32)(1.5)(2.33)^{3/2}$$
$$= 17.7 \text{ cfs}$$

Next, discharge over the third-stage weir is computed. Discharge is zero for water level elevations 560, 561, 562, 562.67, and 563.67.

For water level elevation 564, head is determined to be 0.33 foot. Therefore, discharge is

$$Q = (3.32)(12.5)(0.33)^{3/2}$$
$$= 7.87 \text{ cfs}$$

For water level elevation 565, head is determined to be 1.33 feet. Therefore, discharge is

$$Q = (3.32)(12.5)(1.33)^{3/2}$$
$$= 63.7 \text{ cfs}$$

These results are then summarized in the following table:

W.L. Elev (ft)	4″ Orifice		1.5′ Weir		12.5′ Weir		Total Q (cfs)
	h (ft)	Q (cfs)	H (ft)	Q (cfs)	H (ft)	Q (cfs)	
560	0.0	0.0	—	—	—	—	0.0
561	0.83	0.39	—	—	—	—	0.39
562	1.83	0.59	—	—	—	—	0.59
562.67	2.5	0.68	0.0	0.0	—	—	0.68
563.67	3.5	0.81	1.0	4.98	0.0	0.0	5.79
564	3.83	0.85	1.33	7.64	0.33	7.87	16.36
565	4.83	0.95	2.33	17.7	1.33	63.7	82.4

Finally, check the outflow pipe to be sure it has the capacity to handle the discharge coming into the outflow structure. Treating the outflow pipe as a culvert operating with inlet control, headwater for the maximum Q of 82.4 cfs is found from Chart 2 of Appendix B-1 to be 4.44 feet. This gives a water level elevation inside the outlet structure of

$$558.0 + 4.44 = 562.44$$

as shown below.

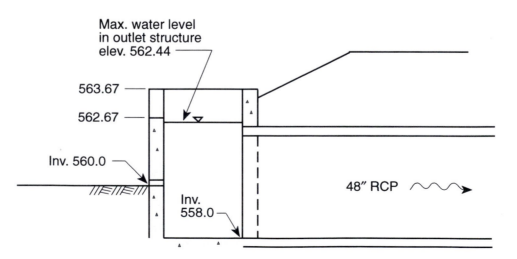

Max. water level
in outlet structure
elev. 562.44

563.67

562.67

Inv. 560.0

Inv.
558.0

48″ RCP

If the water level inside the outlet structure rises above the crest of the second-stage weir, the weir would be submerged and its discharge reduced. This would render the discharge rating somewhat invalid at the highest elevations. Therefore, the outlet pipe should be designed to handle the maximum discharge without causing an excessive backup into the outlet structure.

The 48-inch RCP outlet pipe positioned with its invert at 558.0 is adequate.

However, it should be noted that when the water level rises in the outlet structure, discharge through the orifice is altered. When the orifice becomes submerged, head is measured to the downstream water level, not the center of the orifice, thus reducing h and consequently reducing Q.

Thus, values of Q for the orifice at the higher water levels were computed too high. However, in this case, such an error is not significant, since the reduction of Q is less than 1 cfs when total Q is in the range of 30 cfs and more.

14.3 EMERGENCY SPILLWAY

As a safety feature to prevent detention basins from overflowing, an **emergency spillway** is included in most designs. Emergency spillways consist of an additional outlet set at an elevation higher than all other outlets so that water will not enter unless the impoundment level has risen higher than anticipated for the design storm.

Impoundment level could exceed the design maximum elevation for a variety of reasons; principal among them are the following:

1. A rainfall could occur that exceeds the design storm rainfall.
2. The outlet structure could become blocked, thus preventing stored water from exiting the basin fast enough.

The primary purpose of an emergency spillway is to provide a way for excessive water in the impoundment to exit safely, thus preventing an overtopping of the berm. If the berm is overtopped, it could be breached, or washed out, allowing impounded water suddenly to flood areas downstream of the basin. If a detention basin has no berm and an overtopping of the banks would cause no breach or failure of the sides of the basin, then the need for an emergency spillway is lessened.

A secondary purpose of an emergency spillway is to control any eventual overtopping of the detention basin by directing the flow in a harmless direction, thus preventing uncontrolled flow even if no breach occurs.

Most detention basin designs incorporate one of two general types of emergency spillway:

1. Grassed channel or waterway located separate from the outflow structure.
2. Allowing water to flow into the top of the outflow structure and through the outflow pipe.

Separate grassed channels are used for major detention basins with large maximum impoundments because this is the safest type of emergency spillway. Even if the outflow pipe becomes totally clogged, the grassed channel is free to function and safely convey the excess flow out of the basin. The channel must have an entrance invert below the top of berm, and it must be located in virgin ground beyond the

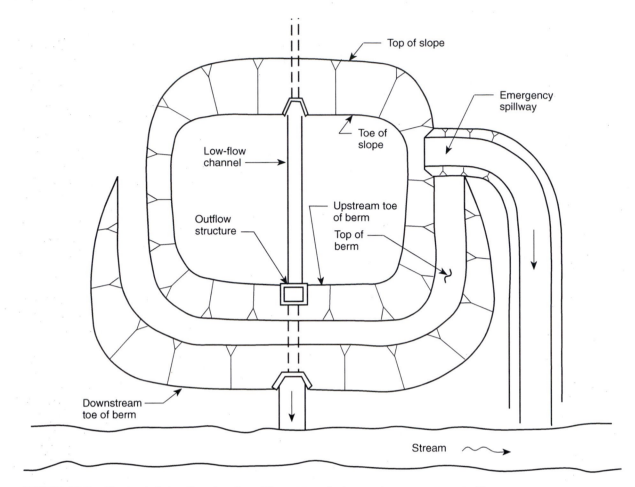

FIGURE 14-7 Typical detention basin with grassed channel emergency spillway.

berm. Normally, the channel cannot be formed by excavating a cut in the berm. This would be feasible only if special measures were employed to protect the berm against erosion.

Figure 14-7 shows a typical emergency spillway arrangement using a grassed swale.

Design criteria for an emergency spillway vary considerably but can be summarized as follows:

1. The invert or crest of the emergency spillway is set at or above the maximum impoundment elevation computed for the design storm.
2. a) The emergency spillway is designed to convey a storm with greater rainfall than the design storm. This larger storm is usually called the *emergency spillway design storm*. The emergency spillway would convey whatever is not handled by the outflow structure.

   or

   b) The emergency spillway is designed to convey the peak discharge of the design storm. This would simulate a situation in which all flow exits the basin through the emergency spillway.
3. The top of berm elevation is set at the elevation of maximum flow through the emergency spillway, plus an additional vertical distance called **freeboard**.

Freeboard provides an extra measure of safety to account for all contingencies such as a storm greater than the design storm or errors in calculations or errors in construction. Freeboard amount can range from zero to one foot or more.

Figure 14-8(a) shows a typical detention basin outlet with separate emergency spillway. Even though the emergency spillway is shown in the same cross section as the outlet structure, it is actually at a different location along the berm. Notice that the crest of the emergency spillway is set at the same elevation as the maximum design water level. This is the impoundment level that will result if the design storm occurs and the basin functions properly.

As soon as the design maximum impoundment level is exceeded, water starts entering the emergency spillway. So the elevation of the emergency spillway cannot be determined until the basin calculations have determined the maximum impoundment level. And the top of berm elevation cannot be determined until the water level in the emergency spillway is computed. Detention basin calculations are presented in the next section.

As we mentioned earlier, the emergency spillway can be incorporated into the outlet structure in certain cases. Figure 14-8(b) depicts this type of arrangement.

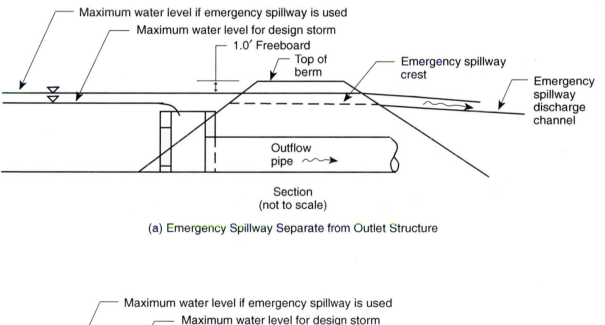

(a) Emergency Spillway Separate from Outlet Structure

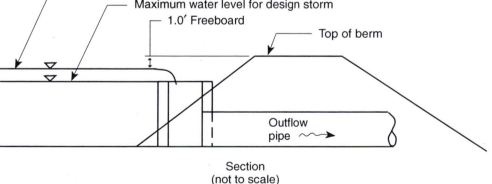

(b) Emergency Spillway Incorporated into Outlet Structure

FIGURE 14-8   Two examples of emergency spillways.

Notice that the top of the outlet structure is set at the same elevation as the maximum design water level. This is because the opening at the top of the structure is being used as the emergency spillway. When the impoundment rises above this level, water starts to pour into the top of the structure, which acts as emergency spillway.

In this type of arrangement, the outflow pipe must handle all outflow, including normal outflow as well as emergency outflow. Therefore, as you might expect, the pipe must be designed larger than in the case of a separate emergency spillway.

In Example 14-4, since the outflow structure handled impoundment levels up to the top of berm, the outlet pipe was as large as it would have to be if the emergency spillway were incorporated into the outlet structure.

14.4 RESERVOIR ROUTING

When runoff enters a detention basin and is temporarily stored and then exits through the outlet structure, the peak rate of outflow is less than the peak rate of inflow. This reduction in peak flow is called *attenuation*, and the procedure for computing the outflow hydrograph when the inflow hydrograph is known is called *routing*. The term *routing* describes a mathematical procedure, not the mapping of a course of movement.

The term *attenuation* was first discussed in Section 10.6 in connection with stormwater flowing in a stream. Whether stormwater flows along a stream or through a detention basin, its hydrograph is attenuated; that is, the hydrograph is lowered and spread out, as shown in Figure 11-14.

Several methods have been devised over the years to compute stream and reservoir (detention basin) routing. For stream routings, the Muskingum Method and the Kinematic Wave Method are widely used. For reservoir routing, the Modified Puls Method is commonly employed.

This routing method relies on the so-called continuity equation, which is a statement of conservation of the mass of water entering and leaving the reservoir or impoundment. (The continuity equation should not be confused with $Q = va$, which goes by the same name in a different context.)

The continuity equation is expressed as

$$\bar{I} - \bar{O} = \frac{\Delta S}{\Delta t} \tag{14-1}$$

where $\bar{I}$ = mean flow into reservoir during time Δt, cfs (m³/s)

$\bar{O}$ = mean outflow from reservoir during time Δt, cfs (m³/s)

ΔS = change in reservoir storage during time Δt, ft³ (m³)

Δt = incremental time period, s

The equation can be considered to be a ledger that keeps account of the balance of water entering, water leaving, and water stored, much like the constantly changing inventory of a warehouse where goods come in and go out and are stored. Numerical solution of the continuity equation is an iteration process in which a small time increment is chosen and the volume balance computed at the end of each time period.

To use the analogy of a warehouse with a time increment of one day, if during the first day 1000 boxes come in and 400 boxes go out, the change in storage is positive 600 boxes. If, during the second day, 500 boxes come in and 700 boxes go out, the change in storage is negative 200 boxes, and the remaining inventory is 400 boxes.

To solve Equation 14-1, first rewrite the equation in a more useful form:

$$\frac{I_1 + I_2}{2} - \frac{O_1 + O_2}{2} = \frac{S_2 - S_1}{\Delta t} \tag{14-2}$$

where the subscripts 1 and 2 denote the beginning and end, respectively, of the chosen time period Δt. Terms in Equation 14-2 may now be rearranged as

$$(I_1 + I_2) + \left[\frac{2S_1}{\Delta t} - O_1\right] = \frac{2S_2}{\Delta t} + O_2 \tag{14-3}$$

In Equation 14-3, all terms on the left-hand side are known from preceding routing computations, while the right-hand terms are unknown and must be determined by storage routing.

Assumptions implicit in this routing method are as follows:

1. The reservoir water surface is horizontal.
2. The outflow is a unique function of storage volume.
3. Outflow rate varies linearly with time during each time period Δt.

In detention basin design, Equation 14-3 is used to compute the outflow hydrograph when the inflow hydrograph is known. This computation constitutes a routing. If the specified detention basin does not produce the desired results, the parameters must be revised and another routing performed. Thus, the process is one of trial and error, just as with culvert design.

Now let us look at Equation 14-3 to see how such an equation can be solved. The first question is: What result do we want the equation to give? The answer is: an outflow hydrograph, that is, a complete list of outflow rates from the detention basin during the design storm. These values are produced by the term O_2 in Equation 14-3. Remember that the equation will be solved many times, once for every chosen time period throughout the storm. Each solution of the equation gives another value O_2, and the total list of such values makes up the outflow hydrograph.

But both S_2 and O_2 are unknowns each time Equation 14-3 is solved. To overcome this problem, we take advantage of the fact that S_2 and O_2 are related to each other, which in effect supplies a second equation, which is needed to solve for two unknowns.

Now, again looking at Equation 14-3, the first term $(I_1 + I_2)$ comes from the inflow hydrograph, which is the runoff hydrograph for the design storm for the watershed tributary to the detention basin. The parameter Δt is an arbitrary time period, which should be chosen as small as practical, remembering that the smaller Δt, the more time periods and the more computations. Δt should be chosen small enough to create at least four or five points on the rising limb of the inflow hydrograph, with one point coinciding with peak inflow.

The parameter S_1 represents the storage volume in the detention basin at the beginning of each time period. It is determined simply by taking the ending storage volume from the preceding time period.

Finally, the parameter O_1 represents the outflow at the beginning of each time period and is determined simply by taking the outflow at the end of the time period preceding.

Row	(1) Time (h)	(2) I_1 (cfs)	(3) $I_1 + I_2$ (cfs)	(4) $\frac{2S}{\Delta t} - O$ (cfs)	(5) $\frac{2S}{\Delta t} + O$ (cfs)	(6) O_2 (cfs)
1						
2						
3						

FIGURE 14-9 Table headings for hand reservoir routing.

To carry out the iterative solution of Equation 14-3, you must therefore start with three elements:

1. Inflow hydrograph
2. Relation of storage volume to elevation in the proposed detention basin
3. Relation of outflow to water level elevation in the proposed detention basin (outflow rating)

On the basis of the duration of the rising limb of the inflow hydrograph, choose a time period, Δt. Then combine the information in items 2 and 3 above to create two new relationships: graphs of O versus $2S/\Delta t + O$ and O versus $2S/\Delta t - O$.

Next, set up a table with headings like those in Figure 14-9.

In column 1, all time values, generated as multiples of Δt, are listed. In column 2, values of the inflow hydrograph corresponding to the time values in column 1 are listed. In column 3, successive pairs of inflow values are summed and listed; that is, in row 1, the sum of the two I_1 values in rows 1 and 2 is listed, and so on. In columns 4 and 5, values of $2S/\Delta t - O$ and $2S/\Delta t + O$ are generated from the appropriate graph or from Equation 14-3. In column 6, values of O_2 are generated, that is, the value of O_2 in row 2 represents the outflow at the end of the time period starting with row 1 and ending at row 2. The use of this routing table is demonstrated in the following example.

Example 14-5

Problem

A detention basin is specified in Figure 14-10, and an inflow hydrograph is shown in Table 14-1. Route the hydrograph through the basin to produce the resulting outflow hydrograph.

Solution

As is shown in Table 14-1, the incremental time period was chosen as $\Delta t = 0.40$ hour, which is equal to 1440 seconds. Now, using the information in Figure 14-10, create a table of values of outflow, O versus $2S/\Delta t - O$ and versus $2S/\Delta t + O$. This is depicted in Table 14-2.

Next, sketch a graph of the above values. The graph is shown in Figure 14-11. Now create a table like the one shown in Figure 14-9, with the inflow hydrograph listed in columns 1 and 2. The table is depicted in Table 14-3.

TABLE 14-1   Inflow Hydrograph for Example 14-5

Time (h)	Inflow (cfs)
0.0	4
0.4	6
0.8	9
1.2	23
1.6	84
2.0	48
2.4	20
2.8	14
3.2	11
3.6	9
4.0	8
4.4	7
4.8	7

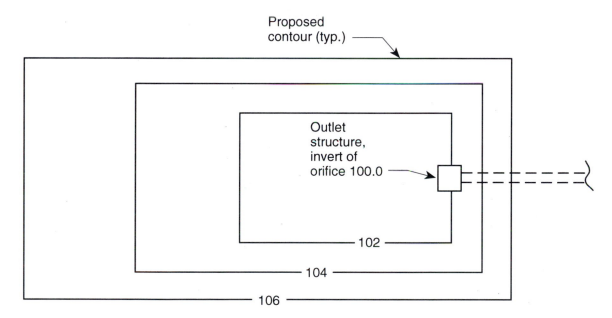

PLAN
(not to scale)

Storage Volume		Discharge Rating	
Elevation (ft)	**Volume (ft³)**	**Elevation (ft)**	**Outflow (cfs)**
100	0	100	0
102	7500	102	2.5
104	36,000	104	24.9
105	60,000	105	67.5
106	90,000	106	122

FIGURE 14-10   Detention basin parameters for Example 14-5.

TABLE 14-2 Parameters Needed for Routing Computation in Example 14-5

O (cfs)	$\dfrac{2S}{\Delta t} - O$ (cfs)	$\dfrac{2S}{\Delta t} + O$ (cfs)
0.0	0.0	0.0
2.5	7.9	12.9
24.9	25.1	74.9
67.5	15.8	151
122	3.0	247

O vs $\dfrac{2S}{\Delta t} + O$

O vs $\dfrac{2S}{\Delta t} - O$

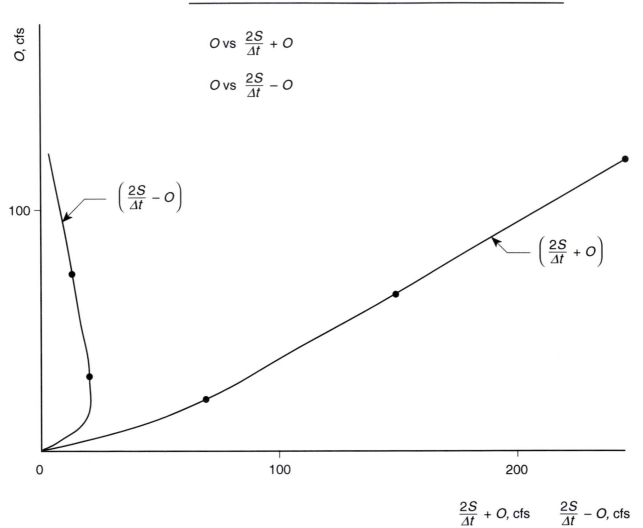

FIGURE 14-11 Graph of O versus $2S/\Delta t + O$ and O versus $2S/\Delta t - O$.

Fill in the appropriate numbers for column 3 by simply adding successive pairs of numbers in column 2. For example, the value in column 3, row 5 is the sum of the numbers in column 2, rows 5 and 6.

The remaining three columns must be generated one row at a time. To begin, consider the first time period, which starts at row 1 and ends at row 2. The two terms

TABLE 14-3   Routing Table for Example 14-5

	(1) Time (h)	(2) I_1 (cfs)	(3) $I_1 + I_2$ (cfs)	(4) $\dfrac{2S}{\Delta t} - O$ (cfs)	(5) $\dfrac{2S}{\Delta t} + O$ (cfs)	(6) O_2 (cfs)
(1)	0.0	4	10	0	0	—
(2)	0.4	6	15	6	10	2
(3)	0.8	9	32	10	21	5
(4)	1.2	23	107	18	42	11
(5)	1.6	84	132	20	125	53
(6)	2.0	48	68	15	152	68
(7)	2.4	20	34	25	83	30
(8)	2.8	14	25	22	59	18
(9)	3.2	11	20	19	47	12
(10)	3.6	9	17	16	39	9
(11)	4.0	8	15	15	33	8
(12)	4.4	7	14	12	30	7
(13)	4.8	7	13	10	26	5

on the left side of Equation 14-3 are found in row 1, columns 3 and 4 and have values 10 and 0, respectively. According to Equation 14-3, these terms are summed to give $2S_2/\Delta t + O_2$, which is column 5, row 2 for the first time period. Therefore, the value 10 goes in that location.

But according to Figure 14-11, when $2S/\Delta t + O$ is 10, $O = 2$ cfs. Therefore, the value 2 goes in column 6, row 2. Figure 14-11 also shows that when $O = 2$ cfs, $2S/\Delta t - O = 6$ cfs. Therefore, the value 6 goes in column 4, row 2.

Now proceed to the second time period, which starts at row 2 and ends at row 3. For this time period, the two terms on the left side of Equation 14-3 are found in row 2, columns 3 and 4, and have values 15 and 6, respectively. Therefore, the sum of these terms (15 + 6 = 21) goes in column 5, row 3. From Figure 14-11, when $2S/\Delta t + O = 21$ cfs, $O = 5$ cfs and $2S/\Delta t - O = 10$ cfs. These values are then written into the appropriate columns of row 3.

Continue this procedure down the table and the values in column 6 become the outflow hydrograph for the routing. Both inflow and outflow hydrographs are plotted in Figure 14-12.   (Answer)

A close look at Figure 14-12 reveals several facts about the routing in Example 14-5. First, notice that the maximum outflow was plotted as approximately 69 cfs even though the maximum O_2 value of the routing is 68 cfs. This is because the sketch reveals that the maximum outflow occurs between computed points.

Next, note that the maximum outflow occurs at the point where the outflow hydrograph crosses the inflow hydrograph. This is a characteristic of reservoir routings.

Also note that the maximum outflow of 69 cfs corresponds to a maximum impoundment elevation of 105.03, which is determined by interpolating the discharge

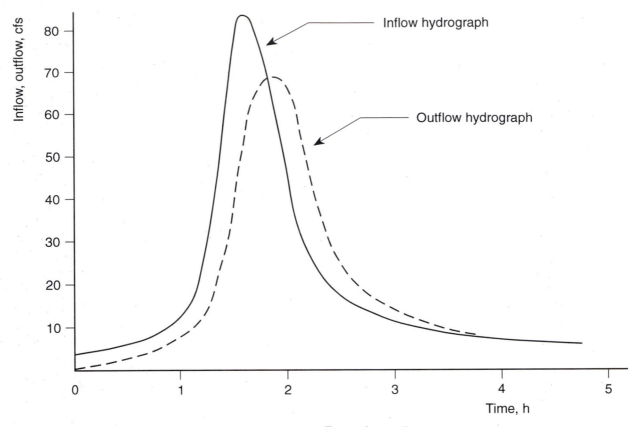

FIGURE 14-12   Inflow and outflow hydrographs for Example 14-5.

rating in Figure 14-10. This elevation would then become the design water level in the detention basin.

Finally, note that the routing resulted in a reduction of peak runoff from 84 cfs (inflow) to 69 cfs (outflow). This is an attenuation of 18 percent.

Example 14-5 illustrates one way to solve Equation 14-3 and perform a reservoir routing by hand. In practice, however, reservoir routings are rarely if ever computed by hand; instead, computers employing any of several available software programs are used. Refer to Appendix E for the names of applicable software.

PROBLEMS

1. Compute an outflow rating chart for a 6-inch-diameter orifice with invert elevation 200.00 ft. Compute outflow values at 1-foot increments to a maximum elevation of 205.00 ft.

2. Compute an outflow rating chart for a 5-foot weir cut into a concrete outflow structure having a 1.0-foot wall thickness. The weir crest is at elevation 100.00 ft. Compute outflow values at 1-foot increments to a maximum elevation of 104.00 ft.

3. Compute an outflow rating chart for the outflow structure shown below. Compute outflow values at 1-foot increments from the orifice invert to the top of the structure. Consider possible constriction caused by flow entering the

outflow pipe. Treat such flow as headwater entering a culvert operating under inlet control.

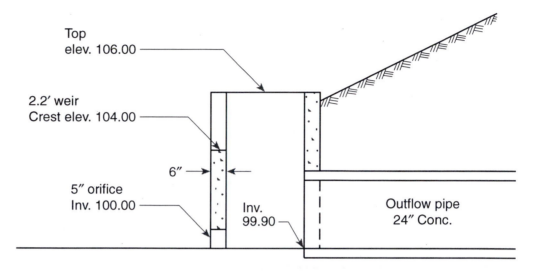

Top elev. 106.00

2.2' weir
Crest elev. 104.00

6"

5" orifice
Inv. 100.00

Inv. 99.90

Outflow pipe
24" Conc.

4. Compute an outflow rating chart for the emergency spillway shown below. Compute outflow values at 1-foot increments from the crest elevation to the top of the berm. Treat the outflow as an entrance to a channel. The emergency spillway is a trapezoidal grass-lined channel with bottom width 10.0 feet and side slopes 3 horizontal to 1 vertical ($n = 0.030$).

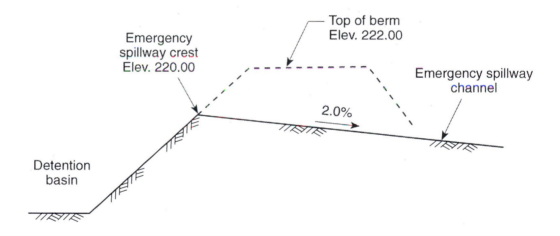

Emergency
spillway crest
Elev. 220.00

Top of berm
Elev. 222.00

Emergency spillway
channel

2.0%

Detention
basin

5. Using the data listed below, compute an inflow hydrograph using the Modified Rational Method. The runoff hydrograph is a triangular hydrograph with base equal to $2.67t_c$. Rout the inflow hydrograph through the detention basin described below. Find the peak inflow and outflow values.

Inflow Hydrograph
Drainage area = 5.0 acres
$c = 0.30$
$t_c = 15$ min.
$i = 6.6$ in/h

Detention Basin

Elevation (ft)	Cum. Volume (c.f.)	Outflow (cfs)
100.00	0	0
102.00	1000	2.5
104.00	2000	3.5
106.00	4000	4.2
108.00	6000	4.9
110.00	8000	5.5

6. Using the data listed below, compute an inflow hydrograph using the NRCS Method. Rout the inflow hydrograph through the detention basin described below. Find the peak inflow and outflow values.

Inflow Hydrograph
Drainage area = 15.0 acres
CN = 60
t_c = 0.50 h
P = 4.4 in
Rainfall Distribution = Type II

Detention Basin

Elevation (ft)	Cum. Volume (c.f.)	Outflow (cfs)
100.00	0	0
102.00	1000	2.5
104.00	2000	3.5
106.00	4000	4.2
108.00	6000	4.9
110.00	8000	5.5

FURTHER READING

Debo, T., and Reese, A. (1995). *Municipal Storm Water Management*. Boca Raton, FL: Lewis Publishers.

Davis, A. P., and McCuen, R. M. (2005). *Stormwater Management for Smart Growth*. New York: Springer Science & Business Media, Inc.

Mays, L. W., ed. (2001). *Stormwater Collection Systems Design Handbook*. New York: McGraw-Hill.

Mays, L. W. (2003). *Urban Stormwater Management Tools*. New York: McGraw-Hill.

U.S. Department of Agriculture (1985). *National Engineering Handbook,* Section 4, Hydrology. Washington, DC: Soil Conservation Service.

U.S. Department of Agriculture (1986). *Urban Hydrology for Small Watersheds,* Technical Release 55. Washington, DC: Soil Conservation Service.

Urban Water Resources Research Council of ASCE and Water Environment Federation (2000). *Design and Construction of Urban Stormwater Management Systems.* New York and Alexandria, VA: ASCE.

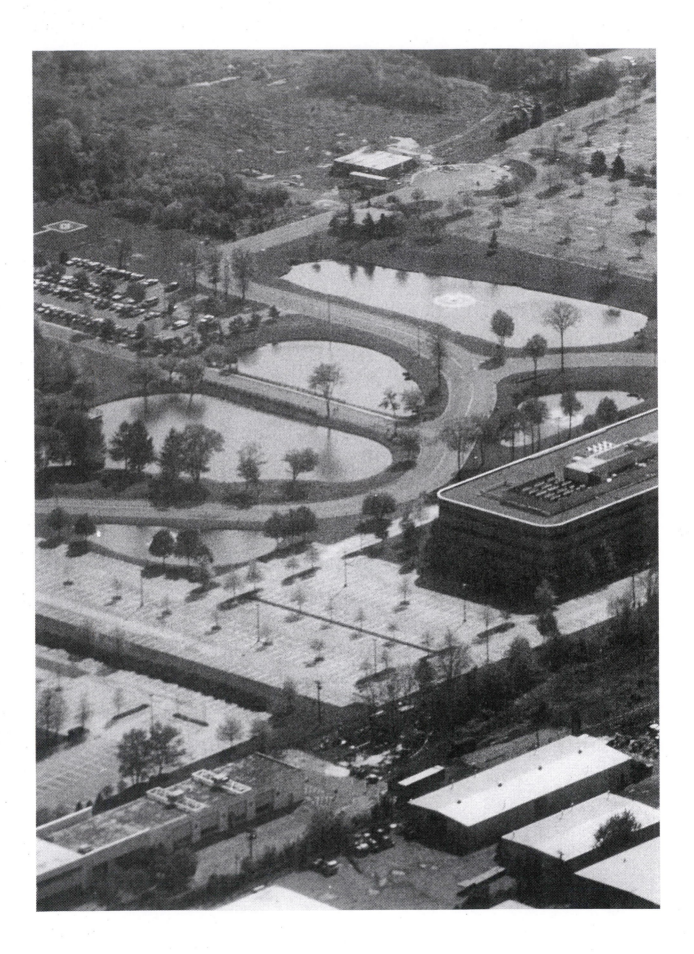

15

DETENTION DESIGN

Stormwater management is a term that is used to describe all endeavors to control runoff in areas affected by development. Typical structures used in stormwater management, such as storm sewers, culverts, and swales, were described in detail earlier in this text. These are used to help convey runoff safely and efficiently away from the development. But another structure, the detention basin, is used to actually reduce the peak rate of flow. In addition, detention basins play a crucial role in controlling the suspended pollutants in stormwater as well as in promoting recharge into the ground. In Chapter 14, we learned the functions of the principal parts of a detention basin.

In this chapter, we will learn how detention basins are employed in the design of stormwater management. The case studies that are presented do not comprise the complete array of detention basin design problems encountered in land development but will give reasonable insight into typical applications. As in previous chapters, design considerations are limited mostly to hydraulic design and do not emphasize other related design factors, such as structural stability and cost.

OBJECTIVES

After completing this chapter, the reader should be able to:

- Explain the difference between on-site and regional detention
- Design a basic detention basin
- Relate detention design to actual case studies

15.1   FUNDAMENTAL CONCEPTS

The use of a detention basin in stormwater management is intended to mitigate the adverse affects of development in the following ways:

1. Control the peak rate of runoff
2. Control the volume of runoff

3. Control the quality of the runoff
4. Promote the recharge of stormwater

When the detention basin temporarily stores stormwater and then releases it slowly, the primary effect is a reduction in peak flow rate leaving the basin, which addresses item 1 above. But the storage and release process also tends to trap pollutants that are suspended in the stormwater, thus addressing item 3 above. During the storage period, some stormwater infiltrates into the ground, thus addressing item 4 above. As stormwater is recharged into the ground, the total volume is reduced, which addresses item 2 above.

The concepts of water quality control and recharge are described in more detail later in this section.

A detention basin functions by storing water in a pond or reservoir, which is usually an open cut in the ground or a series of underground pipes or chambers. The slow release of water is accomplished by an outlet structure or spillway employing an orifice or weir or a combination of flow controlling devices. Figure 15-1 shows schematic sketches of typical detention basin arrangements.

Detention facilities usually are required by local ordinance to be part of the stormwater management measures for all land development. For the purpose of our analysis, we will consider two types of development: residential subdivision and commercial site plans.

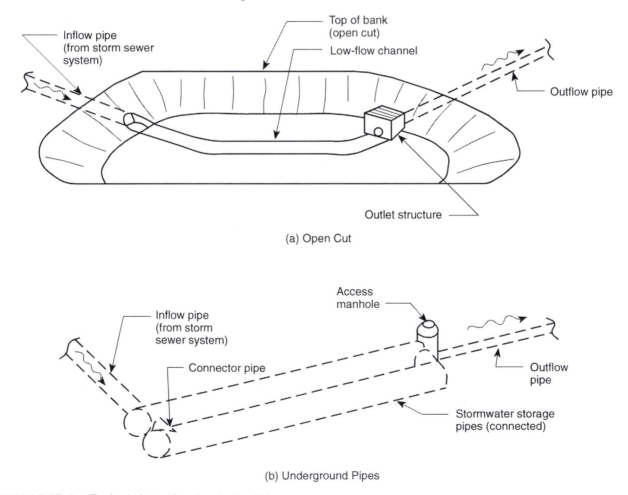

(a) Open Cut

(b) Underground Pipes

FIGURE 15-1   Typical detention basin facilities.

Most detention basins are designed as open cuts in the ground with or without a pond at the bottom. The open cut provides the volume required to store storm-water temporarily during a storm. However, when space on a site is not available, some detention basins are formed by placing large-diameter pipes or other types of chambers underground. The volume provided by the pipes or chambers takes the place of the open cut basin. These types of basins are less desirable because generally pipes provide much less volume than does an open cut, and therefore the cost can skyrocket. Furthermore, underground basins do not possess the pollution-trapping ability of an open cut basin, thus requiring additional measures to control pollution. This causes another increase in cost.

On-Site Detention

On-site detention is intended to protect land in the immediate vicinity of the site from the effects of development. Increased runoff flowing overland directly onto an adjoining property can cause damage by erosion or flooding. Increased runoff flowing into a storm sewer can possibly exceed the pipe capacity. Also, increased runoff flowing into a stream can exceed the capacity of the stream some distance downstream of the site.

Figure 15-2 shows a small on-site detention basin that has become a familiar sight in commercial as well as residential developments. Specific design considerations for on-site detention are discussed in the next section.

Regional Detention

Most detention basins are constructed on individual sites and designed to control the runoff from that site alone. However, calculations performed on a regionwide basis show that individual sites are not always the best place to control the quantity of runoff. In assessing the optimum location for detention facilities, we must focus

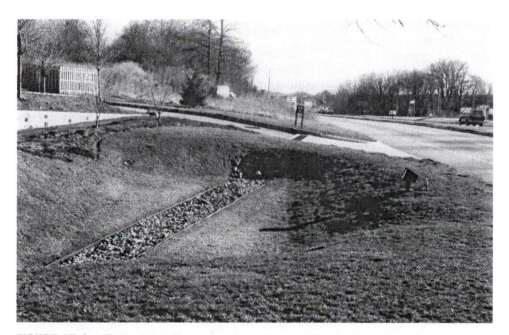

FIGURE 15-2 Typical small on-site detention basin. A riprap low-flow channel runs down the center of the basin.

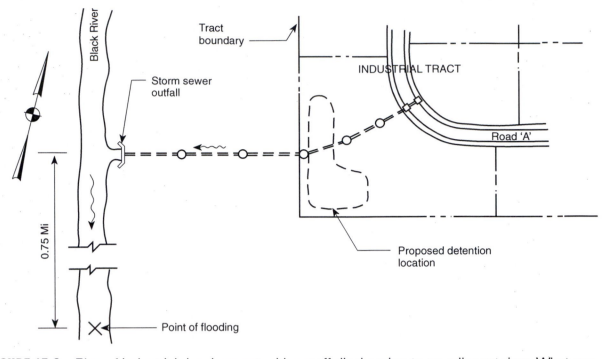

FIGURE 15-3 Plan of industrial development with runoff discharging to an adjacent river. What purpose does the on-site detention basin serve in this case?

on the impact point where we wish to attenuate the stormwater flow. Is it immediately downstream of the site, or is it a mile downstream?

Consider the industrial subdivision shown in Figure 15-3. Stormwater outflow from the subdivision is piped directly to the Black River without affecting any adjacent property. The off-site pipe discharging to the river is designed to convey the 100-year storm flow. Should a detention basin be constructed on-site in accordance with local ordinance? To answer this question, consider the off-site impact. The Black River has capacity to carry the 100-year flood in the project vicinity, but 0.75 mile downstream, low banks result in a flooding condition. The flow contribution of the subdivision to the Black River at the point of flooding is plotted on the hydrograph in Figure 15-4. If no detention basin is constructed, runoff from the site will peak early, and its contribution at the impact point will be relatively low. But if a detention basin is constructed, the outflow will peak in the Black River at a later time, and even though the attenuated flow has a lesser peak contribution than flow with no detention, its contribution at time t_1 when the river flow peaks is greater. Thus, the presence of a detention basin in this case actually aggravates the flooding condition at the most vulnerable point downstream. For this reason, the industrial subdivision should not include a detention basin for stormwater quantity control.

Other land development locations will not present the same downstream conditions as the industrial tract just described. Sometimes on-site detention makes the most sense. Sometimes regional detention is preferable. As shown in Figure 15-5, for example, a watershed tributary to the Blue River could be controlled by 12 on-site detention basins. But detention basins 1 through 6 could be replaced by one regional basin R1 and basins 7 through 11 could be replaced by regional basin R2. Or all 12 basins could be replaced by regional basin R3. This consolidation of detention facilities could be less expensive, require less space, and be easier to maintain than

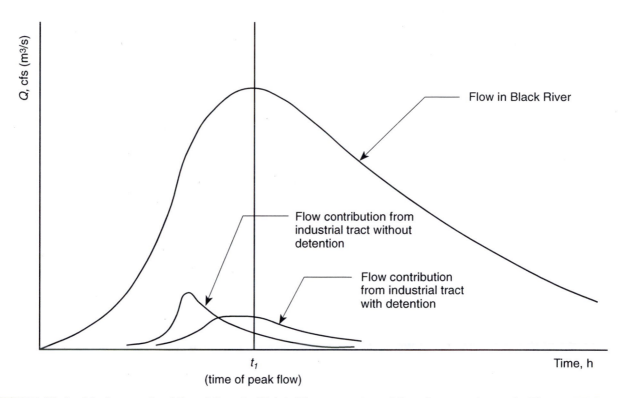

FIGURE 15-4 Hydrograph of flood flow in Black River at point of flooding as shown in Figure 15-3.

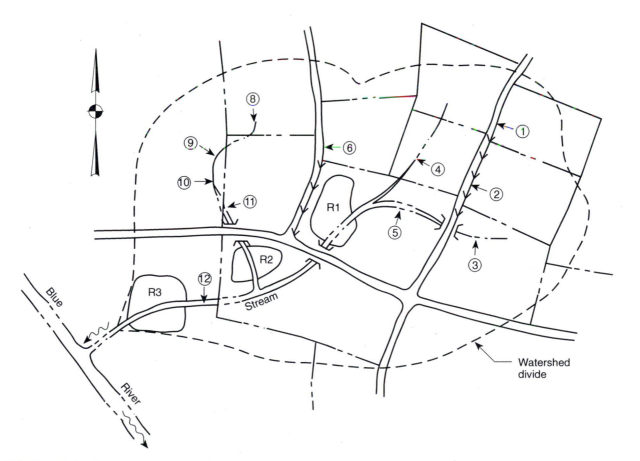

FIGURE 15-5 On-site detention basins versus regional facilities.

individual on-site basins. Of course, before initiating a regional stormwater management system like that in Figure 15-5, all vulnerable impact locations would have to be analyzed. It could be that local flooding within the watershed requires numerous small detention basins. Also, perhaps basins R1 and R3, which are on-stream, will have an adverse effect on fish habitat.

Regional detention is difficult to accomplish but often is more effective and less costly than allowing a proliferation of small on-site facilities. However, the designer has little choice in most cases and must follow local regulations.

Water Quality Control

In addition to controlling the quantity of runoff, detention basins can serve effectively to control the quality as well. When stormwater runs across human-made impervious surfaces, it picks up pollutants, which become suspended in the flow stream. The pollutants typically consist of hydrocarbons, phosphates, nitrates, salts, pesticides, and heavy metals. The mechanism of transport for most pollutants is to adhere to silt particles as the silt is carried along suspended in the stormwater.

Most pollutant transport occurs at the early stage of a rainfall event. Following the initial losses, the first flow of runoff, called **first flush**, picks up the loose dust that has coated the ground since the last rainfall. As the storm progresses and heavier flows of runoff occur, the amount of pollutant transport lessens, making this later runoff much cleaner than the first flush. Since this initial pollutant-carrying discharge is relatively low in flow rate, you can imagine that it does not take a large storm to transport most of the pollutants. It is for this reason, therefore, that the smaller storms such as the one-year storm are typically controlled in an effort to manage pollution.

A detention basin controls pollutants by trapping the silt on which the pollutants ride. As the first flush flow enters into a grass-lined detention basin, the suspended silt is filtered out by the grass; then as the water starts to collect or form a pool, silt particles settle out as they travel through the pool toward the outlet. Trapped pollutants then follow one of these fates: They infiltrate into the ground and lodge in the void spaces between soil particles, or they are absorbed by the grass roots and then harvested with the grass or, if they are volatile, they evaporate.

Not all pollutants are trapped by the typical detention basin. If the basin is constructed to have a permanent pond at its bottom, trap efficiency is increased because the settling process is enhanced. This type of detention basin is called a **wet basin**, **retention basin**, or **sediment basin**. However, studies show that for typical wet basins without extraordinary contrivances, pollutant reduction does not exceed 60 percent. Figure 15-6 shows a schematic sketch of a wet basin.

Infiltration Basin

Another type of detention basin, called an **infiltration basin**, adds a third function to those already discussed. In addition to controlling the quantity and quality of stormwater, it promotes recharge of stormwater to groundwater storage. The advantage of recharge is that it helps to prevent the depletion of groundwater storage. This is very important to drinking water supply.

One of the consequences of land development that has not yet been mentioned is that a greater overall volume of water is converted to runoff and less water infiltrates the ground to become groundwater. Referring to Figure 10-2, we

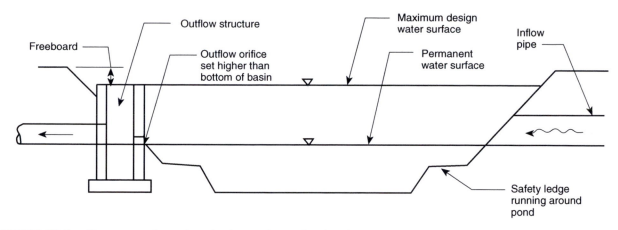

FIGURE 15-6   Cross section of typical wet detention basin.

see that precipitation has three principal fates: overland flow (runoff), subsurface flow, and groundwater.

Land development, because of the addition of impervious surface, upsets this distribution by increasing the percentage of runoff and lessening subsurface flow and groundwater recharge.

So to help reestablish the natural distribution of precipitation, recharge basins employ special measures to intercept some of the runoff and place it into the groundwater. All open-cut detention basins accomplish some groundwater recharge, but the percentage usually is small unless special measures are employed. These measures typically consist of a depression in the ground below the outlet elevation, much like a retention basin, together with excavated porous connections to the ground so that the water retained in the pool infiltrates into it through the excavation. Figure 15-7 shows a schematic diagram of a typical recharge basin.

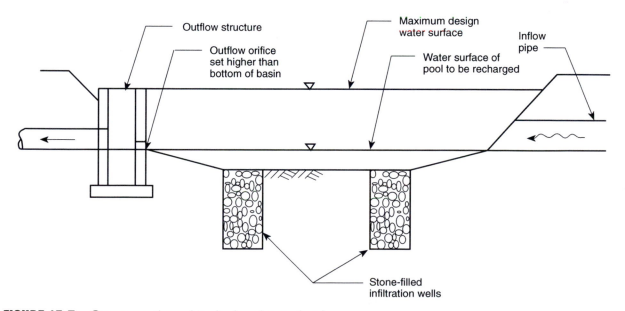

FIGURE 15-7   Cross section of typical recharge basin.

15.2 ON-SITE DETENTION DESIGN

The primary goal of on-site detention is to reduce the peak rate of runoff leaving the site to a level equal to or less than the predevelopment peak rate. This concept can refer to total aggregate runoff or it can refer to runoff leaving the site at a specific location. Figure 15-8 shows an idealized site before and after development. Even though total peak runoff is reduced from 25 cfs to 20 cfs, flow leaving the site has been concentrated. The design depicted in Figure 15-8(b) satisfies the concept of

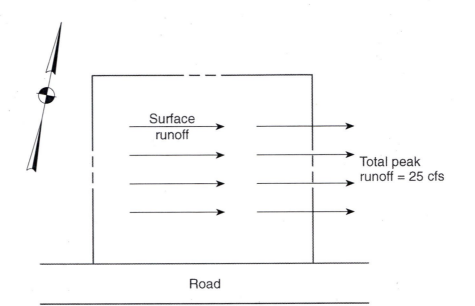

(a) Predevelopment Conditions

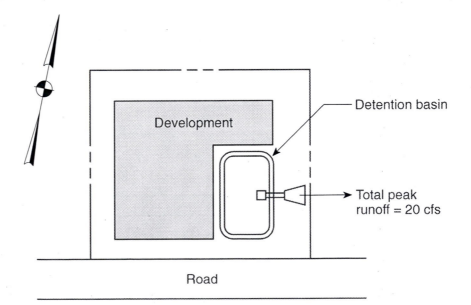

(b) Postdevelopment Conditions

FIGURE 15-8 Comparison of predevelopment and postdevelopment runoff leaving a site.

reducing aggregate runoff but results in an increase in runoff at the point where the detention basin outflow exits the site.

This design would not be chosen if the outlet discharged directly overland as depicted, because it would result in erosion or flooding damage to the adjoining site. However, if the outflow could be connected to an existing storm sewer or if a drainage easement could be obtained on the adjacent site, the design could be chosen because the overall effect is to reduce peak discharge downstream.

Therefore, the designer should ask two questions:

1. Does the design reduce overall peak runoff?
2. Does the design avoid increasing peak runoff leaving the site overland at any point?

The resulting design must satisfy both questions simultaneously.

Note: When computing runoff for both predevelopment and postdevelopment conditions, you may notice that the strict procedure for runoff computation, as described in Chapter 12, can be violated. For example, in Figure 15-8, in computing predevelopment runoff, the point of analysis is chosen as a point on the easterly boundary of the site. Runoff generated on the site does not all flow to a specific point but instead flows to the easterly boundary in general. Despite this anomaly, runoff computations in detention design follow the procedures described in Chapter 12 in all other ways.

Design storms should be chosen to reflect the potential for damage. Although large sites usually need protection against the 100-year storm, protecting against larger storms is rarely cost-effective. However, protection against lesser storms is often very important. This is because detention basins designed for the 100-year storm must necessarily have relatively large outflow devices (orifices and weirs) that allow smaller storms to pass through almost unaffected. Small storms, such as the 2-year storm, can cause significant damage, and they occur much more frequently.

Site Conditions

Topographic conditions peculiar to individual sites affect the approach to detention design. Although the variations found on individual sites are as numerous as the sites, some significant examples can be identified.

First, a significant portion of a site might not be tributary to the detention basin, owing to topographic factors, as shown in Figure 15-9. The area not tributary to, and therefore bypassing, the detention basin can be accounted for in various ways. The design could be based only on the area tributary to the detention basin with the bypass area ignored. Therefore, the runoff hydrographs for both predevelopment and postdevelopment conditions would be based on an area less than the entire site. This can be done because the bypass area does not undergo any changes and does not contribute to the comparison of predevelopment and postdevelopment runoff analysis.

Another way to proceed with the design for the site in Figure 15-9 would be to base the predevelopment hydrograph on the entire site, while the postdevelopment runoff would be based on two hydrographs: one for the area tributary to the detention basin and one for the area that bypasses the detention basin. The bypass

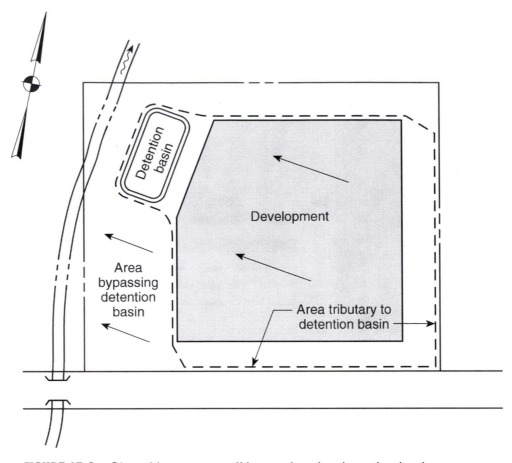

FIGURE 15-9   Site with some runoff bypassing the detention basin.

hydrograph would then be combined (by superposition) with the outflow hydro-graph from the detention basin to compare with predevelopment runoff. This de-sign method is especially relevant if, because of topographic constraints, some of the development is included in the bypass area.

A second site condition involves a ridge line running through a site, forcing it to drain in two distinct directions, such as the site depicted in Figure 15-10. In this case, if a detention basin is placed in the southeast corner of the site, it can control runoff from the easterly half but not the westerly half of the site. It might be nec-essary to place an additional detention basin in the northwest corner. Another so-lution might be to move the ridge line to the westerly portion of the site by grading. However, this can be a very costly solution. Furthermore, if the two halves of the site are in different river basins, the divide for the river basins should not be sig-nificantly altered. Case Study 1 in this chapter addresses the condition of a site that drains in two directions.

A third condition involves a site where, because of topographic factors, some of the runoff leaving the site originates uphill of the site, as shown in Figure 5-11. Because detention basin design is usually limited to controlling runoff originating on the site, off-site runoff does not need to be included in the runoff analysis. How-ever, the off-site runoff is real water and must be considered in sizing the detention basin. The off-site runoff shown in Figure 5-11 can be handled in a variety of ways, including the following examples. First, it could be treated as an undeveloped

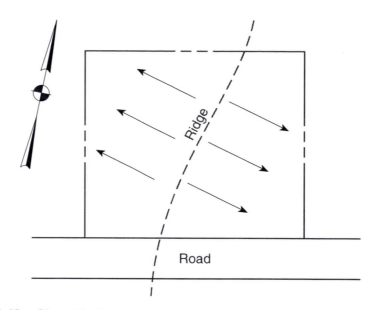

FIGURE 15-10   Site with ridge forcing runoff to flow in two opposite directions.

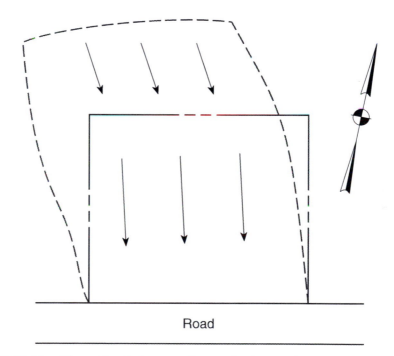
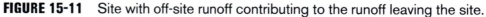

FIGURE 15-11   Site with off-site runoff contributing to the runoff leaving the site.

portion of the site in which it would be included in both predevelopment and post-development runoff. The effect of this approach would be to increase the size of the outlet devices (orifice and weir) in the detention basin but would not significantly increase the size of the impoundment. A second approach is to intercept the off-site runoff by use of a swale or pipe and direct the runoff around the detention basin. In this way, the off-site runoff would not be included in the detention calculations. However, design of the intercepting structure would be required.

15.3   CASE STUDY 1

This case study focuses on the same subdivision located in Atlanta, Georgia, as was discussed in Section 12.6 in relation to storm sewer design. The subdivision, called Tall Pines, is depicted in Figure 12-18. After completing storm sewer design, a detention facility was then designed to complete the stormwater management aspect of the project.

Design Requirements

According to local ordinance, the detention basin design criteria were as follows:

1. Total peak runoff leaving the tract after development cannot exceed total peak runoff leaving the tract before development for the 2-year, 25-year, and 100-year storms, each considered separately, and
2. Method of computation and design parameters are to be in accordance with good engineering practice.

The Modified Rational Method was chosen to be the method of computation, since the project is relatively small and uncomplicated. Computations were performed on a personal computer using hydrologic software called Hydraflow by Intelisolve. The program was used to compute the inflow hydrographs and the detention basin routings.

Before the computing was started, an overall outline was devised. Since predevelopment runoff traveled on the site in two general directions, northerly and southerly, the design process was made a little more involved than it might have been. Peak runoff under predevelopment conditions would have to be computed in two parts: one for all runoff flowing in a northerly direction and one for all runoff flowing south. Figure 15-12 shows the tract under predevelopment conditions divided into the two oppositely directed drainage areas.

Runoff Computations: Predevelopment

Peak runoff for each area was computed using the Rational Method in the usual way except that the drainage areas were not delineated in the usual way. The drainage areas were defined by tract boundaries and not by contour lines, as described in Section 10.2. This results in artificial drainage areas but is accepted practice in determining peak runoff from a tract of land whose boundary does not coincide with a natural drainage basin.

Hydraulic path was delineated as starting at the remotest point in the drainage area and traveling to the farthest downhill point. This procedure also is slightly different from that in Section 10.2 because in this case, we do not have a fixed point of analysis. Runoff crosses tract boundaries at several points, but only one is chosen as the point of analysis—namely, the one that results in the longest hydraulic path.

Therefore, peak runoff under predevelopment conditions was computed as follows:

A. Southerly Area

$A = 6.23$ acres   (measured from plan)
$c = 0.20$ (entirely wooded tract)
$t_c = 14.5$ min   Overland 100′ @ 2.4%, $t = 12.5$ min
                          Shallow conc. 530′ @ 7.7%, $t = 2.0$ min

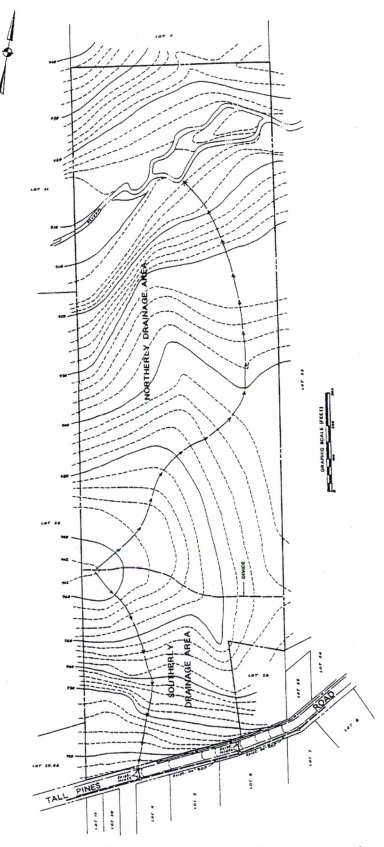

FIGURE 15-12   Map of Tall Pines subdivision, existing conditions. *(Courtesy of Jaman Engineering.)*

Storm (years)	i (in/h)	Q_p (cfs)
2	3.6	4.5
25	6.3	7.8
100	7.5	9.4

Values of i were determined by using the I-D-F curves for Atlanta in Appendix C-3. Values of Q_p were determined by using Equation 11-2.

B. Northerly Area

$A = 22.27$ acres (measured from plan)
$c = 0.20$ (entirely wooded tract)
$t_c = 19.2$ min Overland 100′ @ 3%, $t = 12.0$ min
  Shallow conc. 1300′ @ 3.5%, $t = 7.2$ min

Storm (years)	i (in/h)	Q_p (cfs)
2	3.1	13.9
25	5.4	24.1
100	6.5	28.9

Total peak runoff leaving the tract for predevelopment conditions was then taken as the sum of the southerly and northerly runoffs.

Storm (years)	Q_p (cfs)
2	18.4
25	31.9
100	38.3

These values of Q_p then became the maximum allowable values of peak runoff under postdevelopment conditions.

The location of the detention basin was chosen near the northerly end of the tract as shown in Figure 15-13 because this is a low point and because most of the improved areas drain to this point. Another reason was the proximity of the stream to receive outflow.

The detention basin was designed as an open-cut basin because sufficient land area was available and open cut is much less costly than underground pipes.

Runoff Computations: Postdevelopment

Figure 15-13 shows that the developed tract is divided into three drainage areas:

1. Runoff flowing southerly
2. Runoff tributary to the detention basin
3. Runoff flowing northerly but bypassing the detention basin

Total postdevelopment peak runoff is the sum of the peak runoffs from these three areas. Runoff from Areas 1 and 3 is computed just as was existing runoff, while runoff from Area 2 is equal to outflow from the detention basin.

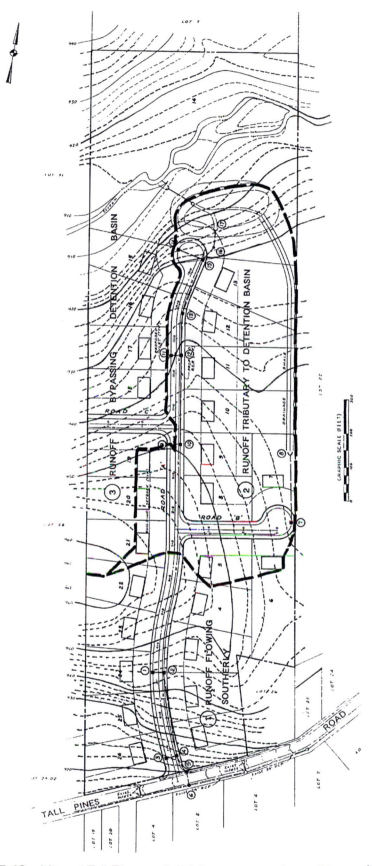

FIGURE 15-13   Map of Tall Pines subdivision, proposed conditions. *(Courtesy of Jaman Engineering.)*

Peak runoff from all three areas increases as a result of development because impervious areas cause the c-value to increase and reduced time of concentration causes the i-value to increase. Since Area 2 is the only area that can have reduced peak runoff (because of the detention basin), it is possible that Areas 1 and 3 could increase sufficiently to exceed total predevelopment runoff on their own without the contribution of Area 2. If this happened, the detention basin would become inadequate because even if it reduced Area 2 runoff to zero, postdevelopment runoff would still exceed predevelopment runoff.

Unfortunately, this is exactly what happened when peak runoff was computed for Areas 1 and 3. This presented a major problem, which had to be solved in order to continue with the project. Possible solutions were listed as follows:

1. Eliminate some of the proposed houses.
2. Regrade the development to cause more lots to drain to the detention basin, that is, increase the size of Area 2 and reduce Areas 1 and 3.
3. Include seepage pits on each lot to intercept runoff from the proposed roofs. This would, in effect, eliminate the roofs from the drainage areas.

Solution 1 was held aside as a last resort. Solution 2 was considered too costly because of the great amount of earthwork involved. Solution 3 proved to be effective because it leads to a reduction of peak runoff from Areas 1 and 3 just sufficient to bring the sum of the two below the total predevelopment peak runoff.

Therefore, two seepage pits were proposed for each lot, and the area of the proposed roofs was subtracted from drainage area values in computing peak runoff.

Peak runoff under postdevelopment conditions was computed as follows:

A. Southerly Area

$A = 6.88$ acres (measured from map minus nine roofs)
$c = 0.33$
 Impervious: 0.66 acre @ $c = 0.9$
 Lawns: 2.26 acres @ $c = 0.3$
 Woods: 3.95 acres @ $c = 0.2$
$t_c = 13.4$ min (see storm sewer design, Section 12.6)

Storm (years)	i (in/h)	Q_p (cfs)
2	3.7	8.4
25	6.5	14.7
100	7.75	17.6

B. Tributary to Detention Basin

$A = 9.46$ acres (measured from map minus 11 roofs)
$c = 0.33$
 Impervious: 1.31 acres @ $c = 0.9$
 Lawns: 2.93 acres @ $c = 0.3$
 Woods: 5.22 acres @ $c = 0.2$
$t_c = 21.0$ min
 t_c to inlet 7 = 12.2 min
 Pipe Segment 7-8, $t = 0.3$ min
 Swale 250′ @ 1.0%,
  $v = 1.1$ fps, $t = 3.8$ min
 Swale 420′ @ 2.1%,
  $v = 2.1$ fps, $t = 4.7$ min
   total = 21.0 min

Storm (years)	i (in/h)	Q_p (cfs)
2	3.0	9.3
25	5.15	16.1
100	6.2	19.3

Note: The hydrograph of runoff from Area 2 was computed by Hydraflow software by Intelisolve using the Modified Rational Method.

C. Northerly Area Bypassing Detention Basin

$A = 11.25$ acres (measured from plan minus four roofs)
$c = 0.21$ Impervious: 0.11 acre @ $c = 0.9$
 Lawns: 0.54 acre @ $c = 0.3$
 Woods: 10.6 acres @ $c = 0.2$
$t_c = 15.6$ min Overland 100′ @ 3%, $t = 12.0$ min
 Shallow conc. 780′ @ 5%, $t = 3.6$ min

Storm (years)	i (in/h)	Q_p (cfs)
2	3.3	7.8
25	6.0	14.2
100	7.1	16.8

Total peak runoff under postdevelopment conditions (before taking into account the detention basin) can be summarized for the three design storms as follows:

Storm (years)	Q_p (cfs) Area 1	Area 2	Area 3	Total Q_p (cfs)
2	8.4	9.3	7.8	25.5
25	14.7	16.1	14.2	45.0
100	17.6	19.3	16.8	53.7

These values are, as expected, greater than corresponding predevelopment runoff values, but they can be reduced to predevelopment values by reducing Area 2 values through use of the detention basin.

For instance, if the 2-year runoff for Area 2 is reduced from 9.3 cfs to 2.2 cfs, then total postdevelopment peak runoff would be reduced to 18.4 cfs, which matches predevelopment peak runoff. Similar reductions can be made for the 25-year and 100-year storms.

Detention Basin Computations

Therefore, the next step was to choose a detention basin size and compute the appropriate routings to determine peak outflow. After a few trial routings were performed, a detention basin as depicted in Figure 15-14 was selected. Parameters for this basin are listed in Tables 15-1 and 15-2.

Routing hydrographs for this detention basin are shown in Figure 15-15.

The routing computations show that the detention basin, as chosen, does a very good job of attenuating the inflow hydrograph. For the 100-year storm, peak inflow

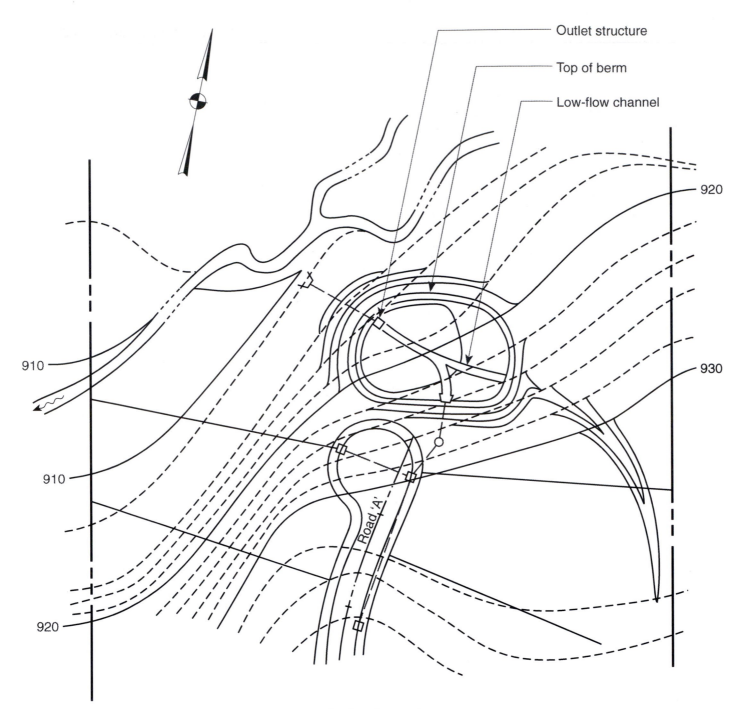

Scale: 1″ = 100′

FIGURE 15-14 Grading plan of proposed detention basin for Tall Pines subdivision. *(Courtesy of Jaman Engineering.)*

TABLE 15-1 Storage Volume Computations for Case Study 1

Elevation (ft)	Area (ft²)	Incremental Volume (ft³)	Cumulative Volume (ft³)
916	0	0	0
917	7,000	3,500	3,500
918	15,000	11,000	14,500
919	16,500	15,750	30,250
920	18,000	17,250	47,500

TABLE 15-2   Outflow Computations for Case Study 1

Elevation (ft)	4″ Orifice (cfs)	6″ Weir (cfs)	Emergency Spillway (cfs)	Total Outflow (cfs)
916	0	—	—	0
917	0.4	—	—	0.4
918	0.6	—	—	0.6
919	0.7	1.7	—	2.4
920	0.8	4.7	38	44

of 19.3 cfs is reduced to peak outflow of 2.2 cfs, an 89 percent attenuation. Similar attenuations are realized for the other two design storms.

The detention basin design summary can be stated by the following table:

Storm (years)	Total Peak Runoff (predevelopment) (cfs)	Total Peak Runoff (postdevelopment) Area 1 (cfs)	Area 2* (cfs)	Area 3 (cfs)	Total (cfs)
2	18.4	8.4	0.6	7.8	16.8
25	31.9	14.7	1.7	14.2	30.6
100	38.3	17.6	2.2	16.8	36.6

Peak outflow from detention basin.

To satisfy the design criterion of zero increase in peak runoff, values in the last column above must be equal to or less than values in the second column. Since this is the case, the detention basin design was accepted.

At this point, two more design tasks remained: emergency spillway and erosion control.

Emergency Spillway

It was decided that because of the low potential downstream hazard of the detention basin, the emergency spillway could be incorporated into the outlet structure. Therefore, the top of the outlet structure, which functions as a weir, was designated as the emergency spillway.

To determine the depth of flow over the emergency spillway, it was assumed that the 100-year peak inflow of 19.3 cfs would enter the emergency spillway with zero flow through the orifice and weir. With the top of the outlet structure treated as a weir, the depth for 19.3 cfs was computed to be 0.50 foot.

The top of the outlet structure was set at elevation 919.0 to be above the 100-year routed water level of 918.9. Therefore, the emergency spillway water level would be 919.5. The top of berm was set 1.0 ft above the emergency water level, which is elevation 920.5. Figure 15-16 shows a schematic drawing of the outlet structure and emergency spillway.

Outfall

Notice that the outflow pipe was designed as a 24-inch concrete pipe. This is because the outflow pipe must be large enough that if full design flow entered the

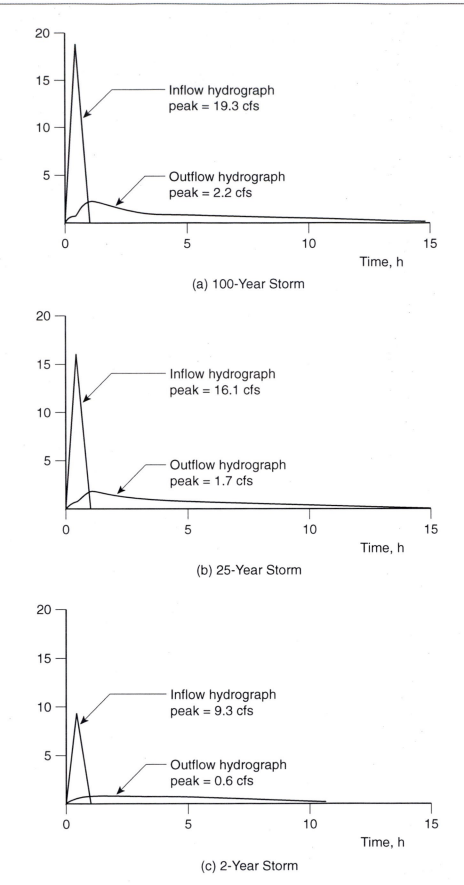

FIGURE 15-15 Routing hydrographs for Case Study 1. The inflow hydrographs represent runoff from Area 2 tributary to the detention basin.

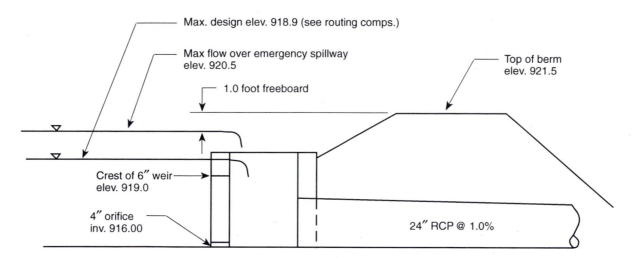

FIGURE 15-16   Schematic drawing of detention basin outlet showing key design elevations.

emergency spillway, the outflow pipe would have sufficient capacity to convey the flow adequately.

Finally, erosion protection at the outfall for the 24-inch outflow pipe was considered. To do this, first the exit velocity was determined for peak 100-year outflow of 2.2 cfs. (The emergency spillway outflow of 19.3 cfs was not used because of the remote possibility of this flow occurring.) By using Chart 39 in Appendix A-4, design velocity was found to be 4.9 fps. (The Manning's *n*-value was assumed to be 0.012.)

Permissible velocity, checked in Appendix A-2 for earth channels with silt loam lining, was found to be 3.0 fps. Since the design velocity exceeded the permissible, a riprap apron was proposed.

To design the riprap lining, first tailwater depth was determined to be 0.4 foot using Chart 39 in Appendix A-4. Then, using Equation 10-1, we have

$$d_{50} = \frac{0.02}{0.4}(2.2/2.0)^{4/3}$$
$$= 0.057 \text{ ft } (0.7 \text{ in})$$

Despite the result of 0.7-inch diameter, the designer proposed 2-inch-diameter crushed stone, 6 inches thick, to provide a more stable lining. Apron length was computed by using Equation 12-2:

$$L_a = \frac{3(2.2)}{2.0^{3/2}}$$
$$= 2.3 \text{ ft}$$

Despite the minimal result of 2.3 feet, the apron length was proposed to be 5.0 feet to provide a more conservative design at minimal extra cost.

15.4 CASE STUDY 2

In this case study, an office site is proposed for a 28-acre tract in northwestern Missouri. The office development, called Liberty Road Associates, consists of a four-story building with parking for 660 cars and is shown in Figure 15-17. A 900-foot-long entrance drive sets the site well back from Martinsville Road, on which the tract fronts.

A stream snakes close to the northwestern corner of the tract, while another stream originates on site and flows northerly across the northern tract boundary. Most of the runoff leaving the site flows into the on-site stream.

Design Requirements

Stormwater management requirements for the development included an on-site detention basin designed in accordance with county regulations:

1. Total peak runoff leaving the tract after development cannot exceed total peak runoff leaving the tract before development for the 2-, 5-, 10-, 25-, 50-, and 100-year storms, each considered separately.
2. Runoff and basin routing computations are to be in accordance with the SCS Method.
3. Emergency spillway design is to be based on routing a storm with 10-inch, 24-hour rainfall.
4. Top of berm elevation is to be based on routing a storm with 17-inch, 24-hour rainfall.

Computations for detention basin design were performed by the Hydro Plus III computer software on a personal computer.

Before the computations were started, a general design outline was devised. Terrain on the tract generally slopes downward from south to north with a high point located about 1000 feet south of the tract. The site is shown in relation to surrounding topography in Figure 15-18. The detention basin location was proposed along the northerly tract boundary as shown in Figure 15-19 because this is a low point on the site and is adjacent to the stream that flows off the site.

The drainage area tributary to the proposed detention basin is delineated in Figure 15-18 and includes land uphill of the tract that drains onto the tract. This area was used to compute both predevelopment and postdevelopment runoff for detention design because it best represents total runoff leaving the tract. Runoff from the easterly portion of the tract on which the access road was proposed was not included in the design because it was considered insignificant in comparison to the rest of the site. However, an analysis of the existing storm sewer system in Martinsville Road was performed to show that sufficient capacity existed to accommodate increased flow from the project access drive.

As shown in Figure 15-19, the detention basin was incorporated into the site as a landscaping feature integral to the building. A permanent pond was designed at the bottom of the basin to serve as a water enhancement for the site. Thus, the basin was designed as a wet detention basin. An internal site driveway was proposed on top of the detention basin berm so that the berm could serve two functions.

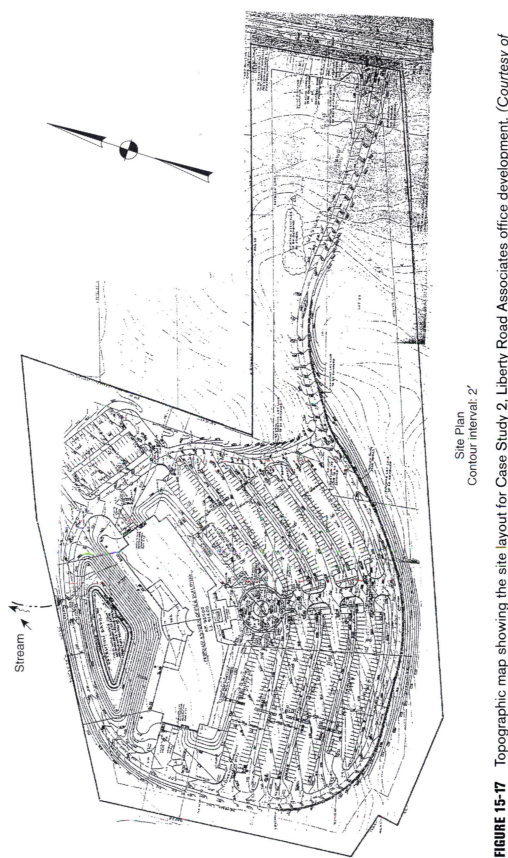

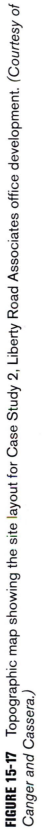

Stream

Site Plan
Contour interval: 2'

FIGURE 15-17   Topographic map showing the site layout for Case Study 2, Liberty Road Associates office development. (*Courtesy of Canger and Cassera.*)

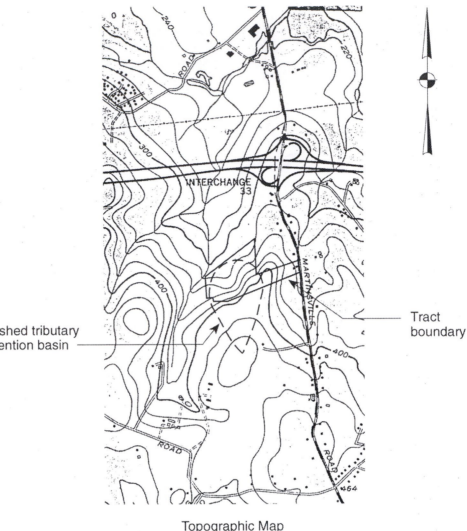

Topographic Map
Scale: 1″ = 2000′ (1:24000)
Contour interval: 20′

FIGURE 15-18   Topographic map showing drainage area used for Liberty Road Associates detention design. *(Courtesy of U.S. Geological Survey.)*

Runoff Computation: Predevelopment

To compute peak runoff under predevelopment conditions, the drainage area used was the area tributary to the detention basin. Although this is a postdevelopment area, it was used so that the predevelopment and postdevelopment drainage areas would be equal and therefore give a fair comparison of runoff.

Figure 15-20 shows predevelopment and postdevelopment watersheds tributary to the stream at the northerly tract boundary. Since the areas are not equal, they cannot be used for a fair comparison for runoff quantities. Therefore, the predevelopment watershed delineation was changed to match the postdevelopment delineation even though this resulted in an artificially drawn watershed.

Hydraulic path was taken as starting at the remotest point of the watershed and traveling to the farthest downhill point, similar to the method used for Case Study 1.

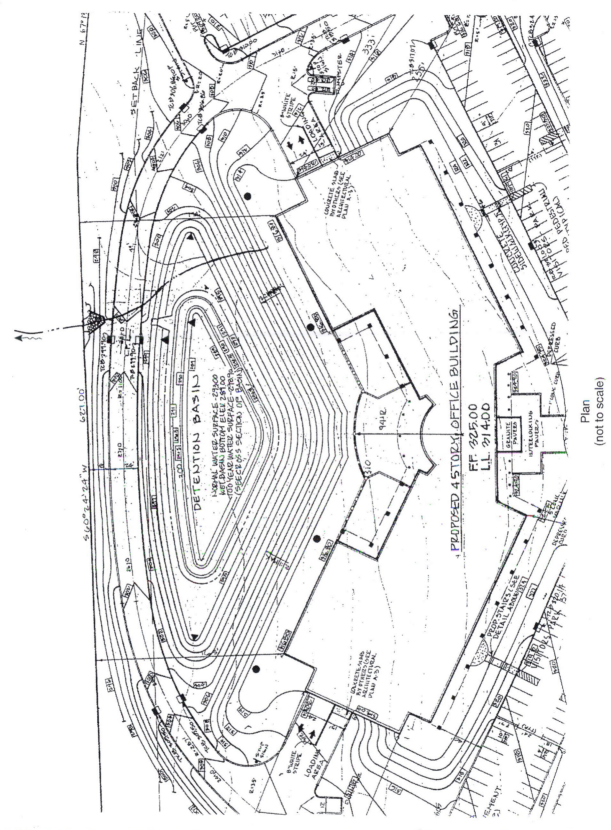

FIGURE 15-19 Plan of detention basin showing proposed contours. *(Courtesy of Canger and Cassera.)*

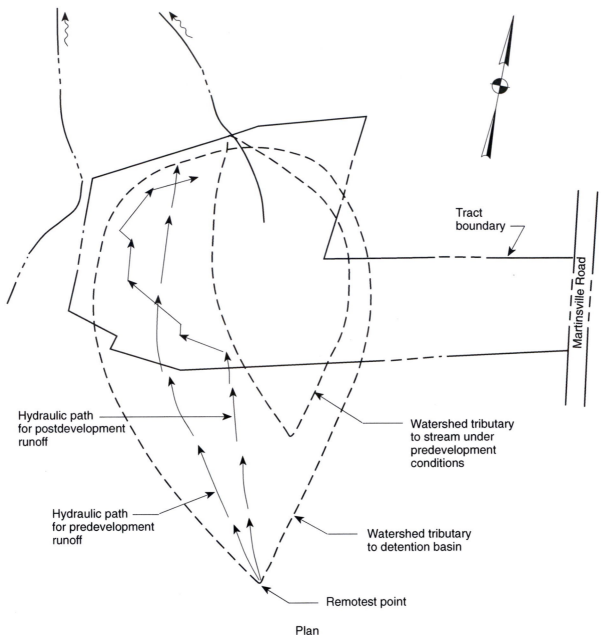

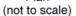

Plan
(not to scale)

FIGURE 15-20 Plan showing a comparison of drainage areas of existing and proposed conditions.

As shown in Figure 15-20, this hydraulic path does not end at the stream, but it does provide the longest time for runoff computation.

Therefore, peak runoff under predevelopment conditions was computed by the NRCS Method as follows:

A_m = 33.45 acres = 0.0523 s.m. (measured from plan)

Curve Number: From the local soil survey, soil types were identified and found to have Hydrologic Soil Group B. The entire watershed was wooded, so from Appendix D-1,

CN = 55

Time of Concentration: From the delineated hydraulic path,

$t_c = 40$ min

Rainfall: Using the various maps in Appendix D-3, rainfall was found for each design storm for the project location.

Storm (years)	Rainfall (in)
100	7.5
50	6.5
25	6.0
10	5.2
5	4.3
2	3.3

Rainfall distribution: From Appendix D-4, rainfall distribution was found to be Type II.

Peak runoff: Using the parameters above, the computer program computed peak runoff as follows:

Storm (years)	q_p (cfs)
100	51.7
50	36.7
25	29.7
10	19.5
5	10.2
2	2.9

These values of peak runoff then became the maximum allowable values of peak runoff under postdevelopment conditions.

Runoff Computations: Postdevelopment

Next, postdevelopment runoff hydrographs were computed by the computer and stored for use in routing computations. NRCS runoff parameters were as follows:

$A_m = 33.45$ acres $= 0.0523$ s.m.   (measured from plan)

Curve Number: Soil cover types are impervious, landscaped, and wooded
      Impervious: 8.5 acres   @ CN = 98
      Landscaped: 12.95 acres   @ CN = 65
      Wooded: 12 acres   @ CN = 55

CN = 70

Time of concentration: From the delineated hydraulic path in Figure 15-20, t_c consists of three components:

Overland flow	32 min
Shallow concentrated flow	3 min
Pipe flow	1.1 min

$t_c = 36$ min

Rainfall: Same as for predevelopment runoff.

Rainfall distribution: Same as for predevelopment runoff.

Peak runoff: Using the parameters above, the computer program computed runoff hydrographs having the following peak values:

Storm (years)	q_p (cfs)
100	98.9
50	78.1
25	68.0
10	52.4
5	35.7
2	19.1

These values are about double predevelopment peak runoff (except the smaller storms, which are as much as six times predevelopment peak runoff). Why are the smaller storm runoffs so much more than corresponding predevelopment runoffs?

Detention Basin Computations

By routing through the detention basin, the runoff rates were attenuated to rates below predevelopment runoff values. The detention basin outflow structure is shown in Figure 15-21, and basin parameters are listed in Figure 15-22.

The routings resulted in the following peak outflow rates and water levels:

(1) Storm (years)	(2) Allowable Outflow (cfs)	(3) Peak Inflow (cfs)	(4) Peak Outflow (cfs)	(5) Max. W.L. Elevation (ft)
100	51.7	98.9	50.0	298.90
50	36.7	78.1	36.4	298.10
25	29.7	68.0	28.7	297.80
10	19.5	52.4	16.8	297.20
5	10.2	35.7	7.0	296.40
2	2.9	19.1	2.3	295.30

To satisfy the design criterion of zero increase in peak runoff, values in column 4 above must be equal to or less than values in column 2. Since this is the case, the detention basin design was accepted.

Inflow and outflow hydrographs for the 100-year storm are plotted in Figure 15-23. Hydrographs for the remaining storms have similar shapes.

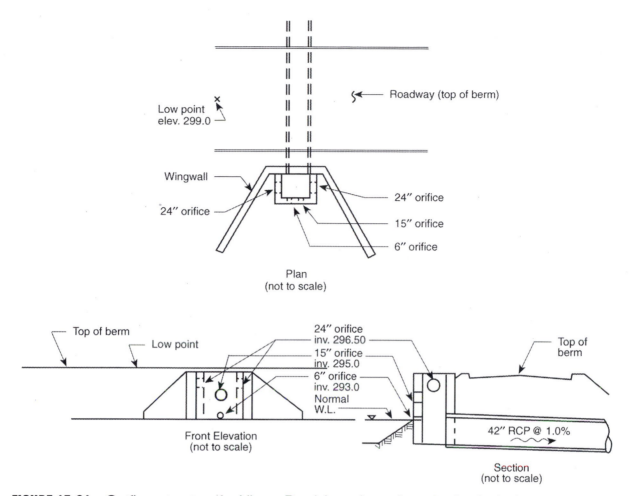

FIGURE 15-21   Outflow structure for Liberty Road Associates detention basin design.

A close inspection of Figure 15-21 reveals that the outflow structure is a three-stage outflow structure. The first stage is a 6-inch orifice, the second stage is a 15-inch orifice, and the third stage consists of two 24-inch orifices on both sides of the structure. The top of the structure contains an access manhole cover that is usually in the closed position. Therefore, the top does not serve hydraulically as another stage. Multiple stages were used because of the multiple storm routings. The outflow rating must be fashioned in such a way as to result in zero increase in runoff for each of the six storms. This can be done efficiently only by manipulating the outflow with multiple stages.

Emergency Spillway

The emergency spillway was incorporated into the berm by providing a low point in the roadway. The elevation of the low point is 299.0, which is just above the maximum 100-year impoundment level of 298.90. Thus, when the water level in the detention basin rises 0.10 feet above the 100-year maximum level, it starts to flow over the emergency spillway.

HYDROLOGIC REPORT FOR LIBERTY ROAD ASSOCIATES STAGE, STORAGE + DISCHARGE

POND IDENTIFIER PROP. DETENTION POND
1 =

ELEV	STORAGE (CU. FT.)	OUTFLOW (CFS)	2S/T+O (CFS)
293.0	0.0	0.0	0.0
293.5	9343.8	0.5	62.8
294.0	19875.0	0.9	133.4
294.5	31593.8	1.1	211.7
295.0	44500.0	1.3	298.0
295.5	58330.0	2.9	391.8
296.0	72816.3	5.4	490.8
296.5	87972.5	7.5	594.0
297.0	103785.0	13.3	705.2
297.5	120240.0	22.5	824.1
298.0	137351.3	33.5	949.2
298.5	155120.0	43.8	1077.9
299.0	173545.0	51.7	1208.7
300.0	212295.0	320.7	1736.0
301.0	253670.0	725.0	2416.1

FIGURE 15-22 Computer printout showing detention basin parameters for Case Study 2.

Normally, an emergency spillway is not allowed to be incorporated as an overtopping of the berm unless sufficient reinforcement of the berm surface is provided. So in this case, the downstream side of the berm was stabilized so that emergency overtopping could take place without eroding the soil and causing a breach or failure of the berm.

A 17-inch storm was routed through the basin to determine freeboard, or the vertical distance from the emergency spillway crest to the top of berm. The routing resulted in a maximum water level elevation of 299.90. This elevation was used to determine the extent of stabilization of the downstream side of the berm.

This berm design was unconventional because the top elevation was varied along its extent, with higher elevations at each end and a low point near the outflow structure. Normally, the berm would be level, and the emergency spillway would be a wide channel cut out of one end. However, in this case, such an arrangement would not have allowed a roadway to traverse the berm, and since the roadway was needed for internal site circulation, the unconventional overtopping proposal was approved.

It is important to note that the only way in which the overtopping emergency spillway was made acceptable was by stabilizing the top of the berm with the paved roadway and stabilizing the downstream side with other materials.

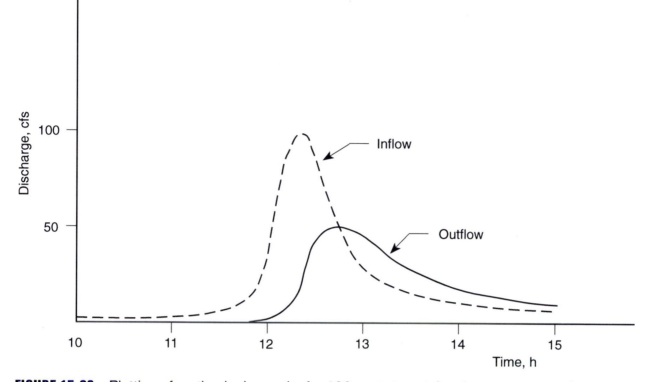

FIGURE 15-23   Plotting of routing hydrographs for 100-year storm taken from computer printout.

Outfall

The last aspect of this detention basin was the selection of the outflow pipe and the outflow apron. The outflow pipe was designed to convey the 100-year outflow with a headwater elevation below the second stage, elevation 295.0. This was accomplished with a 42-inch concrete pipe with invert set at elevation 290.0 as shown in Figure 15-21. Treating the pipe as a culvert with inlet control, a 100-year discharge of 50.0 cfs resulted in $HW = 3.43$ feet, equivalent to a water elevation inside the outflow structure of 293.43, which is below the second stage.

Erosion protection at the outfall of the 42-inch outflow pipe was considered by computing exit velocity for the 100-year outflow of 50.0 cfs. By using Chart 44 in Appendix A-4, design velocity was found to be about 9.0 fps, with a tailwater depth, TW, of 1.65 feet. (The Manning's n-value was assumed to be 0.012.)

The exit velocity of 9.0 fps is well above any permissible velocity found in Appendix A-2. Therefore, a riprap apron was designed. Using Equation 12-1, we have

$$d_{50} = \frac{0.02}{1.65}\left(\frac{50}{3.5}\right)^{4/3}$$
$$= 0.42 \text{ ft (5 in)}$$

Use $d_{50} = 6$ in.

Apron length was computed using Equation 12-2:

$$L_a = \frac{3(50)}{3.5^{3/2}}$$
$$= 22.9 \text{ ft}$$

Despite the computed length of 22.9 feet, the apron was proposed to be 20.0 feet long, since that was the distance from the outfall headwall to the northerly property line.

PROBLEMS

1. Referring to the detention basin shown in Figure 15-24, compute a chart of storage volume values for elevations 100, 101, 102, 102.5, 104, and 106.

2. Compute the outflow rating for the detention basin shown in Figure 15-24. Use the same elevations listed in problem 1. Ignore the constriction caused by the outflow pipe.

3. Using the results of Problems 1 and 2, plot graphs of O versus $2S/\Delta t + O$ and O versus $2S/\Delta t - O$.

4. Using the results of Problems 1 through 3, route the inflow hydrograph listed in Table 15-3 through the detention basin shown in Figure 15-24. From the routing, determine peak outflow and maximum water level.

5. Design a detention basin for the following project. Design storms are the 100-year and 10-year storms. The project is located in Memphis, Tennessee. Use the NRCS Method to compute runoff.

Design Criteria:

For each design storm, peak outflow for proposed conditions is equal to or less than peak inflow for existing conditions. Maximum water level in the detention basin cannot exceed the emergency spillway crest.

Existing Conditions:

Area tributary to detention basin = 20.0 acres

CN = 60

t_c = 0.50 hour

TABLE 15-3 Inflow Hydrograph for Detention Basin Routing

Time (hr)	Inflow (cfs)
0.0	1.2
0.25	1.5
0.50	2.1
0.75	3.2
1.00	11.6
1.25	22.1
1.50	9.8
1.75	4.5
2.00	3.2
2.25	2.7
2.50	2.4
2.75	2.0
3.00	1.8

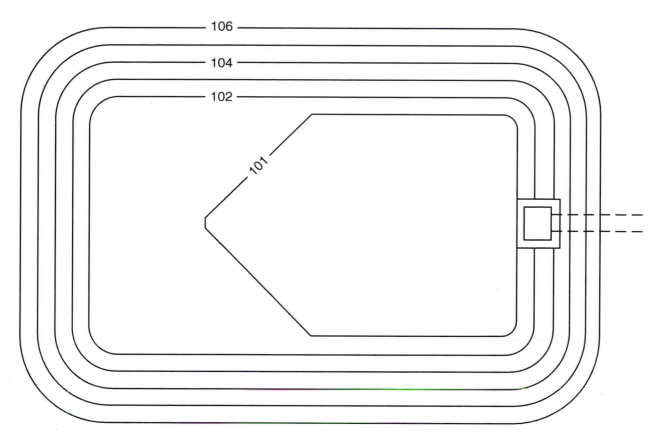

Plan
Scale: 1″ = 30′

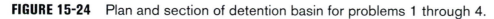

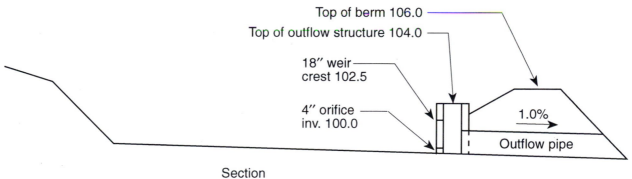

Top of berm 106.0

Top of outflow structure 104.0

18″ weir
crest 102.5

4″ orifice
inv. 100.0

1.0%

Outflow pipe

Section
(not to scale)

FIGURE 15-24 Plan and section of detention basin for problems 1 through 4.

Proposed Conditions:

Area tributary to detention basin = 20.0 acres

CN = 70

t_c = 0.45 hour

Detention Basin:

Grass-lined open cut

Bottom slope = 2.0%

Side slopes = 3 horizontal to 1 vertical

Primary outlet: 4-inch orifice, inv. elev. 650.00 ft

Secondary outlet: Weir (elev. and length to be chosen)

Emergency spillway crest elev.: (Choose an elevation at the maximum 100-year water level.)

Your design will consist of computing inflow hydrographs and then, by trial and error, choosing a detention basin size and a secondary outlet so that the routed inflow hydrographs meet the design criteria. The detention basin size can vary by area and by depth.

6. Design a detention basin for the following project. Design storms are the 100-year and 10-year storms. The project is located in Atlanta, Georgia. Use the Modified Rational Method to compute runoff. The runoff hydrograph is a triangular hydrograph with base equal to $2.67t_c$.

Design Criteria:

For each design storm, peak outflow for proposed conditions is equal to or less than peak inflow for existing conditions. Maximum water level in the detention basin cannot exceed the emergency spillway crest.

Existing Conditions:

Area tributary to detention basin = 10.0 acres

$c = 0.25$

$t_c = 20$ min

Proposed Conditions:

Area tributary to detention basin = 10.0 acres

$c = 0.50$

$t_c = 15$ min

Detention Basin:

Grass-lined open cut

Bottom slope = 2.0%

Side slopes = 3 horizontal to 1 vertical

Primary outlet: 4-inch orifice, inv. elev. 400.00 ft

Secondary outlet: Weir (elev. and length to be chosen)

Emergency spillway crest elev.: (Choose an elevation at the maximum 100-year water level.)

Your design will consist of computing inflow hydrographs and then, by trial and error, choosing a detention basin size and a secondary outlet so that the routed inflow hydrographs meet the design criteria. The detention basin size can vary by area and by depth.

7. Design an open-cut detention basin for the developed tract shown in Figure 15-25 to result in zero increase in peak runoff for the 100-year storm.

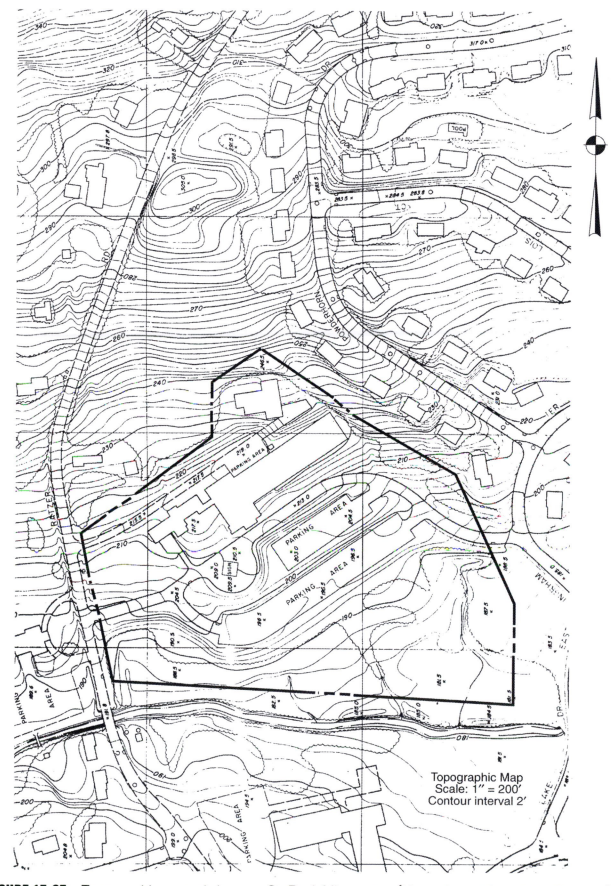

FIGURE 15-25 Topographic map of site near St. Paul, Minnesota. *(Map adapted from Aero Service.)*

Computations are to be by NRCS Method by computer or by hand. Locate the basin on site south of the parking area and discharge at one of the on-site streams. Make all slopes three horizontal to one vertical. Use the following assumptions:

1. Project location: near St. Paul, Minnesota
2. Hydrologic soil group B
3. Predevelopment soil cover on site: wooded, good condition
4. Postdevelopment soil cover on site:

   Impervious
   Lawns, good condition
   Woods, fair condition

FURTHER READING

Debo, T., and Reese, A. (1995). *Municipal Storm Water Management*. Boca Raton, FL: Lewis Publishers.

Davis, A. P., and McCuen, R. M. (2005). *Stormwater Management for Smart Growth*. New York: Springer Science & Business Media.

Mays, L. W., ed. (2001). *Stormwater Collection Systems Design Handbook*. New York: McGraw-Hill.

Mays, L. W. (2003). *Urban Stormwater Management Tools*. New York: McGraw-Hill.

U.S. Department of Agriculture (1985). *National Engineering Handbook, Section 4, Hydrology*. Washington, DC: Soil Conservation Service.

U.S. Department of Agriculture (1986). *Urban Hydrology for Small Watersheds, Technical Release 55*. Washington, DC: Soil Conservation Service.

Urban Water Resources Research Council of ASCE and Water Environment Federation (2000). *Design and Construction of Urban Stormwater Management Systems*. New York and Alexandria, VA: ASCE.

Appendix Contents

DESIGN CHARTS FOR OPEN CHANNEL FLOW

A-1
Roughness Coefficients (Manning's *n*)

I. CLOSED CULVERTS:
- A. Concrete pipe 0.012–0.015
- B. Corrugated-metal pipe or pipe-arch (annular unpaved):
  - 1. 2²⁄₃ by ½ in corrugation riveted pipe 0.024
  - 2. 3 in by 1 in corrugation 0.027
  - 3. 5 in by 1 in corrugation 0.025
  - 4. 6 in by 2 in corrugation (field bolted) 0.033
- C. Vitrified clay pipe 0.012–0.014
- D. Cast-iron pipe, uncoated 0.013
- E. Steel pipe 0.009–0.011
- F. Brick 0.014–0.017
- G. Monolithic concrete:
  - 1. Wood forms, rough 0.015–0.017
  - 2. Wood forms, smooth 0.012–0.014
  - 3. Steel forms 0.012–0.013
- H. Cemented rubble masonry walls:
  - 1. Concrete floor and top 0.017–0.022
  - 2. Natural floor 0.019–0.025
- I. Laminated treated wood 0.015–0.017
- J. Vitrified clay liner plates 0.015
- K. Polyvinyl chloride (PVC) 0.007–0.011

II. OPEN CHANNELS, LINED (Straight Alignment):
- A. Concrete, with surfaces as indicated:
  - 1. Formed, no finish 0.013–0.017
  - 2. Trowel finish 0.012–0.014
  - 3. Float finish 0.013–0.015
  - 4. Float finish, some gravel on bottom 0.015–0.017
  - 5. Gunite, good section 0.016–0.019
  - 6. Gunite, wavy section 0.018–0.022
- B. Concrete, bottom float finished, sides as indicated:
  - 1. Dressed stone in mortar 0.015–0.017
  - 2. Random stone in mortar 0.017–0.020
  - 3. Cement rubble masonry 0.020–0.025
  - 4. Cement rubble masonry, plastered 0.016–0.020
  - 5. Dry rubble (riprap) 0.020–0.030
- C. Gravel bottom, sides as indicated:
  - 1. Formed concrete 0.017–0.020
  - 2. Random stone in mortar 0.020–0.023
  - 3. Dry rubble (riprap) 0.023–0.033
- D. Brick 0.014–0.017
- E. Asphalt:
  - 1. Smooth 0.013
  - 2. Rough 0.016
- F. Wood, planed, clean 0.001–0.013
- G. Concrete-lined excavated rock:
  - 1. Good section 0.017–0.020
  - 2. Irregular section 0.022–0.027

III. OPEN CHANNELS, EXCAVATED (Straight Alignment, Natural Lining):
- A. Earth, uniform section:
  - 1. Clean, recently completed 0.016–0.018
  - 2. Clean, after weathering 0.018–0.020
  - 3. With short grass, few weeds 0.022–0.027
  - 4. In gravelly soil, uniform section, clean 0.022–0.025
- B. Earth, fairly uniform section:
  - 1. No vegetation 0.022–0.025
  - 2. Grass, some weeds 0.025–0.030
  - 3. Dense weeds or aquatic plants in deep channels 0.030–0.035
  - 4. Sides clean, gravel bottom 0.025–0.030
  - 5. Sides clean, cobble bottom 0.030–0.040

  C. Dragline excavated or dredged:
    1. No vegetation 0.028–0.033
    2. Light brush on banks 0.035–0.050
  D. Rock
    1. Based on design section 0.035
    2. Based on actual mean section:
      a. Smooth and uniform 0.035–0.040
      b. Jagged and irregular 0.040–0.045
  E. Channels not maintained, weeds and brush uncut:
    1. Dense weeds, high as flow depth 0.080–0.120
    2. Clean bottom, brush on sides 0.050–0.080
    3. Clean bottom, brush on sides, highest stage of flow 0.070–0.140
    4. Dense brush, high stage 0.100–0.140

IV. HIGHWAY CHANNELS AND SWALES WITH MAINTAINED VEGETATION
  (Values shown are for velocities of 2 and 6 fps.):
  A. Depth of flow up to 0.7 foot:
    1. Bermuda grass, Kentucky bluegrass, buffalo grass:
      a. Mowed to 2 inches 0.070–0.045
      b. Length 4 to 6 inches 0.090–0.050
    2. Good stand, any grass:
      a. Length about 12 inches 0.180–0.090
      b. Length about 24 inches 0.200–0.100
    3. Fair stand, any grass:
      a. Length about 12 inches 0.140–0.080
      b. Length about 24 inches 0.250–0.130
  B. Depth of flow 0.7–1.5 feet:
    1. Bermuda grass, Kentucky bluegrass, buffalo grass:
      a. Mowed to 2 inches 0.050–0.035
      b. Length 4 to 6 inches 0.060–0.040
    2. Good stand, any grass:
      a. Length about 12 inches 0.120–0.070
      b. Length about 24 inches 0.020–0.100
    3. Fair stand, any grass:
      a. Length about 12 inches 0.100–0.060
      b. Length about 24 inches 0.170–0.090

V. STREET AND EXPRESSWAY GUTTERS:
  A. Concrete gutter, troweled finish 0.012
  B. Asphalt pavement:
    1. Smooth texture 0.013
    2. Rough texture 0.016
  C. Concrete gutter with asphalt pavement:
    1. Smooth 0.013
    2. Rough 0.015
  D. Concrete pavement:
    1. Float finish 0.014
    2. Broom finish 0.016
  E. For gutters with small slope, where sediment may accumulate, increase above values of *n* by 0.002

VI. NATURAL STREAM CHANNELS:
  A. Minor streams (surface width at flood stage less 100 ft):
    1. Fairly regular section:
      a. Some grass and weeds, little or no brush 0.030–0.035
      b. Dense growth of weeds, depth of flow materially greater than weed height 0.030–0.050
      c. Some weeds, light brush on banks 0.035–0.050
      d. Some weeds, heavy brush on banks 0.050–0.070
      e. Some weeds, dense willows on banks 0.060–0.080
      f. For trees within channel, with branches submerged at high stage, increase all
        above values by 0.010–0.020
    2. Irregular sections, with pools, slight channel meander; increase values given in
      1.a.–e. about 0.010–0.020
    3. Mountain streams, no vegetation in channel banks usually steep, trees and brush
      along banks submerged at high stage:
      a. Bottom of gravel, cobbles, and few boulders 0.040–0.050
      b. Bottom of cobbles, with large boulders 0.050–0.070

B.   Flood plains (adjacent to natural streams):
   1.   Pasture, no brush:
      a.   Short grass 0.030–0.035
      b.   High grass 0.035–0.050
   2.   Cultivated areas:
      a.   No crop 0.030–0.040
      b.   Mature row crops 0.035–0.045
      c.   Mature field crops 0.040–0.050
   3.   Heavy weeds, scattered brush 0.050–0.070
   4.   Light brush and trees:
      a.   Winter 0.050–0.060
      b.   Summer 0.060–0.080
   5.   Medium to dense brush:
      a.   Winter 0.070–0.110
      b.   Summer 0.100–0.170

(Courtesy of New Jersey Department of Transportation, Design, Manual, Roadway.)

A-2
Permissible Velocities

SOIL TEXTURE	ALLOWABLE VELOCITY (ft/s)
Sand and sandy loam (noncollodial)	2.5
Silt loam (also high lime clay)	3.0
Sandy clay loam	3.5
Clay loam	4.0
Clay, fine gravel, graded loam to gravel	5.0
Cobbles	5.5
Shale	6.0

(Courtesy of New Jersey State Soil Conservation Committee, Standards for Soil Erosion and Sediment Control in New Jersey.)

A-3
Channel Charts for the Solution of Manning's Equation

The following selected design charts provide a direct graphical solution of Manning's equation for various-sized open channels with rectangular and trapezoidal cross section. The channels are assumed to have uniform slope, cross section, and roughness and are not affected by backwater.

Charts 1 through 14 (rectangular channels) are calibrated for a roughness value of 0.015, and Charts 15 through 23 (trapezoidal channels) are calibrated for a roughness value of 0.030. However, by use of the Qn scale, any n-value may be used. Use of the Qn scale is explained below.

You may use the charts to find discharge, velocity, normal depth, and critical depth. Following is a brief outline describing basic use of the charts:

1. **How to Use the Qn Scale.** If $n = 0.015$ for a rectangular channel or $n = 0.030$ for a trapezoidal channel, do not use the Qn scale, but read the discharge directly on the Q scale. However, for all other n values, multiply n by the discharge, Q, and read the resulting Qn value on the Qn scale directly below the Q scale.

2. **How to Find Normal Depth.** If you know discharge, roughness, and slope, find normal depth by entering the value of Q (or Qn), and project a line straight up the graph until you intersect the appropriate slope line. Using the point of intersection, read the normal depth using the series of diagonal lines labeled *NORMAL DEPTH OF FLOW—FEET*. You might need to interpolate between lines.

3. **How to Find Critical Depth.** Critical depth is independent of roughness, so do not use the Qn scale. If you know the discharge, enter the value of Q and project straight up until you intersect the *CRITICAL* curve (dashed line). Using this point of intersection, read normal depth as in Item 2 above. The resulting value of normal depth is critical depth. (Remember that critical depth is a normal depth as well.)

4. **How to Find Velocity.** If you know discharge, roughness, and slope, find velocity by entering the value of Q (or Qn) and project a line straight up until you intersect the appropriate slope line. Using the point of intersection, read the velocity using the series of curves running down and to the left labeled *VELOCITY—FPS*. You might need to interpolate between lines.

5. **How to Find Discharge.** If you know slope, normal depth, and roughness, find discharge by first locating the intersection of the appropriate slope and normal depth lines (interpolating if necessary). From the point of intersection, project a line straight down to the Qn scale and read the value of Qn. Finally, divide the Qn value by n to obtain discharge.

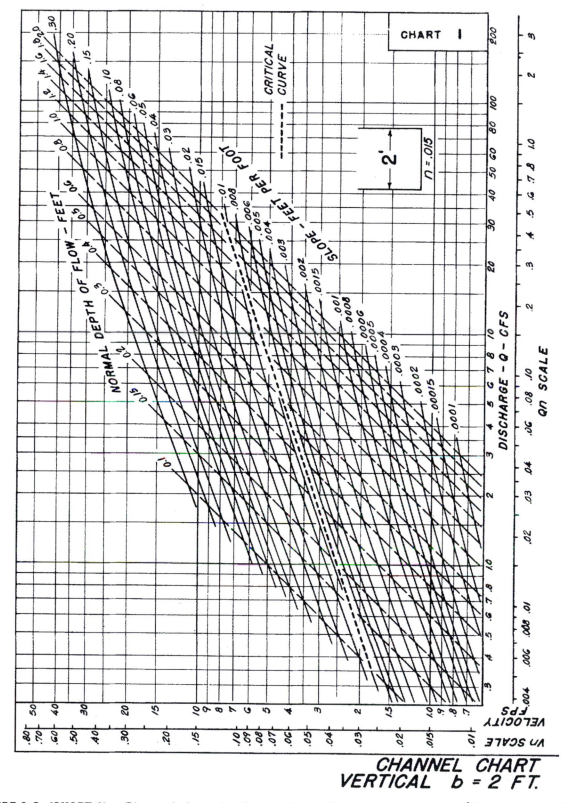

FIGURE A-3. (CHART 1)   Channel charts for the solution of Manning's equation. *(Courtesy of U.S. Department of Commerce, Bureau of Public Roads, Design Charts for Open-Channel Flow.)*

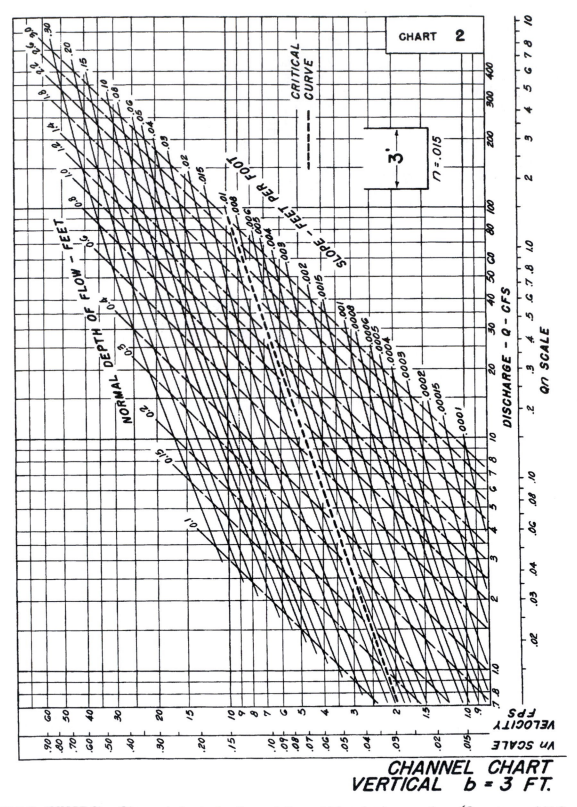

FIGURE A-3. (CHART 2) Channel charts for the solution of Manning's equation. *(Courtesy of U.S. Department of Commerce, Bureau of Public Roads, Design Charts for Open-Channel Flow.)*

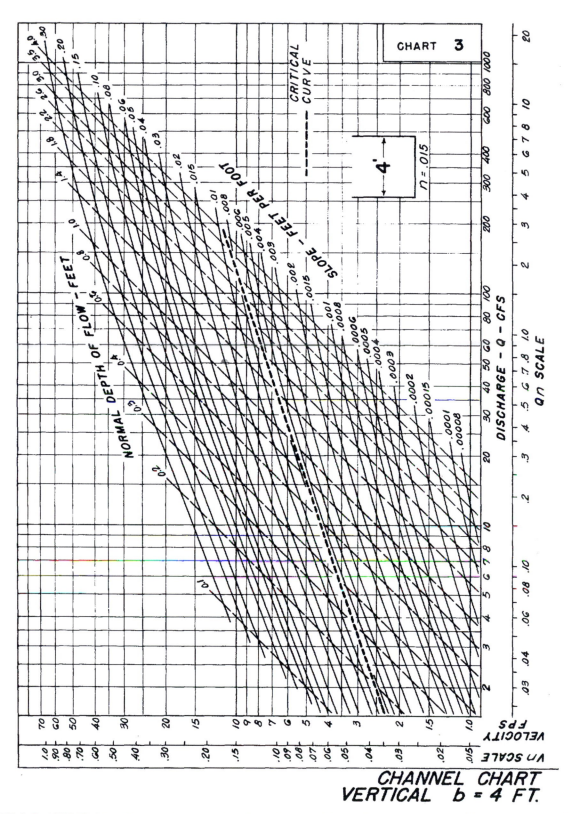

FIGURE A-3. (CHART 3)   Channel charts for the solution of Manning's equation. *(Courtesy of U.S. Department of Commerce, Bureau of Public Roads, Design Charts for Open-Channel Flow.)*

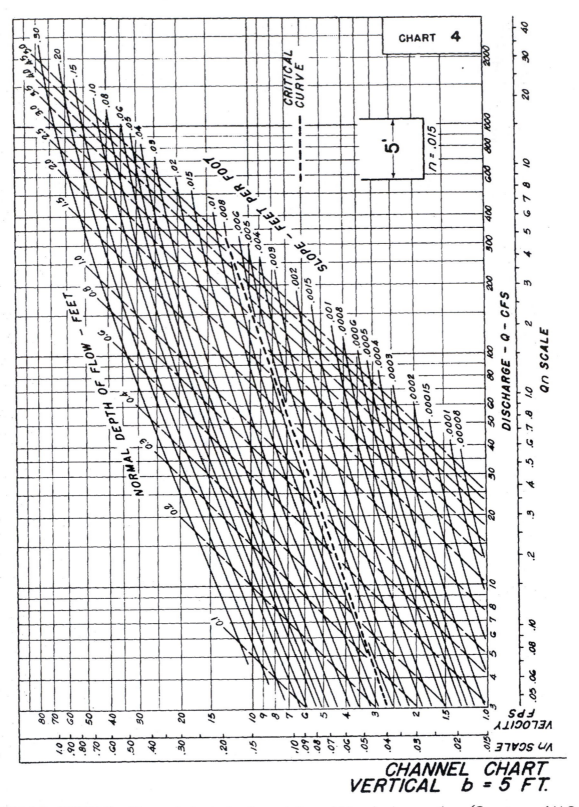

FIGURE A-3. (CHART 4) Channel charts for the solution of Manning's equation. *(Courtesy of U.S. Department of Commerce, Bureau of Public Roads, Design Charts for Open-Channel Flow.)*

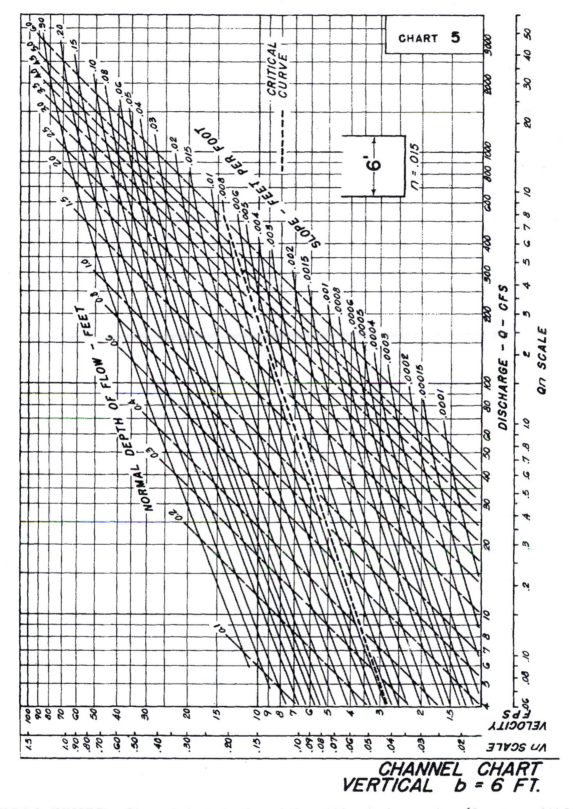

FIGURE A-3. (CHART 5)   Channel charts for the solution of Manning's equation. *(Courtesy of U.S. Department of Commerce, Bureau of Public Roads, Design Charts for Open-Channel Flow.)*

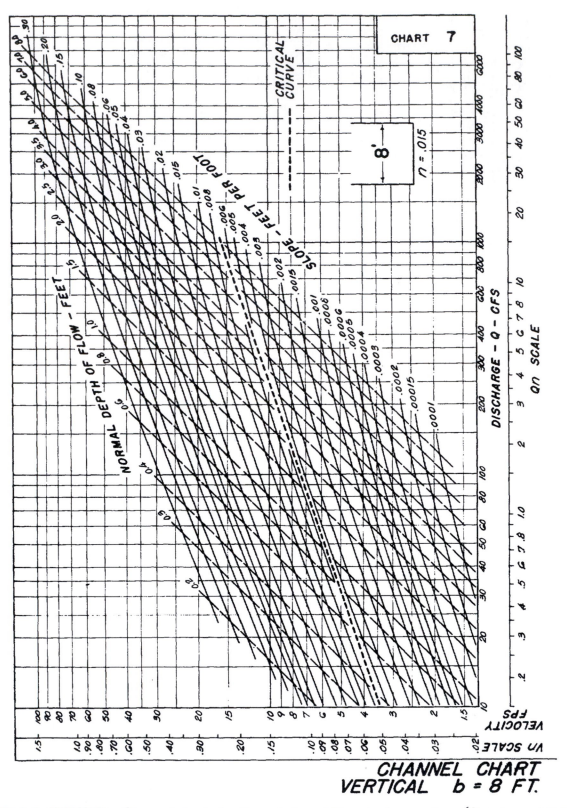

FIGURE A-3. (CHART 7) Channel charts for the solution of Manning's equation. *(Courtesy of U.S. Department of Commerce, Bureau of Public Roads, Design Charts for Open-Channel Flow.)*

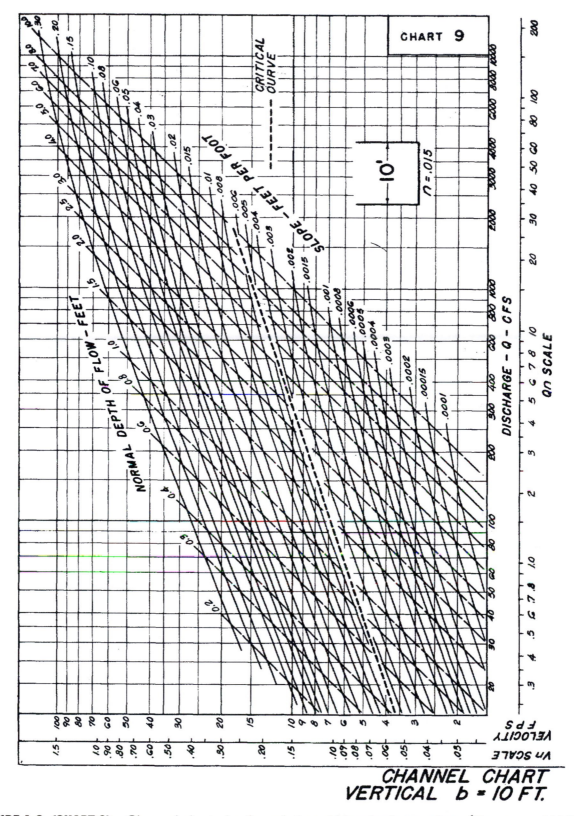

FIGURE A-3. (CHART 9)   Channel charts for the solution of Manning's equation. *(Courtesy of U.S. Department of Commerce, Bureau of Public Roads, Design Charts for Open-Channel Flow.)*

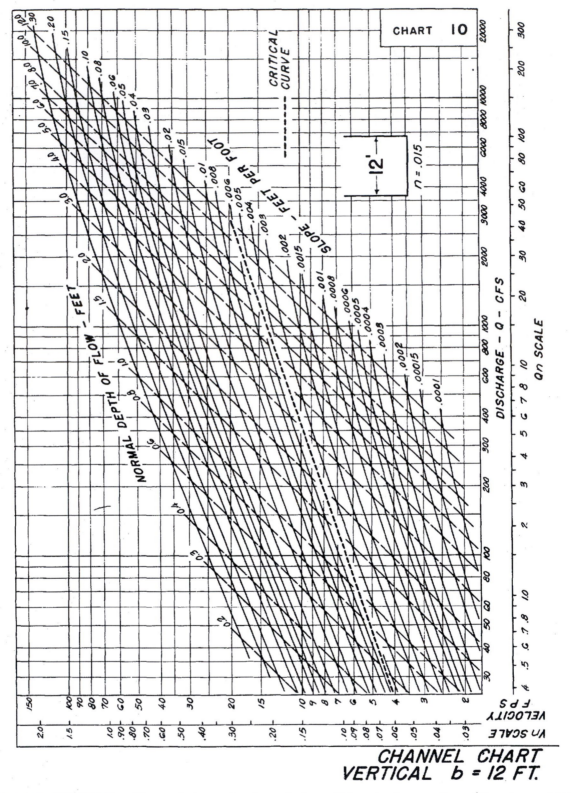

FIGURE A-3. (CHART 10) Channel charts for the solution of Manning's equation. *(Courtesy of U.S. Department of Commerce, Bureau of Public Roads, Design Charts for Open-Channel Flow.)*

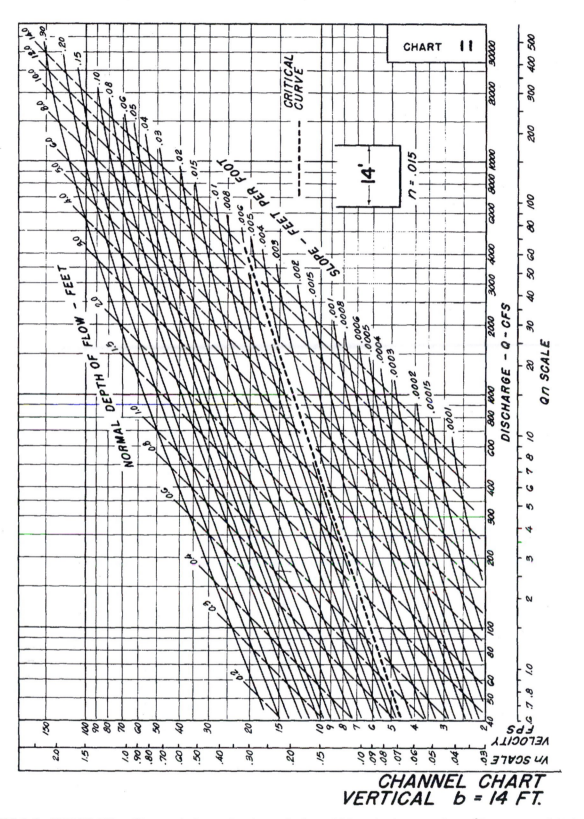

FIGURE A-3. (CHART 11)   Channel charts for the solution of Manning's equation. *(Courtesy of U.S. Department of Commerce, Bureau of Public Roads, Design Charts for Open-Channel Flow.)*

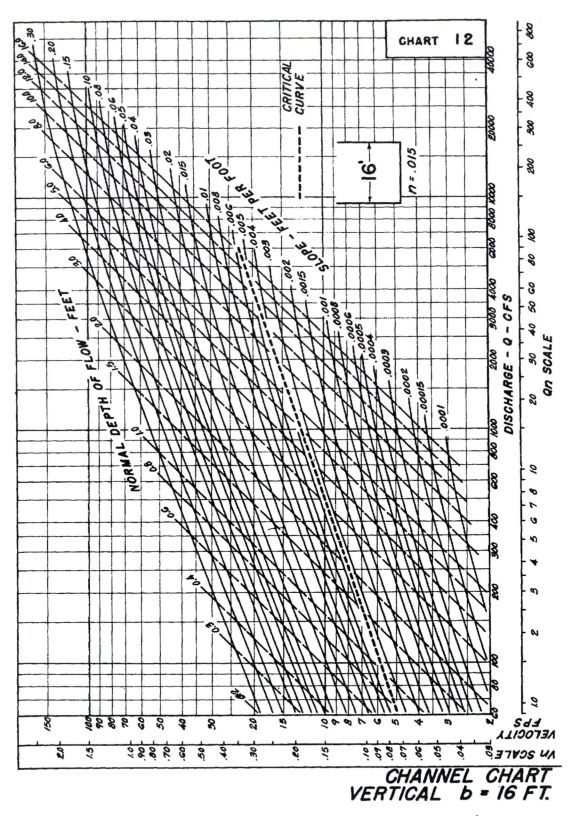

FIGURE A-3. (CHART 12)   Channel charts for the solution of Manning's equation. *(Courtesy of U.S. Department of Commerce, Bureau of Public Roads, Design Charts for Open-Channel Flow.)*

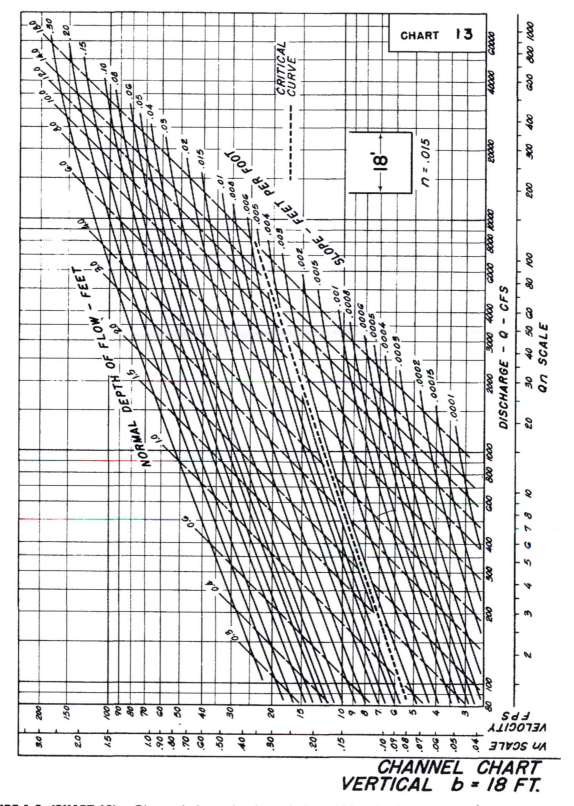

FIGURE A-3. (CHART 13)   Channel charts for the solution of Manning's equation. *(Courtesy of U.S. Department of Commerce, Bureau of Public Roads, Design Charts for Open-Channel Flow.)*

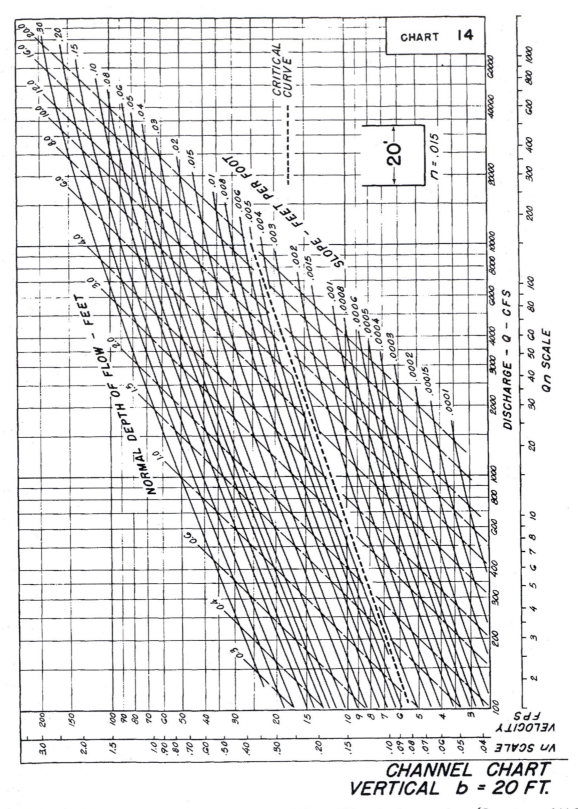

FIGURE A-3. (CHART 14)   Channel charts for the solution of Manning's equation. *(Courtesy of U.S. Department of Commerce, Bureau of Public Roads, Design Charts for Open-Channel Flow.)*

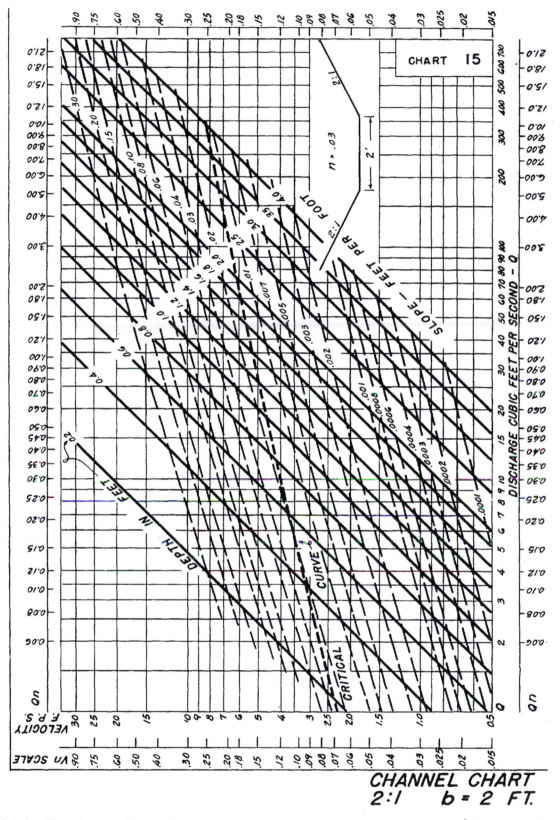

CHANNEL CHART
2:1   b = 2 FT.

FIGURE A-3. (CHART 15)   Channel charts for the solution of Manning's equation. *(Courtesy of U.S. Department of Commerce, Bureau of Public Roads, Design Charts for Open-Channel Flow.)*

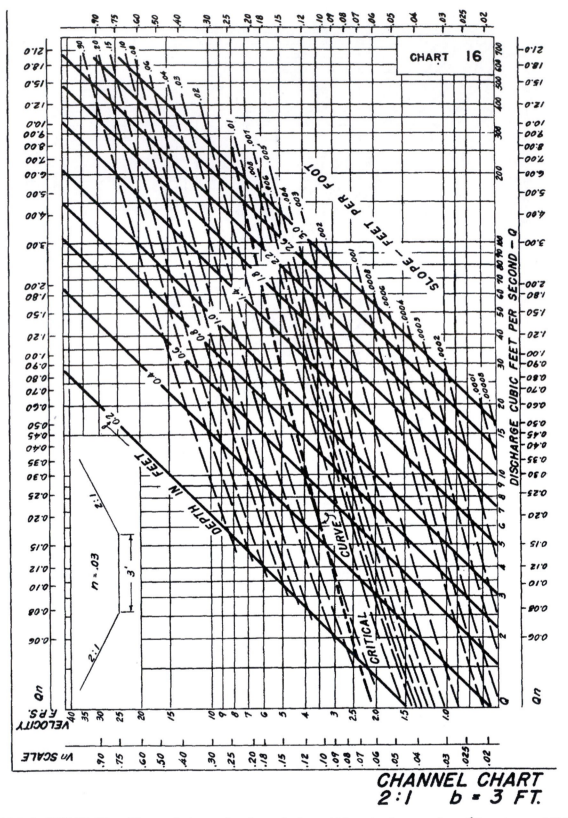

FIGURE A-3. (CHART 16) Channel charts for the solution of Manning's equation. *(Courtesy of U.S. Department of Commerce, Bureau of Public Roads, Design Charts for Open-Channel Flow.)*

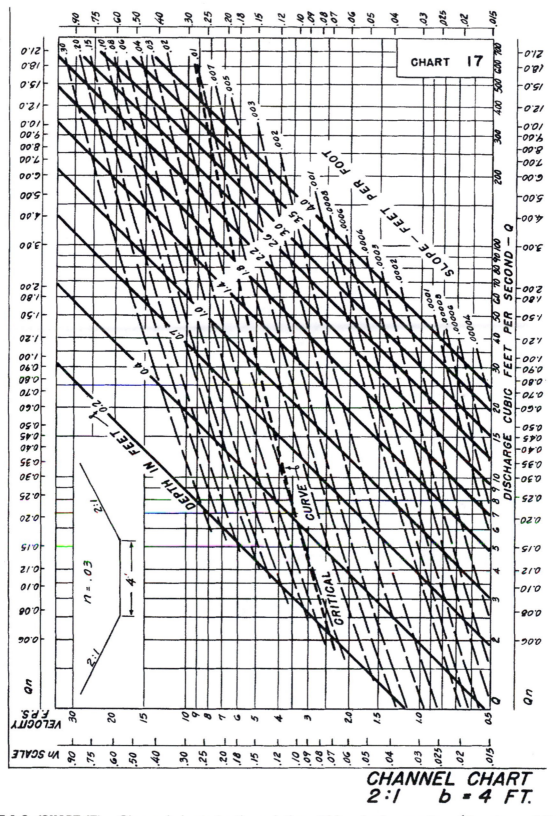

FIGURE A-3. (CHART 17)   Channel charts for the solution of Manning's equation. *(Courtesy of U.S. Department of Commerce, Bureau of Public Roads, Design Charts for Open-Channel Flow.)*

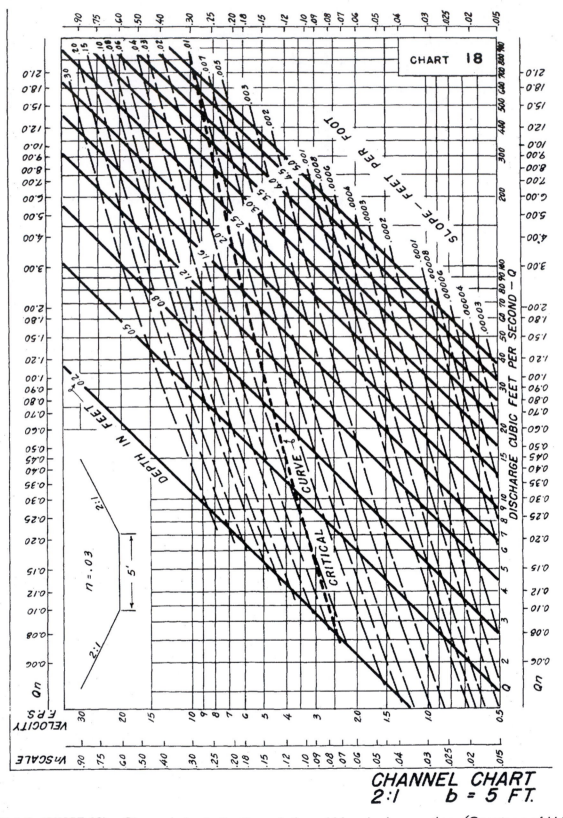

FIGURE A-3. (CHART 18)   Channel charts for the solution of Manning's equation. *(Courtesy of U.S. Department of Commerce, Bureau of Public Roads, Design Charts for Open-Channel Flow.)*

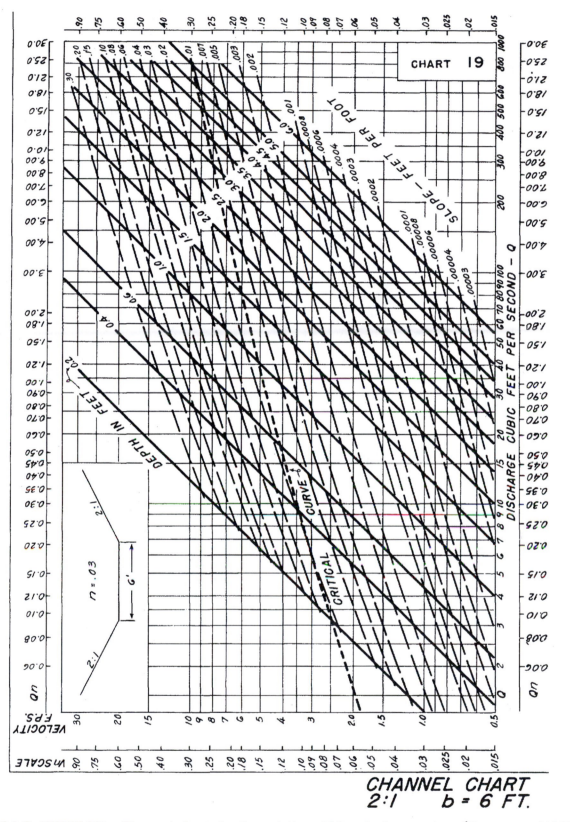

CHANNEL CHART
2:1   b = 6 FT.

FIGURE A-3. (CHART 19) Channel charts for the solution of Manning's equation. *(Courtesy of U.S. Department of Commerce, Bureau of Public Roads, Design Charts for Open-Channel Flow.)*

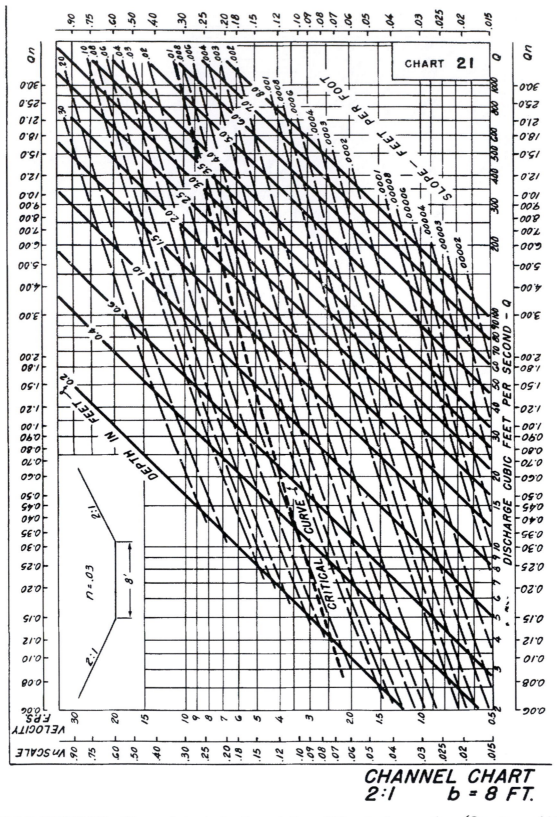

FIGURE A-3. (CHART 21)   Channel charts for the solution of Manning's equation. *(Courtesy of U.S. Department of Commerce, Bureau of Public Roads, Design Charts for Open-Channel Flow.)*

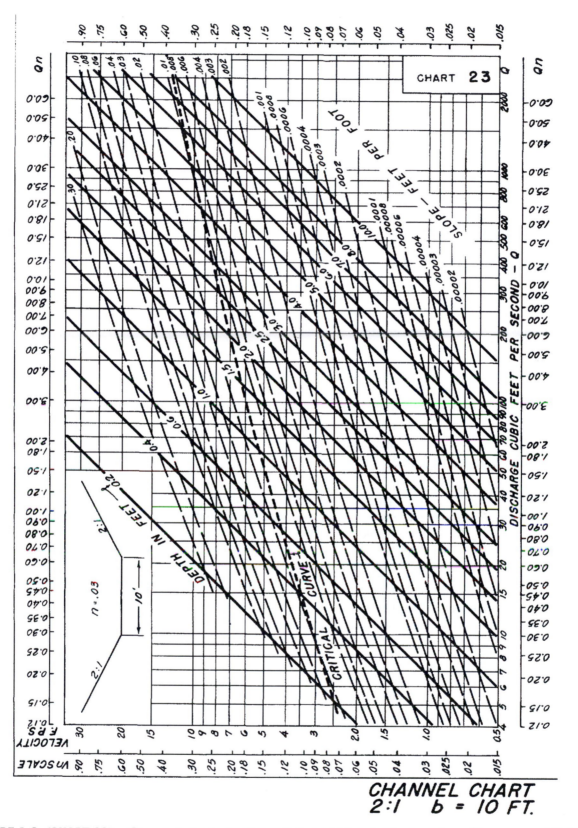

FIGURE A-3. (CHART 23)   Channel charts for the solution of Manning's equation. *(Courtesy of U.S. Department of Commerce, Bureau of Public Roads, Design Charts for Open-Channel Flow.)*

A-4
Pipe Charts for the Solution of Manning's Equation

Charts 35 through 47 provide a direct graphical solution of Manning's equation for circular pipes operating as an open channel (without pressure). The pipes are assumed to have uniform slope, cross section, and roughness and are not affected by backwater.

The charts are calibrated for roughness values of 0.015, 0.012, and 0.024. However, as is explained in Item 1 below, any n-value may be used.

You may use the charts to find discharge, velocity normal depth, and critical depth. Following is a brief outline describing basic use of the charts:

1. **How to Use the Charts for Any n-Value.** If the roughness of your pipe is not one of the three listed above, follow this simple procedure:

    A. Adjust your known value of Q by multiplying by the ratio $\dfrac{n}{0.015}$ to obtain an adjusted value, Q'.
    B. Enter Q' in the discharge scale for $n = 0.015$ and proceed as usual.

    If you are trying to determine discharge, follow this simple procedure:

    A. Using the usual procedure, drop a straight line to the discharge scale for $n = 0.015$.
    B. This value is actually Q', the adjusted discharge.
    C. Find the actual discharge by multiplying Q' by the ratio $\dfrac{0.015}{n}$.

2. **How to Find Normal Depth.** If you know discharge, roughness, and slope, find normal depth by entering the value of Q (or Q') and project a line straight up the graph until you intersect the appropriate slope line. (You might need to interpolate between slope lines.) At the point of intersection, read the normal depth using the series of diagonal lines labeled *NORMAL DEPTH OF FLOW IN PIPE—FEET*. (You might need to interpolate between lines.)

3. **How to Find Critical Depth.** Critical depth is independent of roughness, so do not use the lower Q scales ($n = 0.012, 0.024$). If you know the discharge, enter the value of Q and project straight up until you intersect the *CRITICAL* curve (dashed line). Using this point of intersection, read normal depth as in Item 2 above. The resulting value of normal depth is critical depth. (Remember that critical depth is a normal depth as well.)

4. **How to Find Velocity.** If you know discharge, roughness, and slope, find velocity by entering the value of Q (or Q') and project a line straight up until you intersect the appropriate slope line. (You might need to interpolate between slope lines.) Using this point of intersection, read the velocity using the series of curves running down and to the left labeled *VELOCITY—V—FPS*. (You might need to interpolate between lines.)

5. **How to Find Discharge.** If you know slope, normal depth, and roughness, find discharge by first locating the intersection of the appropriate slope and normal depth lines (interpolating if necessary). From the point of intersection, project a line straight down to the Q scale and read the value of discharge. (If necessary, adjust for a different n-value in accordance with Item 1 above.)

6. **How to Find Pipe Capacity.** Pipe capacity actually is the same as finding discharge when normal depth equals pipe diameter. This value of normal depth is the last line in the series of normal depth lines and occurs at the end of the *hook* of the slope line as shown below.

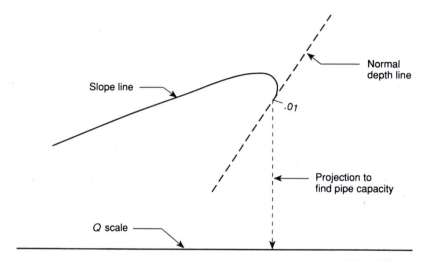

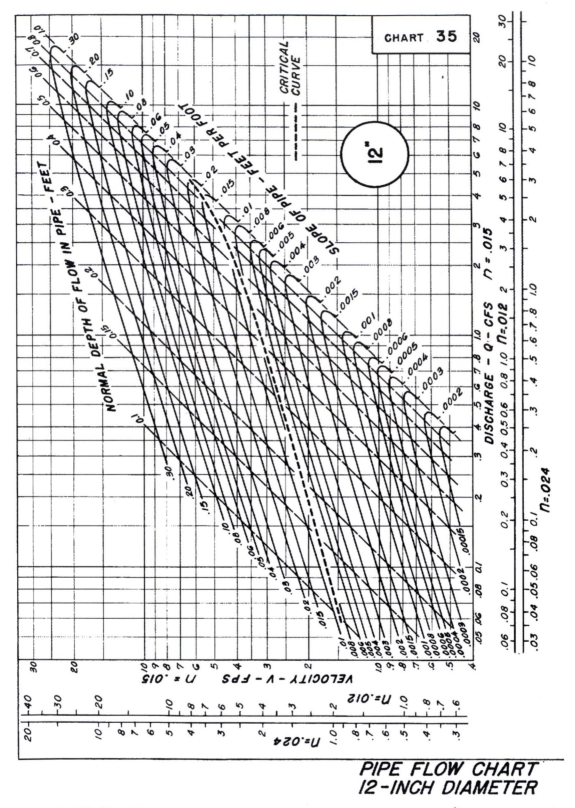

FIGURE A-4. (CHART 35)   Pipe charts for the solution of Manning's equation. *(Courtesy of U.S. Department of Commerce, Bureau of Public Roads, Design Charts for Open-Channel Flow.)*

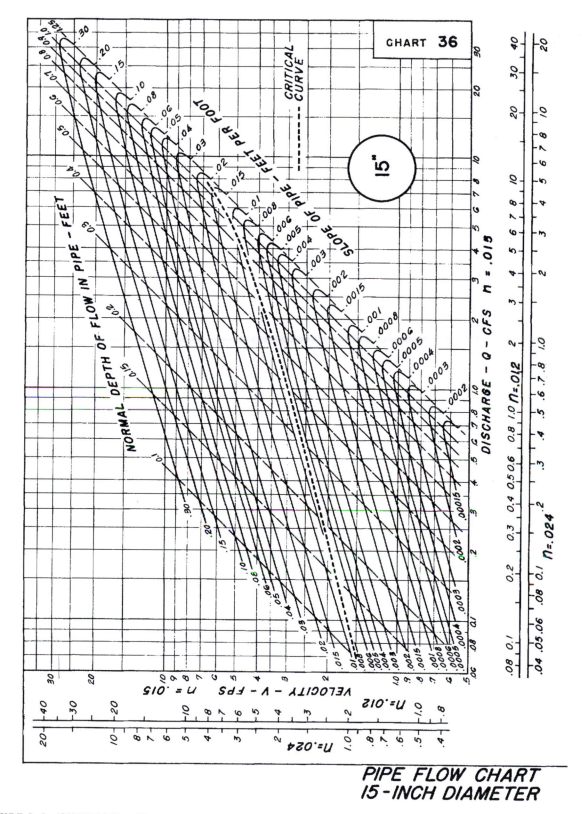

FIGURE A-4. (CHART 36) Pipe charts for the solution of Manning's equation. *(Courtesy of U.S. Department of Commerce, Bureau of Public Roads, Design Charts for Open-Channel Flow.)*

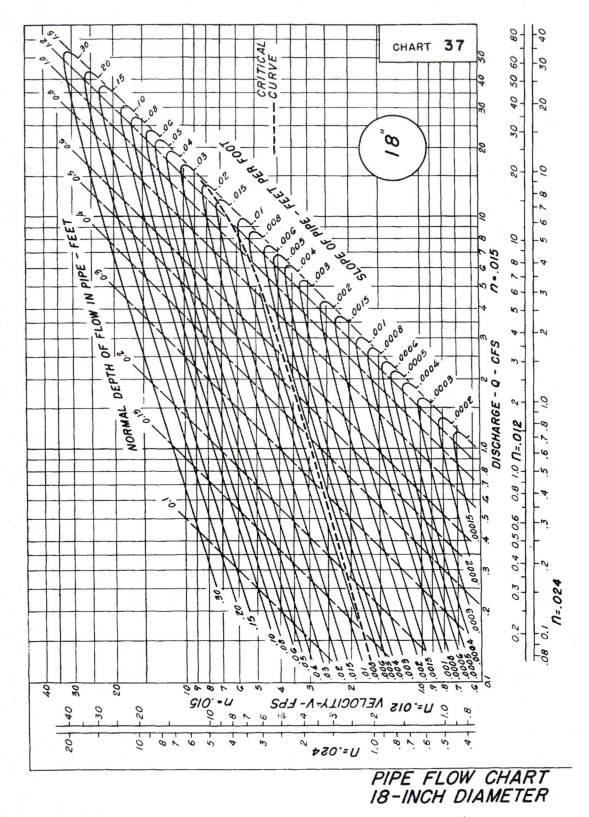

PIPE FLOW CHART
18-INCH DIAMETER

FIGURE A-4. (CHART 37)   Pipe charts for the solution of Manning's equation. (*Courtesy of U.S. Department of Commerce, Bureau of Public Roads, Design Charts for Open-Channel Flow.*)

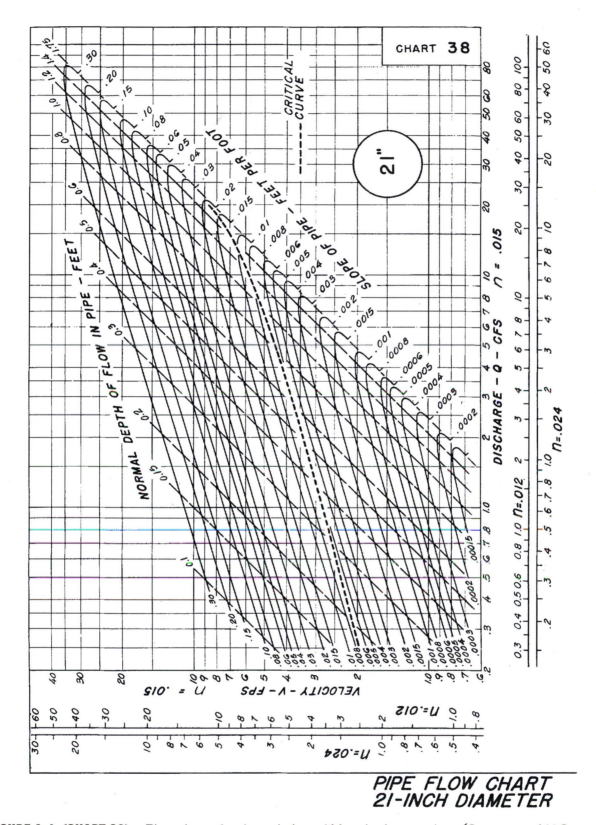

**PIPE FLOW CHART
21-INCH DIAMETER**

FIGURE A-4. (CHART 38)   Pipe charts for the solution of Manning's equation. *(Courtesy of U.S. Department of Commerce, Bureau of Public Roads, Design Charts for Open-Channel Flow.)*

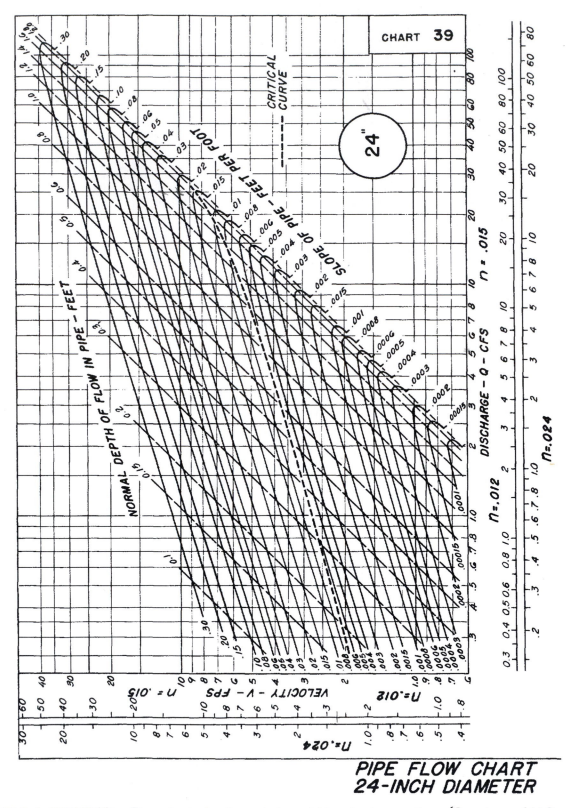

FIGURE A-4. (CHART 39) Pipe charts for the solution of Manning's equation. *(Courtesy of U.S. Department of Commerce, Bureau of Public Roads, Design Charts for Open-Channel Flow.)*

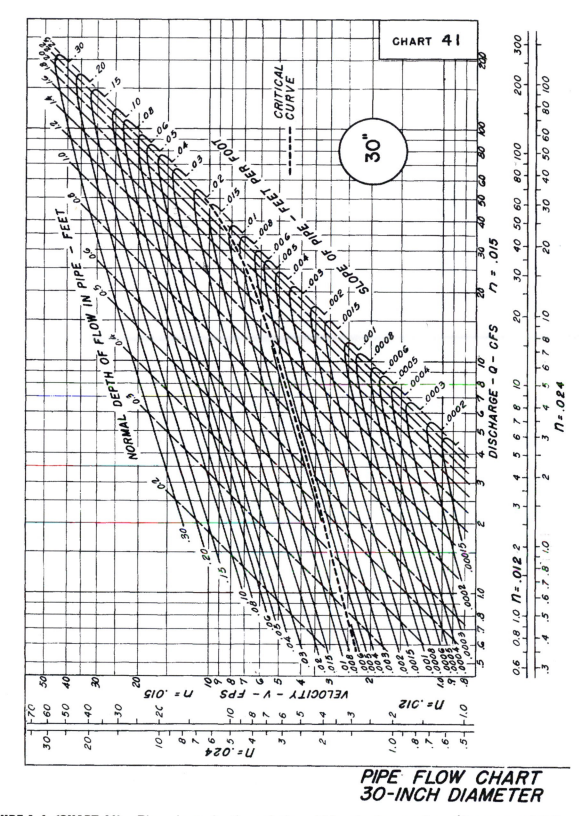

PIPE FLOW CHART
30-INCH DIAMETER

FIGURE A-4. (CHART 41)   Pipe charts for the solution of Manning's equation. (*Courtesy of U.S. Department of Commerce, Bureau of Public Roads, Design Charts for Open-Channel Flow.*)

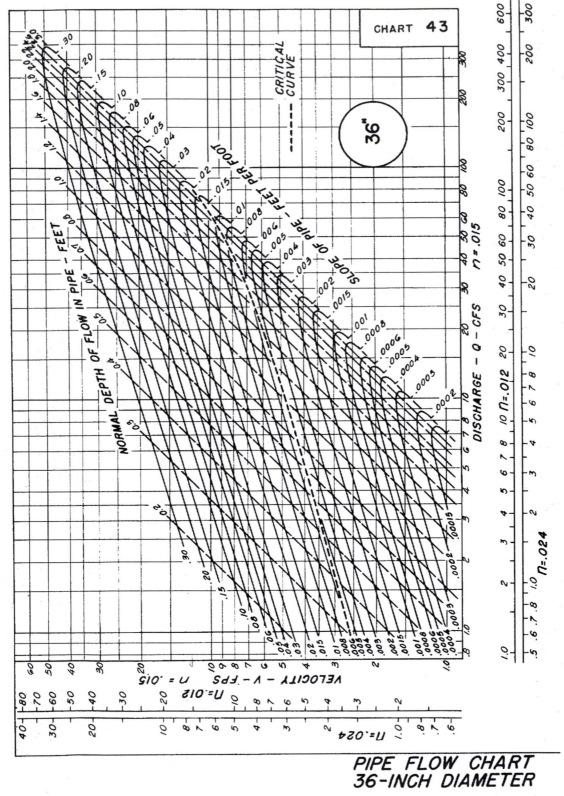

FIGURE A-4. (CHART 43)   Pipe charts for the solution of Manning's equation. *(Courtesy of U.S. Department of Commerce, Bureau of Public Roads, Design Charts for Open-Channel Flow.)*

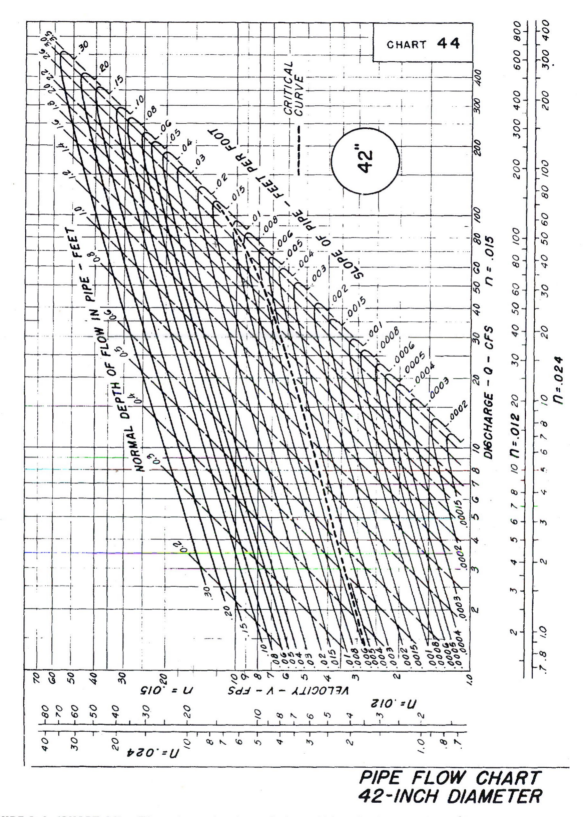

PIPE FLOW CHART
42-INCH DIAMETER

FIGURE A-4. (CHART 44)   Pipe charts for the solution of Manning's equation. (*Courtesy of U.S. Department of Commerce, Bureau of Public Roads, Design Charts for Open-Channel Flow.*)

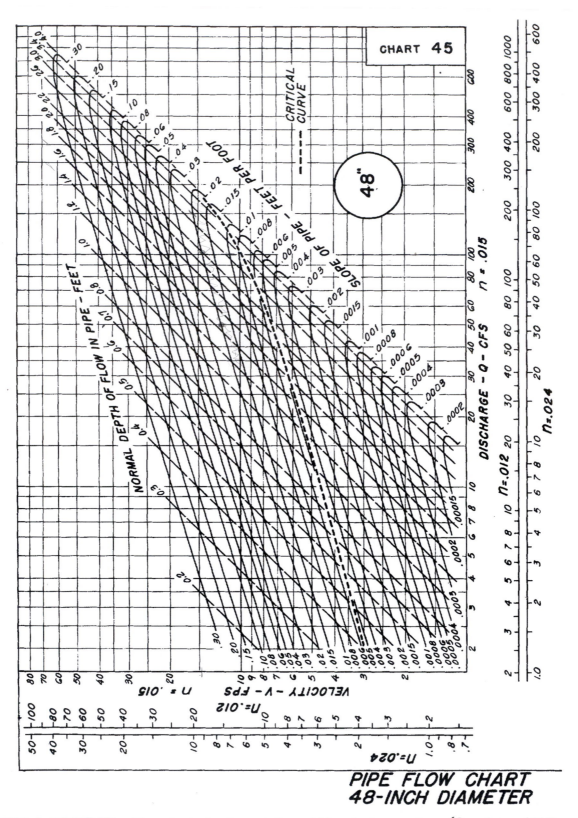

PIPE FLOW CHART 48-INCH DIAMETER

FIGURE A-4. (CHART 45) Pipe charts for the solution of Manning's equation. (*Courtesy of U.S. Department of Commerce, Bureau of Public Roads, Design Charts for Open-Channel Flow.*)

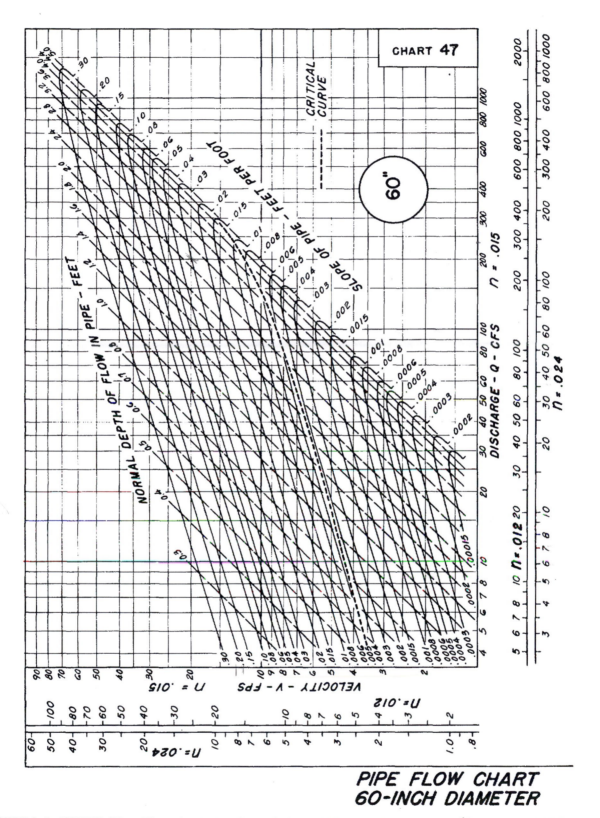

PIPE FLOW CHART
60-INCH DIAMETER

FIGURE A-4. (CHART 47)   Pipe charts for the solution of Manning's equation. *(Courtesy of U.S. Department of Commerce, Bureau of Public Roads, Design Charts for Open-Channel Flow.)*

A-5
Discharge Coefficients, *c*, for Broad-Crested Weirs

Measured Head, H (ft)	Breadth of crest of weir (ft)										
	0.50	0.75	1.00	1.50	2.00	2.50	3.00	4.00	5.00	10.00	15.00
0.2	2.80	2.75	2.69	2.62	2.54	2.48	2.44	2.38	2.34	2.49	2.68
0.4	2.92	2.80	2.72	2.64	2.61	2.60	2.58	2.54	2.50	2.56	2.70
0.6	3.08	2.89	2.75	2.64	2.61	2.60	2.68	2.69	2.70	2.70	2.70
0.8	3.30	3.04	2.85	2.68	2.60	2.60	2.67	2.68	2.68	2.69	2.64
1.0	3.32	3.14	2.98	2.75	2.66	2.64	2.65	2.67	2.68	2.68	2.63
1.2	3.32	3.20	3.08	2.86	2.70	2.65	2.64	2.67	2.66	2.69	2.64
1.4	3.32	3.26	3.20	2.92	2.77	2.68	2.64	2.65	2.65	2.67	2.64
1.6	3.32	3.29	3.28	3.07	2.89	2.75	2.68	2.66	2.65	2.64	2.63
1.8	3.32	3.32	3.31	3.07	2.88	2.74	2.68	2.66	2.65	2.64	2.63
2.0	3.32	3.31	3.30	3.03	2.85	2.76	2.72	2.68	2.65	2.64	2.63
2.5	3.32	3.32	3.31	3.28	3.07	2.89	2.81	2.72	2.67	2.64	2.63
3.0	3.32	3.32	3.32	3.32	3.20	3.05	2.92	2.73	2.66	2.64	2.63
3.5	3.32	3.32	3.32	3.32	2.32	3.19	2.97	2.76	2.68	2.64	2.63
4.0	3.32	3.32	3.32	3.32	3.32	3.32	3.07	2.79	2.70	2.64	2.63
4.5	3.32	3.32	3.32	3.32	3.32	3.32	3.32	2.88	2.74	2.64	2.63
5.0	3.32	3.32	3.32	3.32	3.32	3.32	3.32	3.07	2.79	2.64	2.63
5.5	3.32	3.32	3.32	3.32	3.32	3.32	3.32	3.32	2.88	2.64	2.63

FIGURE A-5. *(Courtesy of Brater & King, Handbook of Hydraulics, John Wiley & Sons, Inc.)*

DESIGN CHARTS FOR CULVERTS

B-1
Culverts with Inlet Control

Instructions for use:

1. How to find headwater depth, *HW*, given *Q* and size and type of culvert:
   a) Locate the height or diameter, *D*, of the culvert on the left-hand scale.
   b) Locate the discharge, *Q*, or *Q/B* for box culverts, on the center scale.
   c) Connect the two points in (a) and (b) above and extend the line to the right until it intersects the *HW/D* scale marked (1).
   d) If the *HW/D* scale marked (1) represents entrance type used, read *HW/D* on scale (1).
   e) If another of the three entrance types listed on the nomograph is used, extend the point of intersection made in (c) above horizontally to scale (2) or (3) and read *HW/D*.

2. How to find discharge, *Q*, per barrel, given *HW* and size and type of culvert:
   a) Compute *HW/D* for given conditions.
   b) Locate *HW/D* on scale (1), (2), or (3) for appropriate entrance type.
   c) If scale (2) or (3) is used, extend *HW/D* point horizontally to scale (1).
   d) Connect point on *HW/D* scale (1) and size of culvert, *D*, on left scale. Read *Q* or *Q/B* on the discharge scale.
   e) If *Q/B* is read in (d) above, multiply by *B* to find *Q*.

CHART 1

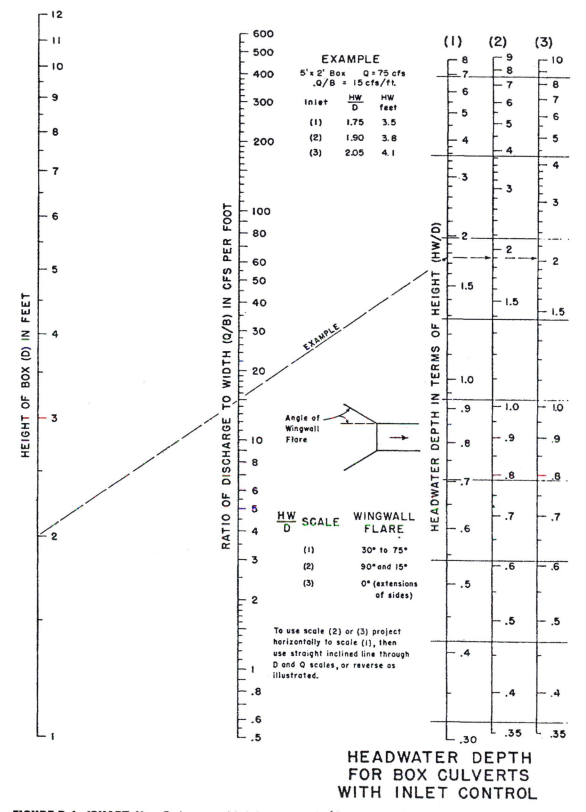

HEADWATER DEPTH FOR BOX CULVERTS WITH INLET CONTROL

FIGURE B-1. (CHART 1) Culverts with inlet control. (*Courtesy of U.S. Department of Transportation, Federal Highway Administration, Hydraulic Charts for the Selection of Highway Culverts.*)

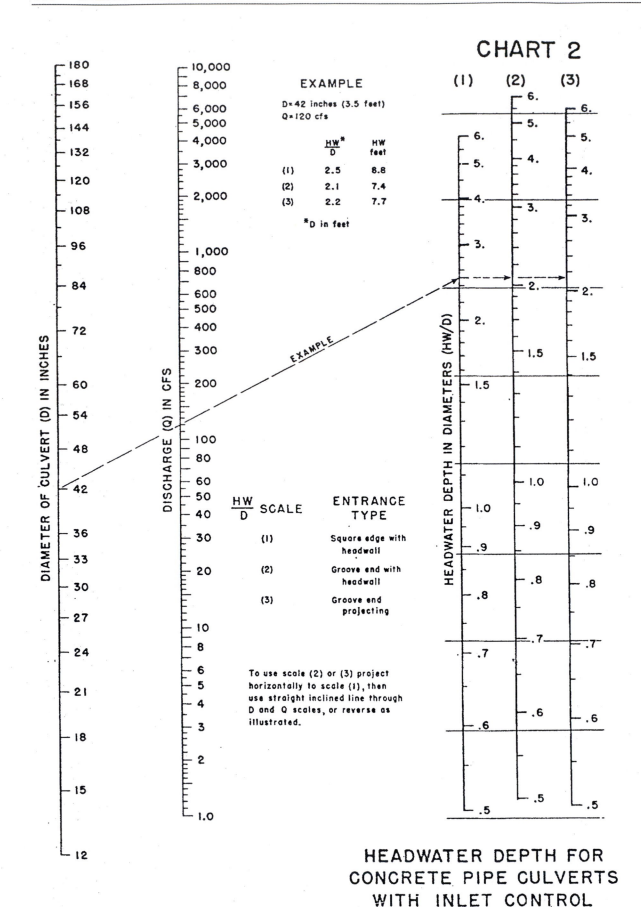

CHART 2

HEADWATER DEPTH FOR CONCRETE PIPE CULVERTS WITH INLET CONTROL

FIGURE B-1. (CHART 2) Culverts with inlet control. *(Courtesy of U.S. Department of Transportation, Federal Highway Administration, Hydraulic Charts for the Selection of Highway Culverts.)*

CHART 5

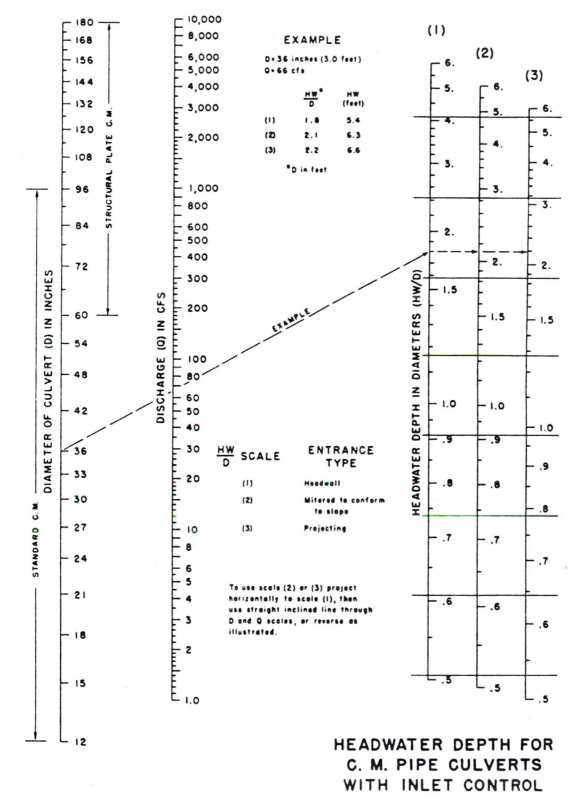

**HEADWATER DEPTH FOR
C. M. PIPE CULVERTS
WITH INLET CONTROL**

FIGURE B-1. (CHART 5)   Culverts with inlet control. *(Courtesy of U.S. Department of Transportation, Federal Highway Administration, Hydraulic Charts for the Selection of Highway Culverts.)*

CHART 7

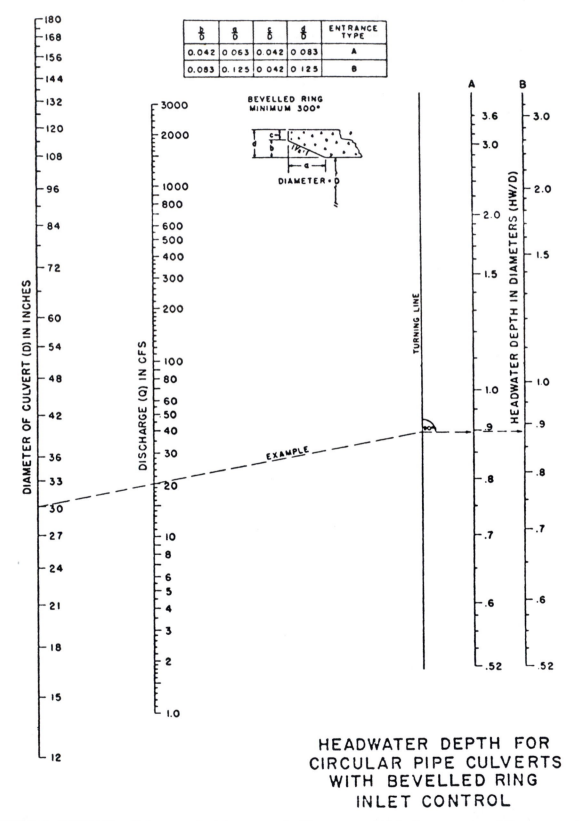

HEADWATER DEPTH FOR
CIRCULAR PIPE CULVERTS
WITH BEVELLED RING
INLET CONTROL

FIGURE B-1. (CHART 7)   Culverts with inlet control. *(Courtesy of U.S. Department of Transportation, Federal Highway Administration, Hydraulic Charts for the Selection of Highway Culverts.)*

B-2
Culverts with Outlet Control

Instructions for use:

1. How to find head, *H*, for a given culvert and discharge, *Q*:
    a) Locate appropriate nomograph for type of culvert selected. Find k_e for entrance type in Appendix B-3.
    b) Locate starting point on length scale. To locate the proper starting point on the length scales, follow the instructions below:
        (1) If the *n*-value for the nomograph corresponds to that of the culvert being used, select the length curve for the proper k_e and locate the starting point at the given culvert length. If a k_e curve is not shown for the selected k_e, see (2) below. If the *n*-value for the culvert selected differs from that of the nomograph, see (3) below.
        (2) For a k_e intermediate between the scales given, connect the given length on adjacent scales by a straight line and select a point on this line spaced between the two chart scales in proportion to the k_e values.
        (3) For a different roughness coefficient, n_1, from that of the chart *n*, use the length scales shown with an adjusted length L_1, calculated by the formula

        $$L_1 = L(n_1/n)^2$$

    c) Locate the size of the culvert barrel on the culvert size scale (second scale from left).
    d) Connect the point on the size scale with the point on the length scale and note where the line passes through the *turning line*. (See Instruction 3 for size considerations for box culvert.)
    e) Locate the given discharge, *Q*, on the discharge scale.
    f) Connect the discharge point with the turning line point, and extend the line to the head scale at the far right side of the nomograph. Read head, *H*, in feet on the head scale.
2. Values of *n* for commonly used culvert materials:
    Concrete——Pipe: 0.012
                Box: 0.012
    Corrugated Metal

	Small Corrugations $(2\frac{2}{3}'' \times \frac{1}{2}'')$	Medium Corrugations $(3'' \times 1'')$	Large Corrugations $(6'' \times 2'')$
Unpaved	0.024	0.027	Varies*
25% paved	0.021	0.023	0.026
Fully paved	0.012	0.012	0.012

*n *varies with diameter shown on charts. The various* n-*values have been incorporated into the nomographs, and no adjustment for culvert length is required.*

3. To use the box culvert nomograph, Chart 8, for full flow for other than square boxes:
    a) Compute the cross-sectional area of the rectangular box.
    b) Locate the area on the area scale.
    c) Connect the point on the area scale to the point on the length scale, and note where the line passes through the turning line.
    d) Connect the discharge with the point on the turning line, and extend the line to the head scale. Read the head in feet on the head scale.

CHART 8

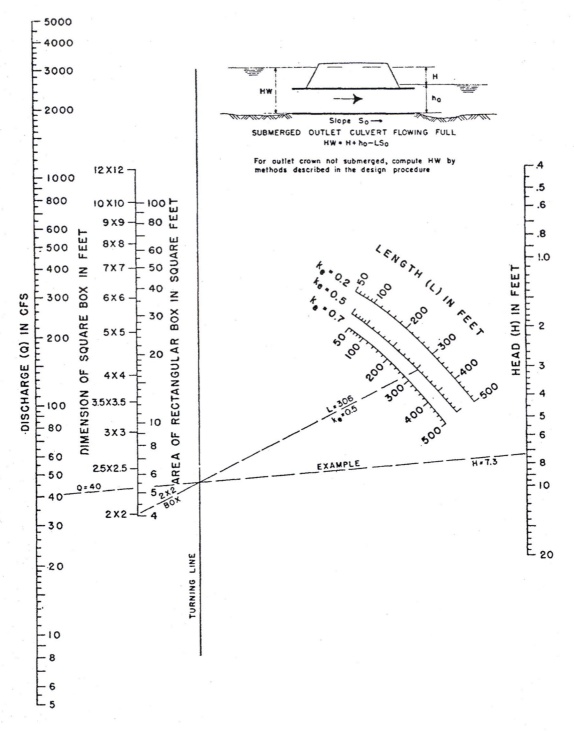

HEAD FOR
CONCRETE BOX CULVERTS
FLOWING FULL
n = 0.012

FIGURE B-2. (CHART 8)   Culverts with outlet control. *(Courtesy of U.S. Department of Transportation, Federal Highway Administration, Hydraulic Charts for the Selection of Highway Culverts.)*

CHART 9

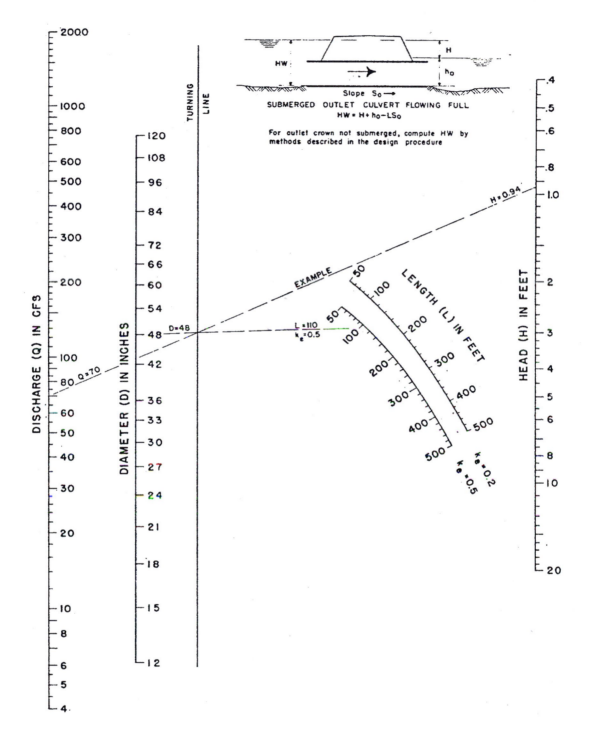

HEAD FOR
CONCRETE PIPE CULVERTS
FLOWING FULL
n = 0.012

FIGURE B-2. (CHART 9)   Culverts with outlet control. *(Courtesy of U.S. Department of Transportation, Federal Highway Administration, Hydraulic Charts for the Selection of Highway Culverts.)*

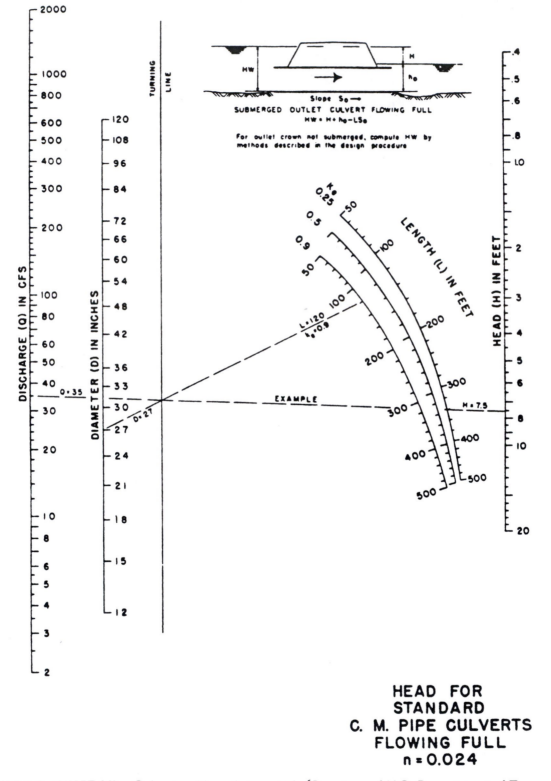

CHART 11

HEAD FOR STANDARD C. M. PIPE CULVERTS FLOWING FULL n = 0.024

FIGURE B-2. (CHART 11)   Culverts with outlet control. *(Courtesy of U.S. Department of Transportation, Federal Highway Administration, Hydraulic Charts for the Selection of Highway Culverts.)*

B-3
Entrance Loss Coefficients

Coefficient k_e to apply to velocity head $\frac{V^2}{2g}$ for determination of head loss at entrance to a structure, such as a culvert or conduit, operating full or partly full with control at the outlet.

$$\text{Entrance head loss } H_e = k_e \frac{V^2}{2g}$$

Type of Structure and Design of Entrance	Coefficient k_e

Pipe, Concrete

Projecting from fill, socket end (groove end)	0.2
Projecting from fill, sq. cut end	0.5
Headwall or headwall and wingwalls	
Socket end of pipe (groove end)	0.2
Square edge	0.5
Rounded (radius = $\frac{1}{12}D$)	0.2
Mitered to conform to fill slope	0.7
*End-Section conforming to fill slope	0.5

Pipe, or Pipe-Arch, Corrugated Metal

Projecting from fill (no headwall)	0.9
Headwall or headwall and wingwalls	
Square edge	0.5
Mitered to conform to fill slope	0.7
*End Section conforming to fill slope	0.5

Box, Reinforced Concrete

Headwall parallel to embankment (no wingwalls)	
Square-edged on 3 edges	0.5
Rounded on 3 edges to radius of $\frac{1}{12}$ barrel dimension	0.2
Wingwalls at 30° to 75° to barrel	
Square-edged at crown	0.4
Crown edge rounded to radius of $\frac{1}{12}$ barrel dimension	0.2
Wingwalls at 10° to 25° to barrel	
Square-edged at crown	0.5
Wingwalls parallel (extension of sides)	
Square-edged at crown	0.7

*"End Section conforming to fill slope," made of either metal or concrete, are the sections commonly available from manufacturers. From limited hydraulic tests, they are equivalent in operation to a headwall in both *inlet* and *outlet* control. Some end sections, incorporating a closed taper in their design have a superior hydraulic performance. These latter sections can be designed by using the information given for the beveled inlet.

FIGURE B-3   Entrance loss coefficients. (*Courtesy of U.S. Department of Transportation, Federal Highway Administration, Hydraulic Charts for the Selection of Highway Culverts.*)

DESIGN CHARTS FOR RATIONAL METHOD

C-1
Values of *c*, Runoff Coefficient

Character of Surface	Runoff Coefficients
Pavement	
Asphalt and concrete	0.70 to 0.95
Brick	0.70 to 0.85
Roofs	0.75 to 0.95
Lawns, sandy soil	
Flat (2 percent)	0.05 to 0.10
Average (2 to 7 percent)	0.10 to 0.15
Steep (> 7 percent)	0.15 to 0.20
Lawns, heavy soil	
Flat (2 percent)	0.13 to 0.17
Average (2 to 7 percent)	0.18 to 0.22
Steep (> 7 percent)	0.25 to 0.35
Composite *c*-values:	
Business	
Downtown	0.70 to 0.95
Neighborhood	0.50 to 0.70
Residential	
Single Family	0.30 to 0.50
Multi-units, detached	0.40 to 0.60
Multi-units, attached	0.60 to 0.75
Residential (suburban)	0.25 to 0.40
Apartment	0.50 to 0.70
Industrial	
Light	0.50 to 0.80
Heavy	0.60 to 0.90
Parks, cemeteries	0.10 to 0.25
Playgrounds	0.20 to 0.35
Railroad yards	0.20 to 0.35
Unimproved	0.10 to 0.30

Note: The ranges of *c*-values presented are typical for return periods of 2–10 years. Higher values are appropriate for larger design storms. Suggested multiplier factors for larger design storms are

Storm	Multiplier
25-year	1.15
50-year	1.20
100-year	1.25

Note: Adjusted *c*-value cannot exceed 1.00.

FIGURE C-1   Values of c, runoff coefficient. *(Courtesy of ASCE & Water Environmental Federation, Design and Construction of Urban Stormwater Management Systems.)*

C-2
Nomograph for Overland Flow Time

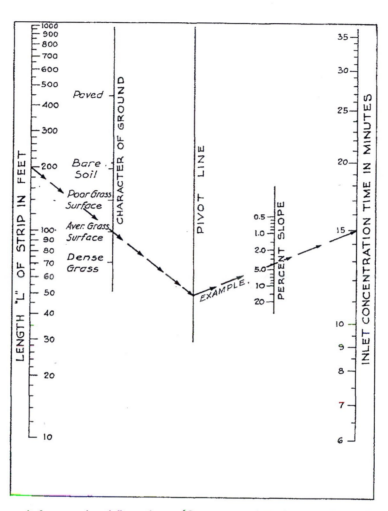

FIGURE C-2   Nomograph for overland flow time. *(Courtesy of E. Seeley, Data Book for Civil Engineers, Vol. 1, John Wiley & Sons, Inc.)*

C-3
Intensity-Duration-Frequency (I-D-F) Curves

<u>Example:</u> For a selected 10-year return period, $P_1 = 2.0$ inches. T_C is calculated as 20 minutes. Therefore, (i) = 4.25 in/h.

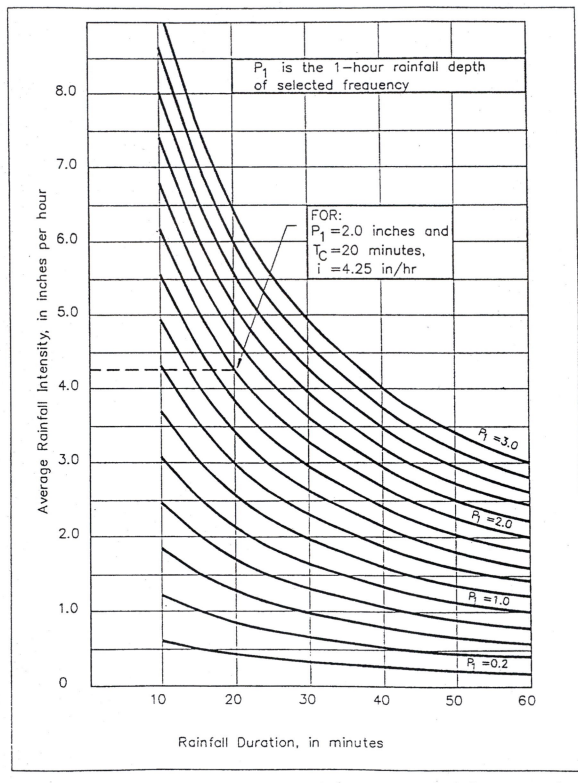

FIGURE C-3. (CHART 1)   IDF curves for Arizona (Zone 6). *(Courtesy of Arizona Department of Transportation.)*

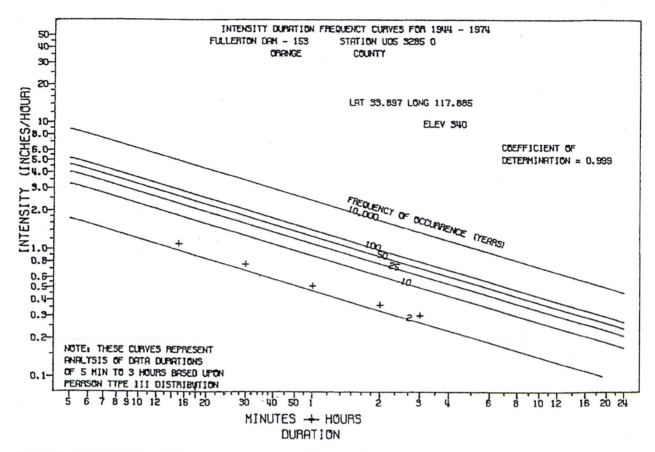

FIGURE C-3. (CHART 2)   IDF curves for Orange County, California. *(Courtesy of California Department of Transportation.)*

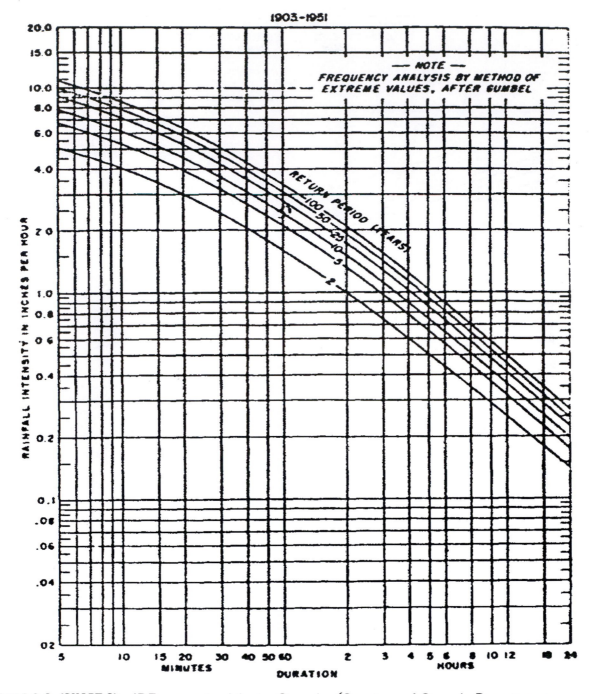

FIGURE C-3. (CHART 3)   IDF curves for Atlanta, Georgia. *(Courtesy of Georgia Department of Transportation.)*

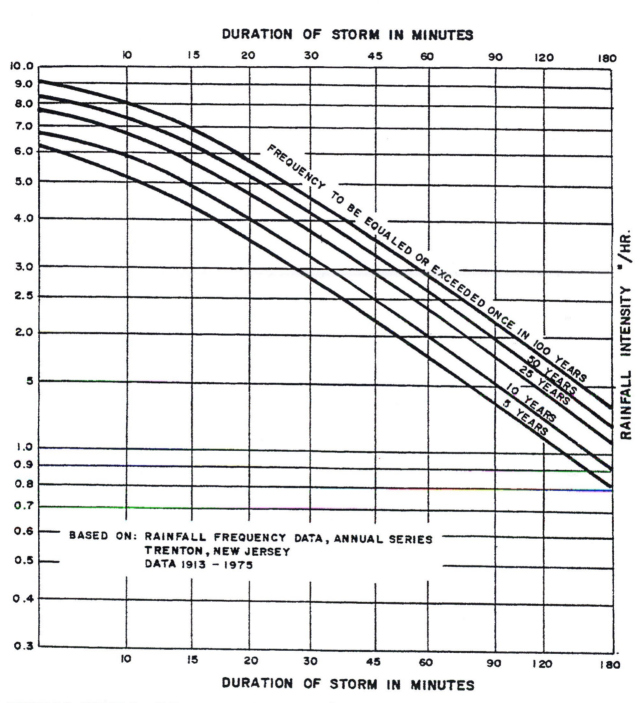

FIGURE C-3. (CHART 4)   IDF curves for New Jersey. *(Courtesy of New Jersey Department of Transportation.)*

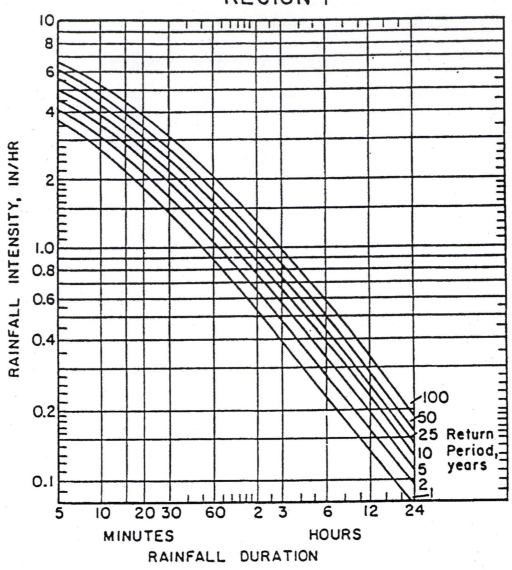

FIGURE C-3. (CHART 5)   IDF curves for Pennsylvania (Region 1). *(Courtesy of Pennsylvania Department of Transportation.)*

DESIGN CHARTS FOR NRCS METHOD

Note: Design charts shown on the following pages are taken from *Technical Release 55* published by the Soil Conservation Service (SCS) in 1986. TR-55 has been replaced by WinTR-55, published by the Natural Resources Conservation Service (NRCS) in 2002. WinTR-55 is available on-line at http://www.wcc.nrcs.usda.gov/hydro. The TR-55 charts are shown for illustration purposes.

D-1
Runoff Curve Numbers

Cover description		Curve numbers for hydrologic soil group			
Cover type and hydrologic condition	Average percent impervious area[2]	A	B	C	D
Fully developed urban areas (vegetation established)					
Open space (lawns, parks, golf courses, cemeteries, etc.)[3]:					
Poor condition (grass cover < 50%)		68	79	86	89
Fair condition (grass cover 50% to 75%)..........		49	69	79	84
Good condition (grass cover > 75%)		39	61	74	80
Impervious areas:					
Paved parking lots, roofs, driveways, etc. (excluding right-of-way)........................		98	98	98	98
Streets and roads:					
Paved; curbs and storm sewers (excluding right-of-way)................................		98	98	98	98
Paved; open ditches (including right-of-way)		83	89	92	93
Gravel (including right-of-way)		76	85	89	91
Dirt (including right-of-way)		72	82	87	89
Western desert urban areas:					
Natural desert landscaping (pervious areas only)[4]...		63	77	85	88
Artificial desert landscaping (impervious weed barrier, desert shrub with 1- to 2-inch sand or gravel mulch and basin borders).		96	96	96	96
Urban districts:					
Commercial and business.........................	85	89	92	94	95
Industrial..	72	81	88	91	93
Residential districts by average lot size:					
1/8 acre or less (town houses).....................	65	77	85	90	92
1/4 acre	38	61	75	83	87
1/3 acre	30	57	72	81	86
1/2 acre	25	54	70	80	85
1 acre	20	51	68	79	84
2 acres	12	46	65	77	82
Developing urban areas					
Newly graded areas (pervious areas only, no vegetation)[5]		77	86	91	94
Idle lands (CN's are determined using cover types similar to those in table 2-2c).					

[1]Average runoff condition, and $I_a = 0.2S$.
[2]The average percent impervious area shown was used to develop the composite CN's. Other assumptions are as follows: impervious areas are directly connected to the drainage system, impervious areas have a CN of 98, and pervious areas are considered equivalent to open space in good hydrologic condition. CN's for other combinations of conditions may be computed using figure 2-3 or 2-4.
[3]CN's shown are equivalent to those of pasture. Composite CN's may be computed for other combinations of open space cover type.
[4]Composite CN's for natural desert landscaping should be computed using figures 2-3 or 2-4 based on the impervious area percentage (CN = 98) and the pervious area CN. The pervious area CN's are assumed equivalent to desert shrub in poor hydrologic condition.
[5]Composite CN's to use for the design of temporary measures during grading and construction should be computed using figure 2-3 or 2-4, based on the degree of development (impervious area percentage) and the CN's for the newly graded pervious areas.

FIGURE D-1. (CHART 1)   Runoff curve numbers. *(Courtesy of Soil Conservation Service, Technical Release 55.)*

Cover description		Curve numbers for hydrologic soil group—			
Cover type	Hydrologic condition	A	B	C	D
Pasture, grassland, or range—continuous forage for grazing.[2]	Poor	68	79	86	89
	Fair	49	69	79	84
	Good	39	61	74	80
Meadow—continuous grass, protected from grazing and generally mowed for hay.	—	30	58	71	78
Brush—brush-weed-grass mixture with brush the major element.[3]	Poor	48	67	77	83
	Fair	35	56	70	77
	Good	[4]30	48	65	73
Woods—grass combination (orchard or tree farm).[5]	Poor	57	73	82	86
	Fair	43	65	76	82
	Good	32	58	72	79
Woods.[6]	Poor	45	66	77	83
	Fair	36	60	73	79
	Good	[4]30	55	70	77
Farmsteads—buildings, lanes, driveways, and surrounding lots.	—	59	74	82	86

[1]Average runoff condition, and $I_a = 0.2S$.

[2]*Poor:* <50% ground cover or heavily grazed with no mulch.
Fair: 50 to 75% ground cover and not heavily grazed.
Good: >75% ground cover and lightly or only occasionally grazed.

[3]*Poor:* <50% ground cover.
Fair: 50 to 75% ground cover.
Good: >75% ground cover.

[4]Actual curve number is less than 30; use CN = 30 for runoff computations.

[5]CN's shown were computed for areas with 50% woods and 50% grass (pasture) cover. Other combinations of conditions may be computed from the CN's for woods and pasture.

[6]*Poor:* Forest litter, small trees, and brush are destroyed by heavy grazing or regular burning.
Fair: Woods are grazed but not burned, and some forest litter covers the soil.
Good: Woods are protected from grazing, and litter and brush adequately cover the soil.

FIGURE D-1. (CHART 2)   Runoff curve numbers. *(Courtesy of Soil Conservation Service, Technical Release 55.)*

D-2
Hydrologic Soil Groups for Selected Soil Types

Aabab	D	Lamington	D
Alluvial land	C	Lansing	B
Amwell	C	Lehigh	C
Avoca	B	Linkville	B
Bartley	C	Louisa	B
Belmill	B	Lynchburg	C
Bigbee	A	Madden	C
Boonton	C	Madrid	B
Broadwell	B	Maplecrest	B
Bucks	B	McDaniel	B
Califon	C	Menlo	D
Chancelor	C	Minoa	C
Chesire	B	Mirkwood	D
Conic	C	Modesto	C
Continental	C	Moundhaven	A
Custer	D	Muskingum	C
Delaney	A	Narragansett	B
Dickerson	D	Netcong	B
Dundee	C	Nobscot	A
Eastland	B	Nuff	C
Edneyville	B	Okeetee	D
Exeter	C	Outlet	C
Fairchild	C	Oxbow	C
Freedom	C	Parker	B
Fulerton	B	Penn	C
Georgetown	D	Pompton	B
Gleason	B	Preakness	C
Goosebury	B	Punsit	C
Gravel pits	A	Rayburn	D
Grigston	B	Reading	B
Haledon	C	Riverhead	B
Hamel	C	Rodessa	D
Haven	B	Santa Fe	D
Herty	D	Scarboro	D
Hotsprings	B	Shellbluff	B
Hungry	C	Snelling	B
Idlewild	D	Summers	B
Isabella	B	Tarrytown	C
Jardin	D	Terril	B
Jigsaw	C	Troutdale	C
Jonesville	B	Urban land	(varies)
Joplin	C	Utica	B
Kaplan	D	Vercliff	C
Kehar	D	Vinsad	C
Kilkenny	B	Washington	B
Kirkville	C	Whitecross	D
Kreamer	C	Yardley	C
Lambert	B	Zynbar	B

FIGURE D-2   Hydrologic soil groups for selected soil types. *(Courtesy of Soil Conservation Service, Technical Release 55.)*

D-3
24-Hour Rainfall Amounts by Return Period

The following maps are reproduced from the *Rainfall Atlas of the United States*, Technical Paper No. 40 by the U.S. Weather Bureau. The maps show isopluvial lines (lines of equal rainfall depth) for 100-, 50-, 25-, 10-, 5-, and 2-year, 24-hour rainfalls throughout the contiguous 37 states east of 103° W longitude.

Also included are selected maps from the National Oceanic and Atmospheric Administration (NOAA) Atlas 2 for Arizona and Southern California for the 100-year, 24-hour rainfall.

Both TP40 and Atlas 2 have been superceded by NOAA Atlas 14, which is available in electronic form only. NOAA Atlas 14 can be accessed on-line at http://hdsc.nws.noaa.gov.

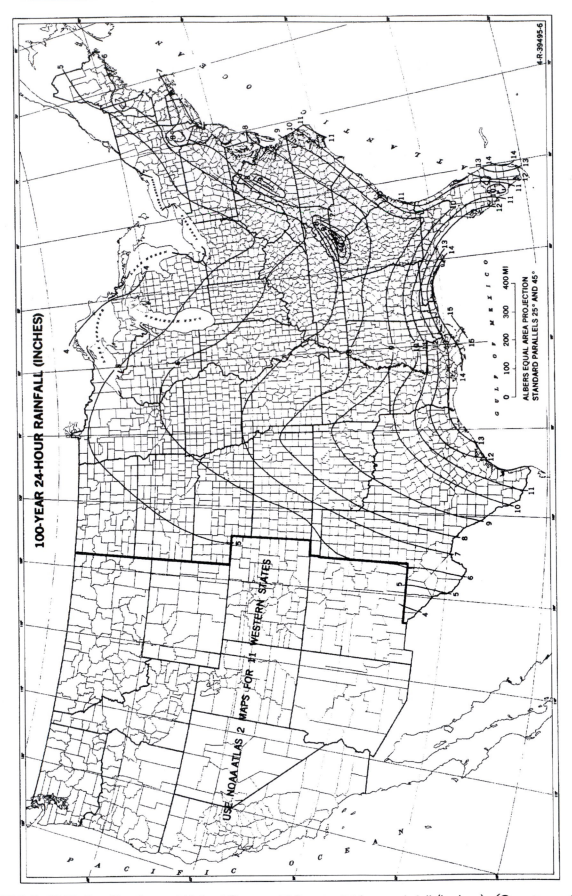

FIGURE D-3. (MAP 1)   Continental United States, 100-year, 24-hour rainfall (inches). *(Courtesy of U.S. Weather Bureau, Rainfall Atlas of the United States.)*

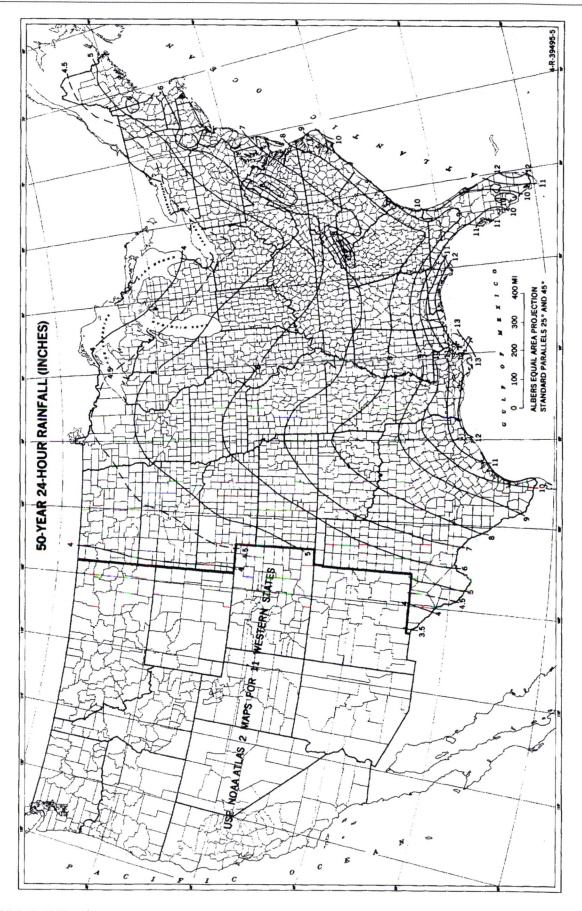

FIGURE D-3. (MAP 2)   Continental United States, 50-year, 24-hour rainfall (inches). *(Courtesy of U.S. Weather Bureau, Rainfall Atlas of the United States.)*

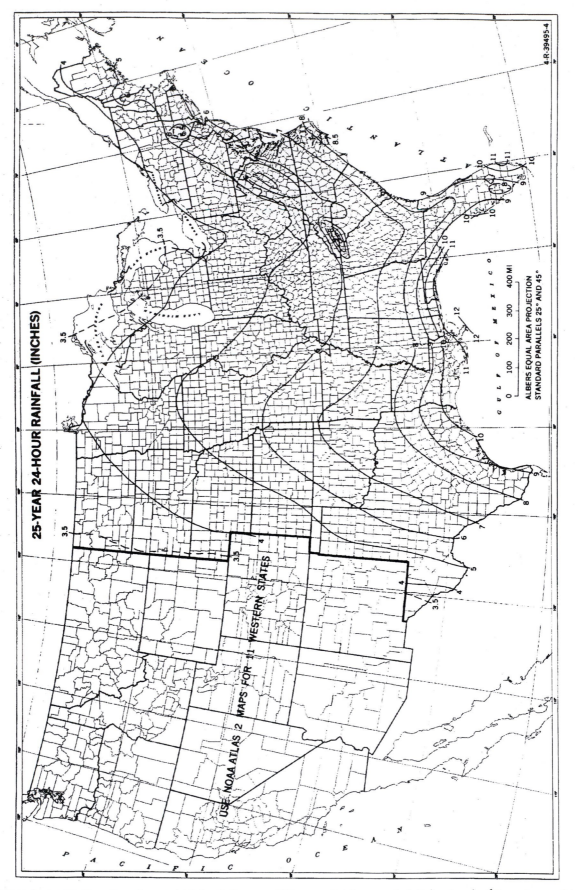

FIGURE D-3. (MAP 3) Continental United States, 25-year, 24-hour rainfall (inches). *(Courtesy of U.S. Weather Bureau, Rainfall Atlas of the United States.)*

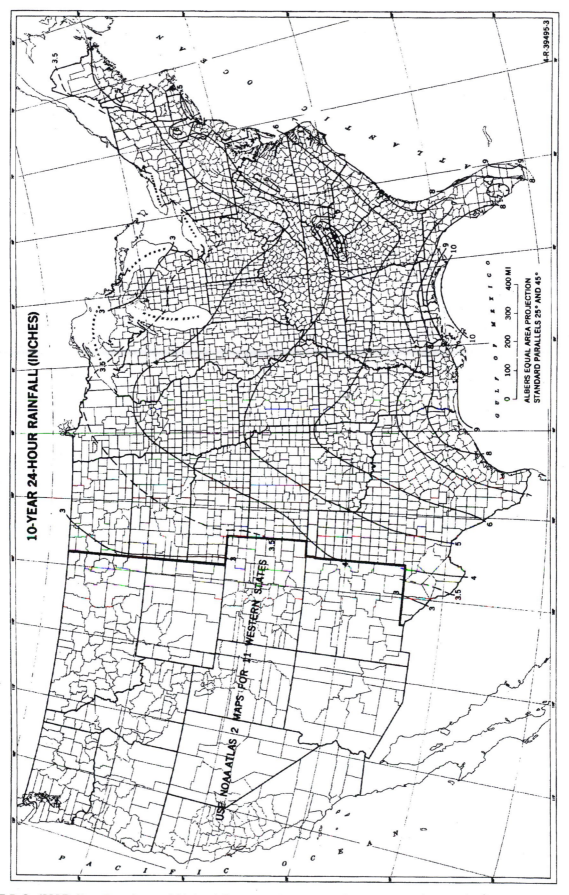

FIGURE D-3. (MAP 4)   Continental United States, 10-year, 24-hour rainfall (inches). *(Courtesy of U.S. Weather Bureau, Rainfall Atlas of the United States.)*

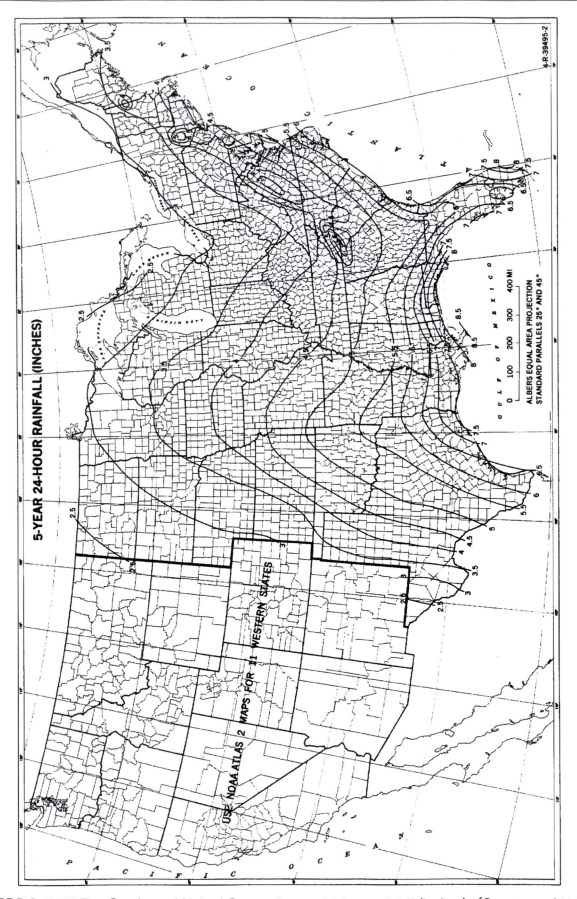

FIGURE D-3. (MAP 5) Continental United States, 5-year, 24-hour rainfall (inches). *(Courtesy of U.S. Weather Bureau, Rainfall Atlas of the United States.)*

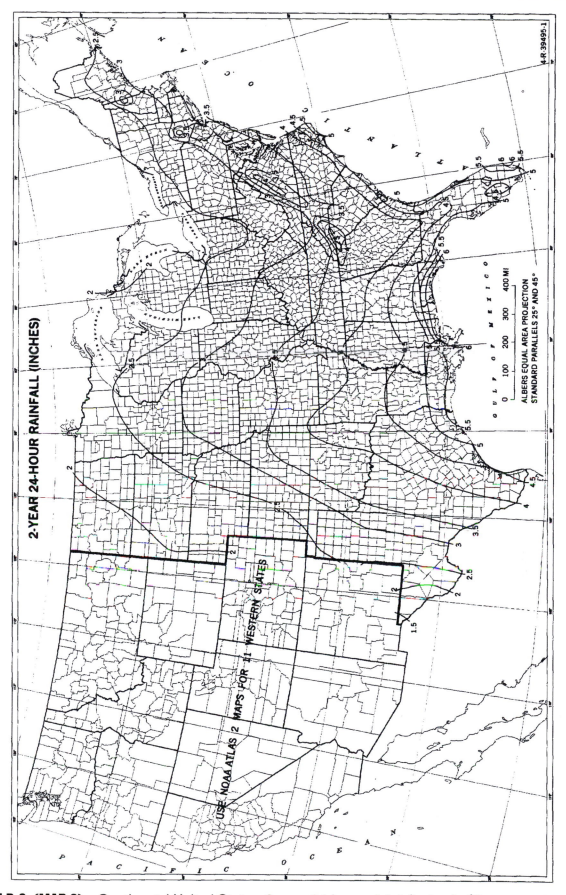

FIGURE D-3. (MAP 6)   Continental United States, 2-year, 24-hour rainfall (inches). *(Courtesy of U.S. Weather Bureau, Rainfall Atlas of the United States.)*

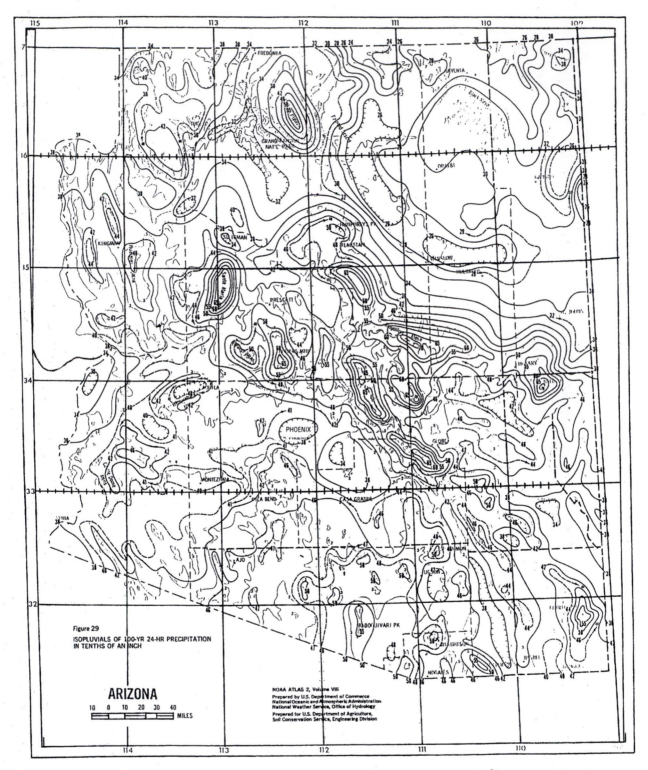

FIGURE D-3. (MAP 7)   Arizona, 100-year, 24-hour rainfall (tenths of an inch). *(Courtesy of NOAA Atlas 2, Volume VIII.)*

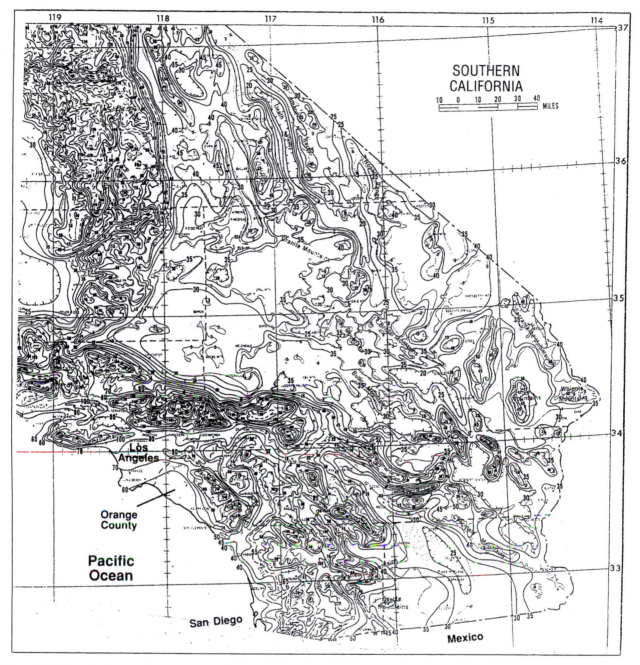

FIGURE D-3. (MAP 8)   Southern California, 100-year, 24-hour rainfall (tenths of an inch). *(Courtesy of NOAA Atlas 2, Volume XI.)*

D-4
Approximate Geographical Boundaries for NRCS Rainfall Distributions

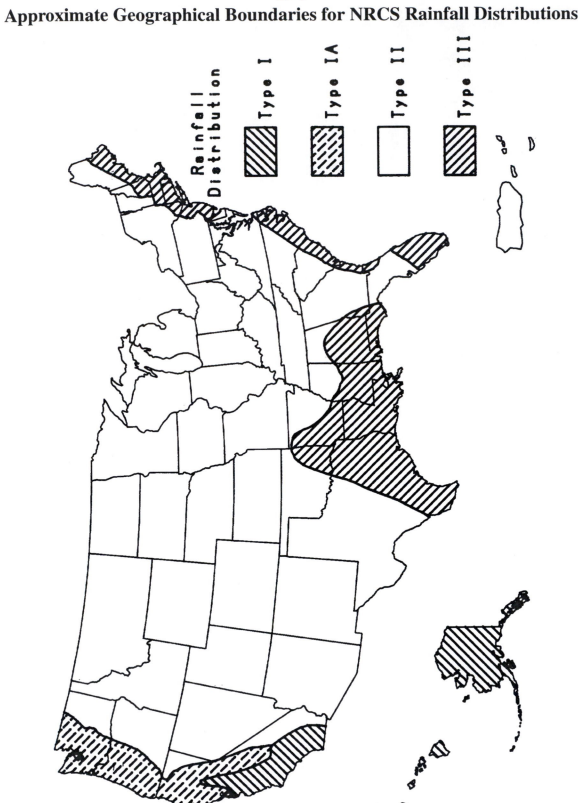

FIGURE D-4 Approximate geographical boundaries for NRCS rainfall distributions. *(Courtesy of Soil Conservation Service, Technical Release 55.)*

D-5
Unit Peak Discharge (q_u)

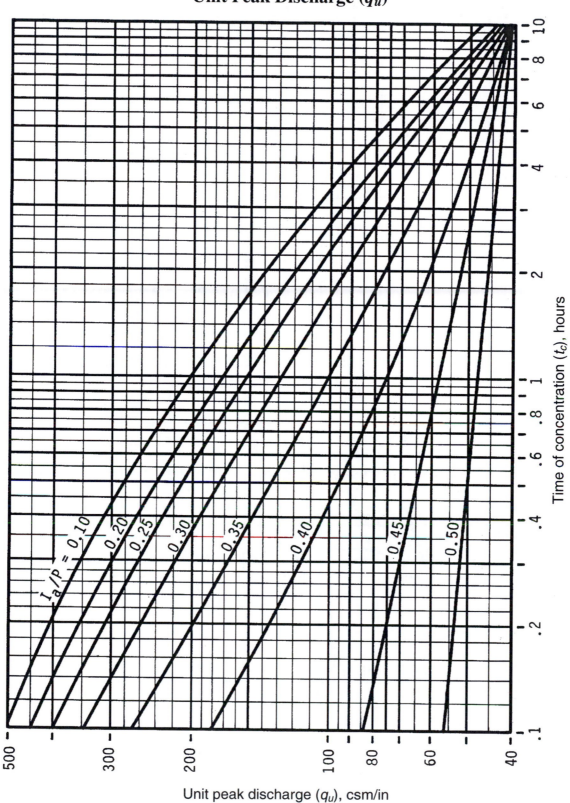

FIGURE D-5. (CHART 1)   Unit peak discharge (q_u) for NRCS type I rainfall distribution. *(Courtesy of Soil Conservation Service, Technical Release 55.)*

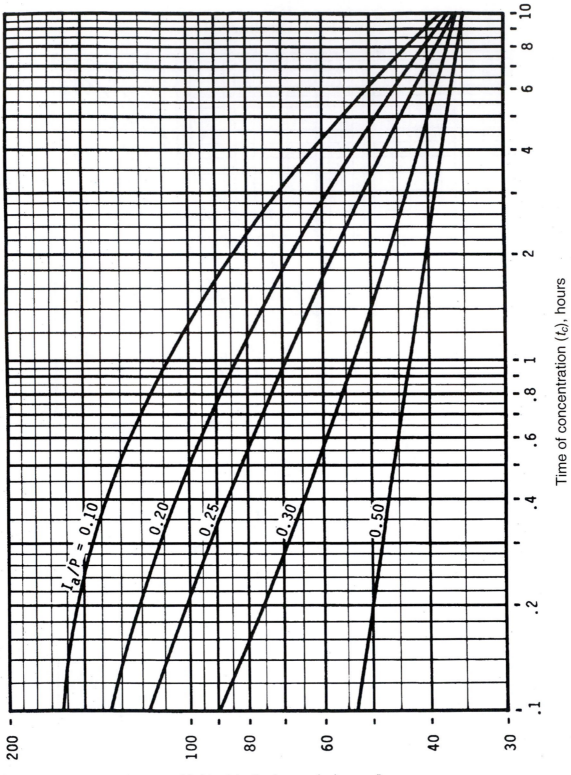

FIGURE D-5. (CHART 2) Unit peak discharge (q_u) for NRCS type IA rainfall distribution. *(Courtesy of Soil Conservation Service, Technical Release 55.)*

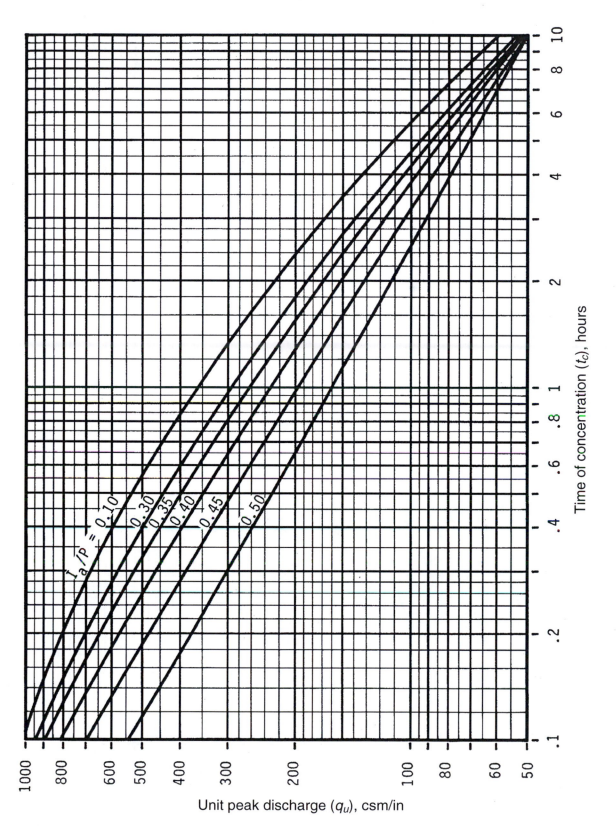

FIGURE D-5. (CHART 3)   Unit peak discharge (q_u) for NRCS type II rainfall distribution. *(Courtesy of Soil Conservation Service, Technical Release 55.)*

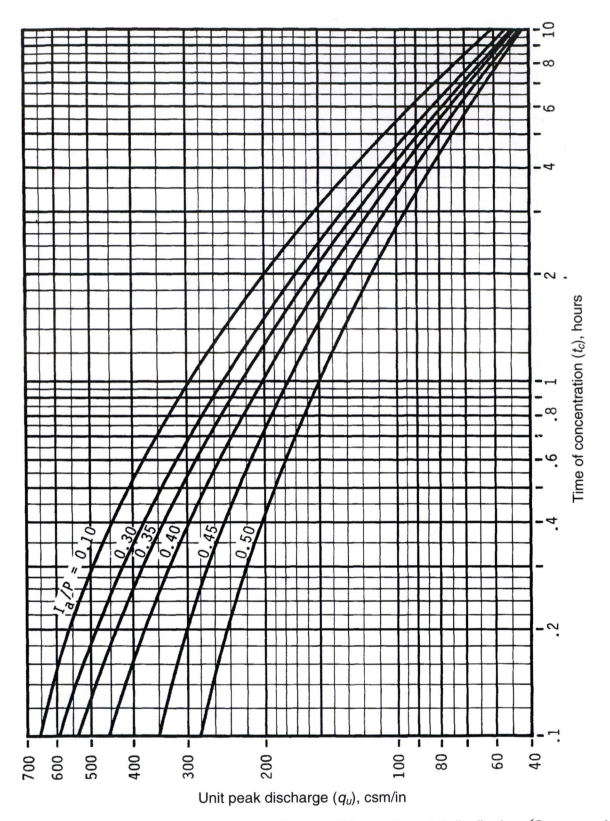

FIGURE D-5. (CHART 4) Unit peak discharge (q_u) for NRCS type III rainfall distribution. *(Courtesy of Soil Conservation Service, Technical Release 55.)*

D-6
Tabular Hydrograph Unit Discharges (csm/in)
for Type II Rainfall Distributions

HYDROGRAPH TIME (HOURS)

IA/P = 0.10   TC = 0.4 HR

TRVL TIME (HR)	11.0	11.3	11.6	11.9	12.0	12.1	12.2	12.3	12.4	12.5	12.6	12.7	12.8	13.0	13.2	13.4	13.6	13.8	14.0	14.3	14.6	15.0	15.5	16.0	16.5	17.0	17.5	18.0	19.0	20.0	22.0	26.0
0.0	18	25	36	77	141	271	468	592	574	431	298	216	163	104	77	63	55	49	44	38	34	31	28	25	22	21	20	18	16	14	12	0
.10	18	24	34	67	116	219	385	574	557	473	357	216	196	119	84	67	57	51	46	39	35	32	25	25	23	21	20	18	16	14	12	0
.20	15	20	28	44	59	97	179	316	454	523	489	309	178	112	81	65	56	49	42	37	37	33	30	26	23	21	20	19	17	14	12	0
.30	15	20	27	41	53	82	147	260	389	478	486	401	210	129	89	69	58	51	43	38	38	33	30	27	24	21	20	19	17	14	12	0
.40	13	17	23	33	38	48	71	121	214	331	429	467	308	189	120	66	85	66	56	41	35	31	28	24	24	22	20	19	17	15	12	1
.50	12	16	22	31	36	44	62	102	176	279	379	438	339	218	137	94	71	59	42	35	30	28	25	25	24	23	21	19	15	12	0
.75	10	13	18	24	26	30	35	45	65	106	170	251	326	341	245	164	112	81	59	48	39	33	30	26	22	20	20	18	15	12	1
1.0	8	10	13	17	19	21	24	27	31	37	50	75	118	251	360	376	292	205	138	83	60	45	36	32	28	25	22	21	16	12	1
1.5	6	7	9	12	13	14	15	17	19	21	23	26	31	56	121	224	311	333	293	192	115	66	45	36	31	28	25	22	17	13	4
2.0	5	5	6	8	8	10	11	12	12	14	16	20	27	43	85	159	243	306	264	154	74	47	37	32	28	25	21	19	15	9
2.5	4	4	4	5	4	7	7	8	9	9	13	16	20	27	46	85	184	285	262	147	74	47	38	32	28	23	22	19	15	11
3.0	1	2	3	4	4	4	5	6	7	8	10	12	14	17	23	47	109	227	268	160	83	50	38	32	25	21	16	11

IA/P = 0.30   TC = 0.4 HR

TRVL TIME (HR)	11.0	11.3	11.6	11.9	12.0	12.1	12.2	12.3	12.4	12.5	12.6	12.7	12.8	13.0	13.2	13.4	13.6	13.8	14.0	14.3	14.6	15.0	15.5	16.0	16.5	17.0	17.5	18.0	19.0	20.0	22.0	26.0
0.0	0	0	4	26	113	296	480	495	413	306	234	186	127	100	84	74	67	61	54	49	45	41	37	33	31	29	28	25	21	19	0
.10	0	0	2	18	81	224	395	462	430	347	272	121	172	121	96	82	66	51	60	55	46	42	34	30	29	28	25	22	19	0
.20	0	0	2	13	59	169	320	414	424	373	305	172	134	103	82	67	59	51	47	43	39	34	30	29	25	22	19	0
.30	0	0	1	9	42	127	255	361	403	383	274	181	99	83	73	63	55	48	44	40	36	33	30	29	26	23	19	0
.40	0	0	1	6	30	94	202	308	372	379	298	203	141	106	87	76	65	56	49	44	40	36	31	29	26	23	19	0
.50	0	0	1	4	21	70	158	258	334	364	270	187	133	102	85	70	60	51	46	41	37	30	26	24	19	1
.75	0	0	0	2	8	30	76	145	219	321	305	241	177	130	102	78	55	47	38	34	30	27	25	19	1
1.0	0	0	1	1	6	15	42	150	267	308	272	209	154	103	79	62	51	45	41	37	33	31	28	25	19	1
1.5	0	0	1	0	10	51	136	226	274	263	195	131	85	62	51	45	41	36	33	29	26	20	6
2.0	0	0	0	0	1	31	86	162	239	252	162	93	64	52	45	41	37	32	28	21	15
2.5	0	0	0	0	0	0	9	33	112	202	235	155	92	64	52	47	41	33	30	29	23	18
3.0	0	0	0	0	0	0	2	21	76	182	221	148	90	63	51	45	36	31	29	24	18

IA/P = 0.50   tc = 0.4 HR

TRVL TIME (HR)	11.0	11.3	11.6	11.9	12.0	12.1	12.2	12.3	12.4	12.5	12.6	12.7	12.8	13.0	13.2	13.4	13.6	13.8	14.0	14.3	14.6	15.0	15.5	16.0	16.5	17.0	17.5	18.0	19.0	20.0	22.0	26.0
0.0	0	0	0	7	59	168	245	257	213	186	163	128	109	96	88	81	75	67	62	58	54	50	45	43	41	39	35	31	28	0
.10	0	0	0	5	41	125	205	213	198	154	123	106	94	86	79	71	64	60	56	51	46	43	42	40	36	32	28	0
.20	0	0	0	3	28	93	168	240	216	220	205	164	131	110	97	88	81	72	65	60	55	51	46	43	42	38	34	28	0
.30	0	0	0	2	20	69	135	189	216	209	155	126	107	95	86	77	69	62	57	53	48	44	42	41	39	35	28	0
.40	0	0	0	1	14	50	106	161	202	193	133	112	98	89	78	70	62	58	53	48	44	41	40	37	33	29	1
.50	0	0	0	1	9	37	83	135	174	194	140	117	102	91	80	71	63	58	54	49	45	42	41	37	33	31	20
.75	0	0	0	0	3	15	40	76	147	171	146	124	107	90	73	68	60	51	46	43	38	34	32	28	26
1.0	0	0	0	0	2	7	21	78	141	173	167	125	101	86	73	63	53	48	44	42	39	35	28	27
1.5	0	0	0	0	0	1	26	71	121	153	159	113	89	72	63	57	53	48	44	40	37	33	29	7
2.0	0	0	0	0	0	0	3	37	83	135	174	117	83	64	58	53	49	45	48	42	39	33	31	20
2.5	0	0	0	0	0	0	0	3	15	40	112	102	68	60	57	51	47	53	34	45	40	34	32	26
3.0	0	0	0	0	0	0	0	0	0	7	21	40	73	101	138	117	63	58	48	44	42	35	34	27

RAINFALL TYPE = II

FIGURE D-6. (CHART 1) Tabular hydrograph unit discharges (csm/in) for type II rainfall distribution (t_c = 0.4 hour). *(Courtesy of Soil Conservation Service, Technical Release 55.)*

FIGURE D-6. (CHART 2) Tabular hydrograph unit discharges (csm/in) for type II rainfall distribution ($t_c = 0.5$ hour). (Courtesy of Soil Conservation Service, Technical Release 55.)

TRVL TIME (HR)	11.0	11.3	11.6	11.9	12.0	12.1	12.2	12.3	12.4	12.5	12.6	12.7	12.8	13.0	13.2	13.4	13.6	13.8	14.0	14.3	14.6	15.0	15.5	16.0	16.5	17.0	17.5	18.0	19.0	20.0	22.0	26.0
										IA/P = 0.10				* * * TC =0.5 HR * * *														IA/P = 0.10				
0.0	17	23	32	57	94	170	308	467	529	507	402	297	226	140	96	74	61	53	47	41	36	32	29	26	23	21	20	19	16	14	12	0
.10	16	22	30	51	80	140	252	395	484	499	434	343	265	162	108	80	65	55	49	42	36	33	29	26	23	21	20	19	16	14	12	0
.20	14	19	25	38	47	69	116	207	332	434	477	449	378	238	149	101	77	62	53	45	39	34	30	27	24	22	20	19	17	14	12	0
.30	13	18	24	35	43	60	97	170	278	382	446	448	401	270	171	114	83	66	56	46	40	34	31	27	24	22	20	19	17	15	12	0
.40	12	15	21	29	33	40	53	83	141	233	332	408	434	361	243	157	107	79	64	51	43	36	32	28	25	22	21	20	17	15	12	0
.50	11	15	20	28	31	37	48	71	118	194	286	367	412	378	271	178	119	86	68	53	44	37	32	29	25	23	21	20	17	15	12	0
.75	9	11	14	19	21	24	27	31	37	49	74	118	182	319	374	328	244	169	117	76	56	43	35	31	28	25	22	21	18	16	12	0
1.0	7	9	12	16	17	19	21	24	27	32	40	55	83	188	309	359	322	245	172	102	68	49	38	32	29	26	23	21	19	16	12	1
1.5	5	7	8	11	12	13	14	15	17	19	21	23	27	43	89	175	269	322	309	225	140	77	49	38	32	29	25	23	20	17	13	5
2.0	3	4	6	7	8	8	9	10	10	11	12	14	15	18	23	35	65	123	202	297	280	181	88	52	39	33	29	26	21	19	14	10
2.5	2	3	4	5	5	6	6	7	7	8	9	9	10	12	15	18	24	36	66	150	244	278	171	87	52	39	33	29	23	20	15	11
3.0	1	1	2	3	3	4	4	4	5	5	6	6	7	7	9	11	13	16	20	37	86	198	263	182	96	56	40	33	26	21	16	11
										IA/P = 0.30				* * * TC =0.5 HR * * *														IA/P = 0.30				
0.0	0	0	0	1	9	53	157	314	433	439	379	299	237	159	118	95	81	71	65	56	50	46	42	38	34	31	30	28	25	22	19	0
.10	0	0	0	0	1	6	37	117	248	372	416	391	330	218	150	113	92	79	70	60	53	47	43	39	35	32	30	29	26	22	19	0
.20	0	0	0	0	1	4	26	87	194	313	382	388	349	244	167	122	97	82	72	62	54	48	43	39	35	32	30	29	26	22	19	0
.30	0	0	0	0	0	0	3	19	64	151	259	341	372	316	223	156	117	94	80	67	58	50	45	41	36	33	31	29	26	23	19	0
.40	0	0	0	0	0	0	2	13	47	116	211	298	354	328	245	172	127	100	83	69	59	51	45	41	37	33	31	29	26	23	19	0
.50	0	0	0	0	0	0	1	9	34	89	170	255	341	303	225	161	120	96	76	64	54	47	42	38	34	31	30	27	24	19	0	
.75	0	0	0	0	0	0	0	1	4	14	41	89	152	270	305	268	207	155	118	87	70	57	48	44	39	35	32	30	27	24	19	0
1.0	0	0	0	0	0	0	0	0	2	7	22	98	212	295	285	237	181	120	88	67	53	46	42	38	34	31	28	25	19	2		
1.5	0	0	0	0	0	0	0	0	0	0	0	5	30	95	183	249	265	217	152	96	66	53	46	41	37	34	30	26	20	8		
2.0	0	0	0	0	0	0	0	0	0	0	0	0	3	18	59	125	221	245	182	105	69	54	47	42	38	32	28	22	16			
2.5	0	0	0	0	0	0	0	0	0	0	0	0	1	5	21	84	174	230	172	103	69	54	46	42	34	30	23	18				
3.0	0	0	0	0	0	0	0	0	0	0	0	0	0	1	13	56	157	217	163	101	68	53	46	37	31	25	18					
										IA/P = 0.50				* * * TC =0.5 HR * * *														IA/P = 0.50				
0.0	0	0	0	0	0	2	26	89	170	217	229	200	179	144	119	104	93	85	78	70	64	59	55	51	46	43	41	40	36	32	28	0
.10	0	0	0	0	0	1	18	65	135	190	216	205	170	137	115	101	91	83	74	67	61	56	52	47	44	42	40	36	32	28	0	
.20	0	0	0	0	0	1	12	47	106	162	198	203	178	145	121	105	94	85	76	68	61	57	52	48	44	42	40	37	32	28	0	
.30	0	0	0	0	0	0	1	8	34	82	135	177	194	168	139	117	102	92	80	71	63	58	54	49	45	43	41	37	33	28	0	
.40	0	0	0	0	0	0	0	6	25	63	111	155	189	174	146	122	106	94	82	73	64	58	54	50	45	43	41	37	33	28	0	
.50	0	0	0	0	0	0	0	4	18	48	90	133	184	177	152	128	110	97	84	74	65	59	55	50	45	43	41	38	33	28	0	
.75	0	0	0	0	0	0	0	1	7	22	47	80	142	169	164	144	124	108	91	79	68	61	56	51	47	44	42	38	34	28	0	
1.0	0	0	0	0	0	0	0	0	1	3	11	51	112	155	166	154	134	109	91	76	65	59	54	49	45	43	39	35	28	2		
1.5	0	0	0	0	0	0	0	0	0	0	0	2	16	50	97	136	154	145	121	95	75	64	58	54	49	45	41	37	29	10		
2.0	0	0	0	0	0	0	0	0	0	0	0	0	0	4	18	47	86	134	146	125	94	75	64	58	53	49	42	39	31	21		
2.5	0	0	0	0	0	0	0	0	0	0	0	0	0	0	3	11	44	95	140	127	97	77	65	58	54	45	41	33	26			
3.0	0	0	0	0	0	0	0	0	0	0	0	0	0	0	1	7	29	36	135	122	95	76	65	58	49	43	35	27				

RAINFALL TYPE = II   * * t_c = 0.5 HR * * *

HYDROGRAPH TIME (HOURS)

TRVL TIME (HR)	11.0	11.3	11.6	11.9	12.0	12.1	12.2	12.3	12.4	12.5	12.6	12.7	12.8	13.0	13.2	13.4	13.6	13.8	14.0	14.3	14.6	15.0	15.5	16.0	16.5	17.0	17.5	18.0	19.0	20.0	22.0	26.0
IA/P = 0.10														* * * TC =1.0 HR * * *														IA/P = 0.10				
0.0	11	15	20	29	35	47	72	112	168	231	289	329	357	313	239	175	133	103	83	63	50	40	33	29	26	23	21	20	17	15	12	0
.10	10	13	17	24	27	33	42	62	95	144	202	260	306	340	293	222	165	126	98	72	56	43	35	30	27	24	22	20	18	15	12	0
.20	10	13	17	23	26	30	38	54	82	123	176	232	281	332	303	238	179	136	105	76	59	45	35	30	27	24	22	20	18	16	12	1
.30	9	12	16	22	24	28	35	48	70	105	152	205	256	323	310	254	193	146	113	81	61	46	36	31	27	24	22	20	18	16	12	1
.40	8	11	14	19	21	23	27	32	42	61	91	132	181	276	318	294	237	181	138	95	70	51	39	32	28	25	23	21	18	16	12	1
.50	8	10	13	18	20	22	25	30	38	53	78	114	159	253	311	300	251	195	149	102	74	53	40	33	29	25	23	21	18	16	12	1
.75	7	8	11	14	16	17	19	21	25	30	38	53	76	146	228	284	293	256	208	143	99	66	46	36	31	27	24	22	19	17	13	2
1.0	5	7	8	11	12	13	14	16	17	19	22	25	31	57	111	188	256	286	272	208	144	90	56	41	33	29	26	23	20	17	13	4
1.5	4	5	6	8	8	9	10	11	12	13	14	15	17	22	33	59	107	171	231	268	235	157	88	56	41	33	29	25	21	18	14	8
2.0	2	3	4	5	5	6	6	7	7	8	9	9	10	12	15	19	27	44	78	157	231	252	167	96	59	42	34	29	23	20	15	11
2.5	1	2	2	3	4	4	4	5	5	6	6	7	7	8	10	12	15	19	27	58	120	214	241	159	94	59	42	34	26	21	16	11
3.0	0	1	1	2	2	3	3	3	4	4	4	5	5	6	7	8	10	12	14	22	44	113	214	231	152	91	58	42	29	23	17	12
IA/P = 0.30														* * * TC =1.0 HR * * *														IA/P = 0.30				
0.0	0	0	0	0	1	4	16	42	83	137	195	243	271	292	227	178	143	117	98	79	66	55	47	42	38	34	31	30	27	23	19	0
.10	0	0	0	0	0	0	3	12	32	66	113	168	218	279	260	213	169	136	113	88	72	59	49	43	39	35	32	30	27	24	19	1
.20	0	0	0	0	0	0	2	9	24	52	93	143	193	271	271	225	180	145	119	92	75	60	50	44	39	35	32	30	27	24	19	1
.30	0	0	0	0	0	0	1	6	18	41	75	120	169	246	264	234	191	153	125	96	78	62	51	44	40	36	33	31	27	24	19	1
.40	0	0	0	0	0	0	0	1	4	14	32	61	100	190	251	259	222	181	146	109	86	67	53	46	41	37	33	31	28	25	19	2
.50	0	0	0	0	0	0	0	1	3	10	24	49	83	168	237	254	230	191	155	115	90	69	54	47	42	37	34	31	28	25	19	2
.75	0	0	0	0	0	0	0	0	0	1	4	12	25	76	150	213	239	228	198	149	112	82	61	50	44	39	35	32	29	26	20	4
1.0	0	0	0	0	0	0	0	0	0	0	0	1	2	15	51	113	182	226	234	197	150	104	72	56	47	42	38	34	30	27	20	7
1.5	0	0	0	0	0	0	0	0	0	0	0	0	0	0	4	18	51	104	162	220	210	158	102	71	56	47	42	37	31	28	22	13
2.0	0	0	0	0	0	0	0	0	0	0	0	0	0	0	0	1	5	20	49	121	187	209	152	100	70	55	47	41	34	29	23	17
2.5	0	0	0	0	0	0	0	0	0	0	0	0	0	0	0	0	0	2	7	32	87	171	199	146	98	69	54	46	37	31	24	18
3.0	0	0	0	0	0	0	0	0	0	0	0	0	0	0	0	0	0	0	0	2	13	62	158	192	151	103	73	56	41	34	26	18
IA/P = 0.50														* * * TC =1.0 HR * * *														IA/P = 0.50				
0.0	0	0	0	0	0	0	1	7	21	42	71	101	126	160	154	138	123	110	100	87	77	67	60	55	50	46	43	41	38	34	28	1
.10	0	0	0	0	0	0	0	1	5	15	33	58	87	134	156	149	134	120	108	93	82	71	62	57	52	47	44	42	38	34	28	1
.20	0	0	0	0	0	0	0	1	4	12	26	48	74	123	153	153	137	123	111	95	84	72	63	57	52	47	44	42	38	34	28	1
.30	0	0	0	0	0	0	0	0	3	9	20	38	62	111	143	150	140	127	114	98	86	73	63	58	53	48	45	42	39	35	28	1
.40	0	0	0	0	0	0	0	0	0	2	6	16	31	75	120	145	148	137	123	106	91	77	66	59	54	49	45	43	39	35	29	2
.50	0	0	0	0	0	0	0	0	0	1	5	12	25	64	109	139	146	139	127	108	94	79	67	60	55	50	46	43	39	36	29	3
.75	0	0	0	0	0	0	0	0	0	0	2	5	12	39	78	115	136	140	134	117	101	84	70	62	56	51	47	44	40	36	29	4
1.0	0	0	0	0	0	0	0	0	0	0	0	0	1	7	26	59	96	125	139	133	117	97	78	66	59	54	49	46	41	37	29	8
1.5	0	0	0	0	0	0	0	0	0	0	0	0	0	0	2	9	26	54	86	123	133	119	95	77	66	59	54	49	43	39	31	17
2.0	0	0	0	0	0	0	0	0	0	0	0	0	0	0	0	0	3	10	25	64	104	129	116	93	76	65	58	53	45	41	33	24
2.5	0	0	0	0	0	0	0	0	0	0	0	0	0	0	0	0	0	0	2	10	34	84	125	117	96	78	66	59	49	43	35	27
3.0	0	0	0	0	0	0	0	0	0	0	0	0	0	0	0	0	0	0	0	1	6	32	89	122	114	94	77	66	53	45	37	27

RAINFALL TYPE = II　　　　* * t_c = 1.0 HR * * *

FIGURE D-6. (CHART 3) Tabular hydrograph unit discharges (csm/in) for type II rainfall distribution (t_c = 1.0 hour). *(Courtesy of Soil Conservation Service, Technical Release 55.)*

TRVL TIME (HR)	11.0	11.3	11.6	11.9	12.0	12.1	12.2	12.3	12.4	12.5	12.6	12.7	12.8	13.0	13.2	13.4	13.6	13.8	14.0	14.3	14.6	15.0	15.5	16.0	16.5	17.0	17.5	18.0	19.0	20.0	22.0	26.0
IA/P = 0.10														* * * TC =1.25 HR * * *														IA/P = 0.10				
0.0	10	13	18	25	29	38	54	81	118	163	213	256	284	311	266	212	163	129	104	78	61	47	37	31	27	24	22	20	18	16	12	1
.10	10	13	17	23	27	34	47	69	102	143	189	234	267	297	274	226	175	138	111	82	64	48	38	31	27	24	22	20	18	16	12	1
.20	9	11	15	20	22	26	31	42	60	88	124	168	212	280	292	261	212	166	131	95	72	53	40	33	28	25	23	21	18	16	12	1
.30	8	11	14	19	21	24	29	38	53	76	108	148	190	263	288	268	224	177	140	101	76	55	41	34	29	25	23	21	18	16	12	2
.40	8	10	13	18	20	23	27	34	46	66	94	130	170	245	282	273	235	188	149	107	80	58	42	34	29	26	23	21	19	16	12	2
.50	7	9	12	16	17	19	22	25	31	41	58	82	114	190	256	279	262	222	178	127	93	65	46	36	31	27	24	22	19	17	13	2
.75	6	8	10	14	15	17	19	21	25	31	41	56	78	139	207	254	265	245	208	152	110	75	51	39	32	28	25	22	19	17	13	3
1.0	5	6	8	10	11	13	14	15	17	19	22	26	33	60	109	173	230	261	255	208	153	100	64	46	36	30	26	24	20	18	13	5
1.5	3	4	5	7	7	8	9	9	10	11	12	13	15	19	27	45	79	130	186	247	239	180	108	68	48	37	31	27	22	19	14	10
2.0	2	3	4	5	6	6	7	7	8	8	9	10	11	13	16	22	35	59	98	171	236	236	156	95	62	44	35	30	23	20	15	11
2.5	1	2	2	3	4	4	4	5	5	5	6	6	7	8	10	12	14	19	28	58	114	197	226	163	102	65	46	36	26	21	16	11
3.0	0	1	1	2	2	2	2	3	3	3	4	4	4	5	6	7	9	10	13	19	35	88	184	218	169	109	70	49	31	24	18	12
IA/P = 0.30														* * * TC =1.25 HR * * *														IA/P = 0.30				
0.0	0	0	0	0	0	2	9	25	50	86	130	174	208	253	235	201	164	136	115	92	76	61	51	44	39	35	32	30	27	24	19	1
.10	0	0	0	0	0	0	1	6	19	40	71	110	153	217	247	227	191	157	131	103	84	66	53	46	41	36	33	31	28	24	19	2
.20	0	0	0	0	0	0	1	4	14	31	58	93	133	202	239	231	199	165	138	108	87	68	55	47	41	37	33	31	28	25	19	2
.30	0	0	0	0	0	0	0	1	3	10	24	46	77	152	210	236	222	190	158	122	97	74	58	49	43	38	34	32	28	25	20	3
.40	0	0	0	0	0	0	0	0	2	8	19	37	64	134	196	232	225	198	166	127	101	77	59	50	43	38	35	32	28	25	20	3
.50	0	0	0	0	0	0	0	0	0	2	6	14	30	82	151	206	228	217	189	146	113	85	64	52	45	40	36	33	29	26	20	5
.75	0	0	0	0	0	0	0	0	0	1	2	7	15	49	105	164	205	218	205	166	129	95	69	55	47	41	37	33	29	26	20	6
1.0	0	0	0	0	0	0	0	0	0	0	0	0	1	9	32	77	134	185	214	203	166	120	83	63	52	45	39	35	30	27	21	10
1.5	0	0	0	0	0	0	0	0	0	0	0	0	0	0	2	11	33	72	121	184	203	171	117	82	62	51	44	39	32	29	22	15
2.0	0	0	0	0	0	0	0	0	0	0	0	0	0	0	0	0	1	7	21	67	132	194	174	123	86	64	52	45	35	31	24	18
2.5	0	0	0	0	0	0	0	0	0	0	0	0	0	0	0	0	0	0	2	13	46	121	187	166	119	84	63	52	39	32	25	18
3.0	0	0	0	0	0	0	0	0	0	0	0	0	0	0	0	0	0	0	0	1	8	44	129	180	160	116	83	63	44	35	27	18
IA/P = 0.50														* * * TC =1.25 HR * * *														IA/P = 0.50				
0.0	0	0	0	0	0	0	1	5	13	26	44	68	91	125	142	142	128	117	107	94	83	72	63	57	52	47	44	42	38	34	28	2
.10	0	0	0	0	0	0	0	0	3	10	20	36	57	100	129	140	136	125	114	100	88	76	65	59	54	49	45	43	39	35	29	3
.20	0	0	0	0	0	0	0	0	2	7	16	30	48	90	122	139	139	127	117	102	90	77	66	60	54	49	45	43	39	35	29	3
.30	0	0	0	0	0	0	0	0	0	2	5	12	24	59	98	126	137	134	125	109	96	82	69	61	56	51	46	44	40.	36	29	4
.40	0	0	0	0	0	0	0	0	0	1	4	10	19	51	89	119	134	136	127	112	98	83	70	62	56	51	47	44	40	36	29	5
.50	0	0	0	0	0	0	0	0	0	1	3	7	15	43	79	112	131	135	129	114	100	35	71	63	57	52	47	44	40	36	29	6
.75	0	0	0	0	0	0	0	0	0	0	0	1	3	15	39	71	102	123	130	125	112	94	78	67	60	54	49	46	41	37	29	9
1.0	0	0	0	0	0	0	0	0	0	0	0	0	1	4	17	40	71	101	121	129	121	103	84	71	62	56	51	47	42	38	30	13
1.5	0	0	0	0	0	0	0	0	0	0	0	0	0	0	0	3	10	26	51	92	119	125	105	86	72	63	57	52	44	40	32	23
2.0	0	0	0	0	0	0	0	0	0	0	0	0	0	0	0	0	1	3	11	35	72	112	122	103	85	71	63	56	47	42	34	26
2.5	0	0	0	0	0	0	0	0	0	0	0	0	0	0	0	0	0	0	1	7	24	66	111	119	101	83	71	62	51	44	36	27
3.0	0	0	0	0	0	0	0	0	0	0	0	0	0	0	0	0	0	0	0	1	4	23	71	110	116	99	82	70	55	46	37	27

RAINFALL TYPE = II * * t_c = 1.25 HR * * *

FIGURE D-6. (CHART 4) Tabular hydrograph unit discharges (csm/in) for type II rainfall distribution (t_c = 1.25 hours). *(Courtesy of Soil Conservation Service, Technical Release 55.)*

HYDROGRAPH TIME (HOURS)

TRVL TIME (HR)	11.0	11.3	11.6	11.9	12.0	12.1	12.2	12.3	12.4	12.5	12.6	12.7	12.8	13.0	13.2	13.4	13.6	13.8	14.0	14.3	14.6	15.0	15.5	16.0	16.5	17.0	17.5	18.0	19.0	20.0	22.0	26.0
IA/P = 0.10														* * * TC =1.5 HR * * *														IA/P = 0.10				
0.0	9	11	15	21	25	31	41	58	82	112	147	184	216	255	275	236	198	159	129	98	76	57	43	35	30	25	23	21	18	16	12	1
.10	8	10	13	18	20	23	28	37	51	72	98	131	166	226	265	254	226	187	151	113	86	63	46	37	31	26	23	21	19	16	13	2
.20	8	10	13	17	19	22	26	33	45	63	87	116	149	212	259	259	233	197	160	119	90	66	48	38	32	27	24	22	19	16	13	2
.30	7	9	12	16	18	21	24	30	40	55	76	103	134	197	244	255	238	206	169	125	95	68	49	38	32	27	24	22	19	17	13	2
.40	7	8	11	14	15	17	19	23	28	36	49	67	91	151	208	247	252	230	196	146	109	77	54	41	34	29	25	22	19	17	13	3
.50	6	8	10	13	15	16	18	21	26	33	43	59	80	136	194	238	249	235	204	154	115	81	56	42	34	29	25	23	20	17	13	3
.75	5	7	8	11	12	13	14	16	18	21	25	32	42	76	125	179	222	240	233	193	148	102	67	48	38	32	27	24	20	18	13	5
1.0	4	5	7	8	9	10	11	12	13	14	16	18	22	34	59	101	152	201	236	230	193	135	86	59	44	35	30	26	21	18	14	7
1.5	3	4	5	6	6	7	8	8	9	10	11	12	13	16	22	34	58	95	141	203	226	197	131	84	58	43	35	29	23	20	15	10
2.0	1	2	3	4	4	5	5	6	6	7	7	8	9	10	12	16	22	34	56	110	172	218	187	126	82	57	43	34	25	21	16	11
2.5	1	1	2	2	3	3	3	4	4	4	5	5	6	7	8	9	11	14	18	34	69	141	210	190	133	87	60	44	30	23	17	12
3.0	0	0	1	1	2	2	2	2	3	3	3	3	4	5	5	6	8	9	11	16	27	66	149	204	181	128	85	58	35	25	18	12
IA/P = 0.30														* * * TC =1.5 HR * * *														IA/P = 0.30				
0.0	0	0	0	0	0	1	6	15	31	53	80	112	144	193	225	208	186	157	134	108	89	70	56	48	42	37	34	31	28	25	20	2
.10	0	0	0	0	0	0	1	4	12	25	43	68	97	157	198	219	203	178	151	120	98	77	60	50	44	38	35	32	28	25	20	3
.20	0	0	0	0	0	0	0	1	3	9	19	35	57	114	168	201	213	196	171	135	108	84	64	53	46	40	36	33	29	26	20	4
.30	0	0	0	0	0	0	0	1	2	7	15	29	48	100	155	193	210	200	177	140	113	87	66	54	46	41	36	33	29	26	20	5
.40	0	0	0	0	0	0	0	0	2	5	12	23	39	87	141	184	207	202	182	146	117	89	68	55	47	41	36	33	29	26	20	5
.50	0	0	0	0	0	0	0	0	0	1	4	9	18	51	101	153	190	205	197	164	131	99	73	58	49	43	38	34	30	26	20	7
.75	0	0	0	0	0	0	0	0	0	0	2	4	9	30	68	116	160	189	197	179	147	110	80	62	52	45	39	35	30	27	21	8
1.0	0	0	0	0	0	0	0	0	0	0	0	0	1	5	20	49	92	138	175	195	178	137	97	72	57	48	42	37	31	28	21	12
1.5	0	0	0	0	0	0	0	0	0	0	0	0	0	0	1	7	21	47	85	145	187	178	133	95	71	57	48	42	34	29	23	16
2.0	0	0	0	0	0	0	0	0	0	0	0	0	0	0	0	0	1	4	13	45	97	162	180	138	99	74	58	49	38	32	25	18
2.5	0	0	0	0	0	0	0	0	0	0	0	0	0	0	0	0	0	0	1	8	31	89	161	174	133	97	72	58	42	34	26	18
3.0	0	0	0	0	0	0	0	0	0	0	0	0	0	0	0	0	0	0	0	1	5	29	98	160	169	129	95	71	48	37	28	19
IA/P = 0.50														* * * TC =1.5 HR * * *														IA/P = 0.50				
0.0	0	0	0	0	0	0	0	3	8	16	27	42	59	92	116	128	130	121	112	100	90	78	67	60	55	50	46	43	39	35	29	4
.10	0	0	0	0	0	0	0	2	6	12	22	35	51	84	110	125	128	123	114	102	91	79	68	61	55	50	46	43	39	35	29	4
.20	0	0	0	0	0	0	0	0	1	4	10	18	29	60	91	114	126	128	120	108	97	83	71	63	57	52	47	44	40	36	29	5
.30	0	0	0	0	0	0	0	0	1	3	8	14	24	52	83	108	123	126	122	110	98	85	72	63	57	52	48	44	40	36	29	6
.40	0	0	0	0	0	0	0	0	0	1	2	6	12	31	60	90	112	124	126	116	104	90	75	66	59	54	49	45	41	37	29	8
.50	0	0	0	0	0	0	0	0	0	0	2	4	9	26	53	83	106	121	125	118	106	91	77	67	60	54	49	46	41	37	29	8
.75	0	0	0	0	0	0	0	0	0	0	1	2	5	16	36	62	88	108	119	122	112	97	81	69	62	56	51	47	42	38	30	11
1.0	0	0	0	0	0	0	0	0	0	0	0	0	0	3	10	26	49	75	98	118	121	108	90	76	66	59	54	49	43	39	31	16
1.5	0	0	0	0	0	0	0	0	0	0	0	0	0	0	1	3	11	25	45	80	107	118	106	89	75	65	59	53	45	41	32	23
2.0	0	0	0	0	0	0	0	0	0	0	0	0	0	0	0	0	1	4	11	32	63	100	115	104	87	74	65	58	48	42	34	26
2.5	0	0	0	0	0	0	0	0	0	0	0	0	0	0	0	0	0	0	1	4	16	48	94	113	105	89	76	66	53	45	36	27
3.0	0	0	0	0	0	0	0	0	0	0	0	0	0	0	0	0	0	0	0	0	3	15	54	96	111	103	88	75	58	48	38	28

RAINFALL TYPE = II * * t_c = 1.5 HR * * *

FIGURE D-6. (CHART 5) Tabular hydrograph unit discharges (csm/in) for type II rainfall distribution ($t_c = 1.5$ hours). *(Courtesy of Soil Conservation Service, Technical Release 55.)*

HYDROGRAPH TIME (HOURS)

TRVL TIME (HR)	11.0	11.3	11.6	11.9	12.0	12.1	12.2	12.3	12.4	12.5	12.6	12.7	12.8	13.0	13.2	13.4	13.6	13.8	14.0	14.3	14.6	15.0	15.5	16.0	16.5	17.0	17.5	18.0	19.0	20.0	22.0	26.0

*** TC = 2.0 HR ***

IA/P = 0.10

TRVL TIME																																
0.0	7	9	12	16	18	21	27	36	49	64	82	104	127	171	201	226	208	193	171	132	105	79	58	45	36	30	26	23	20	17	13	3
.10	6	8	10	14	15	17	25	33	43	57	74	94	139	179	204	218	205	188	150	118	88	63	48	38	32	27	24	20	17	13		
.20	6	8	10	13	14	16	20	23	29	39	51	66	84	128	169	198	213	207	192	157	123	91	65	49	39	33	28	24	20	17	13	4
.30	6	7	9	12	12	15	18	21	27	35	45	59	76	117	159	191	211	208	196	163	128	95	68	51	40	33	30	25	20	18	13	4
.40	5	6	8	11	11	13	17	20	24	31	41	53	87	128	167	197	209	205	180	145	106	75	55	45	36	30	26	23	21	18	14	5
.50	5	6	7	10	10	13	16	18	22	28	37	48	78	118	158	190	208	204	185	151	111	77	57	44	36	32	27	24	21	18	14	5
.75	4	6	6	9	9	11	13	15	18	22	27	35	58	91	129	164	191	202	187	167	125	87	63	48	38	32	26	24	21	18	14	8
1.0	4	4	6	7	8	10	11	12	14	18	28	46	74	110	147	178	201	193	156	108	76	56	43	35	30	23	19	8				

*** TC = 2.0 HR ***

IA/P = 0.30

TRVL TIME																																
0.0	3	3	3	5	5	5	6	6	7	8	8	9	10	12	16	23	36	57	86	137	178	195	160	113	79	58	45	36	26	21	16	11
.10	2	2	2	3	3	4	4	5	5	5	6	6	7	10	16	19	35	67	112	169	190	154	110	78	57	44	39	30	23	16	11	
.20	1	1	2	2	3	3	3	3	3	4	4	4	5	7	8	16	28	52	105	152	185	170	149	107	76	56	38	35	26	18	12	
.30	0	0	1	1	1	1	2	2	2	2	2	3	3	4	6	12	18	41	74	110	161	180	152	108	80	45	30	19	12			

*** TC = 2.0 HR ***

IA/P = 0.50

TRVL TIME																																
0.0	0	0	1	1	1	1	4	8	11	19	43	77	113	163	173	140	114	85	67	55	47	41	37	30	27	21	21	17				
.10	0	0	0	0	3	5	6	13	37	68	104	171	165	144	111	87	69	56	46	42	34	30	27	22	18							
.20	0	0	0	0	2	4	11	21	40	62	104	152	160	132	102	77	62	55	47	41	35	30	28	22	19							
.30	0	0	0	0	1	3	7	14	23	46	86	122	150	136	111	84	71	58	49	43	37	31	29	23	19							

*** tc = 2.0 HR ***

RAINFALL TYPE = II

FIGURE D-6. (CHART 6) Tabular hydrograph unit discharges (csm/in) for type II rainfall distribution ($t_c = 2.0$ hours). *(Courtesy of Soil Conservation Service, Technical Release 55.)*

COMPUTER SOFTWARE APPLICATIONS FOR STORMWATER MANAGEMENT (SELECTED LIST)

Software specifically designed for use in stormwater management is available from a number of vendors, including both private companies and public agencies. All vendors can be accessed on the World Wide Web. The representative list of software that follows is not intended to imply any rating of the software packages. A more comprehensive list can be accessed on-line at www.engsoftwarecenter.com.

Software	*Vendor*
Watershed Modeling	
HEC-1	U.S. Corps of Engineers
TR-20	Natural resources Conservation Service
WinTR-55	Natural resources Conservation Service
HydroCAD	HydroCAD Software Solutions
Hydorflow Hydrograph	Interlisolve
PondPak	Haestad Methods
WMS	ems-i
Stream Modeling	
HEC-RAS	U.S. Corps of Engineers
FlowMaster	Haestad Methods
WSPRO	Boss International

Storm Sewer Modeling

Hrdraflow Storm Sewers	Intelisolve
StormCAD	Haestad Methods

Culvert Analysis

CulvertMaster	Haestad Methods
CAP	U.S. Geological Survey

Symbols

The following symbols representing mathematical quantities are defined as they are used in this text. Units are given in the English system followed by metric units in parentheses. Parameters used in the SCS Method are defined in English units only.

a = cross-sectional area, ft^2 (m^2)

A = drainage area, acres (m^2), used in Rational Method

        = area over which pressure acts, ft^2 (m^2)

A_m = watershed drainage area, mi^2, used in NRCS Method

B = bottom width of a channel or culvert, ft (m)

c = entrance coefficient (dimensionless) used in orifice equation

        = runoff coefficient (dimensionless) used in Rational Method

        = discharge coefficient (dimensionless) used in weir equation

CN   = curve number (dimensionless) used in NRCS Method

d = distance, ft (m)

d_{50} = median stone size, ft (m), used for riprap

D = diameter of pipe, ft (m)

        = time duration of a unit rainfall, hours

D_c = critical depth, ft (m)

D_e = depth of water at the entrance to a channel, ft (m)

D_h = hydraulic depth, ft (m)

D_n = normal depth, ft (m)

D_r = depth of water in a reservoir used for flow entering a channel, ft (m)

D_0 = maximum pipe or culvert width, ft (m)

E = specific energy, ft (m)

ε = roughness, ft (m), used in connection with Bernoulli's equation (ε is the Greek letter *epsilon*)

f = friction factor (dimensionless) used in Bernoulli's equation

F = force, pounds (N)

g = acceleration of gravity, 32.2 ft/s^2 (9.81 m/s^2)

γ = specific weight of water, 62.4 lb/ft^3 (9.8×10^3 N/m^3) (γ is the Greek letter *gamma*)

h = vertical height of water surface above an arbitrary datum, ft (m)

h_e = entrance head loss, ft (m)

h_f = friction head loss, ft (m)

h_i = eddy head loss, ft (m)

h_l = total head loss, ft (m)

H = head above crest, ft (m), used in weir equation

HW = headwater depth, ft (m)

i = rainfall intensity, in/h (m/s), used in Rational Method

I = flow into a reservoir, cfs (m^3/s)

I_a = initial abstraction or losses, inches, used in NRCS Method

k_e = entrance loss coefficient (dimensionless) used with culverts

K = kinetic energy, ft-pounds (N-m)

L = length of pipe or culvert, ft (m)

    = length of flow, ft, used in NRCS Method overland travel time

    = effective crest length, ft (m), used in weir equation

    = length of a hydraulic jump, ft (m)

L' = measured crest length, ft (m), used with sharp crested weirs

L_a = apron length, ft (m)

m = mass, slugs (kg)

μ = absolute viscosity, lb-s/ft^2 (kg-s/m^2) (μ is the Greek letter *mu*)

n = roughness factor (dimensionless) used in Manning's equation

    = roughness coefficient (dimensionless) used in NRCS Method overland travel time

    = number of contractions (dimensionless) used with sharp crested weirs

υ = kinematic viscosity, ft^2/s (m^2/s) (υ is the Greek letter *nu*)

= viscosity of water, 1×10^{-5} ft^2/s (9.29×10^{-7} m^2/s) (υ is the Greek letter *nu*)

N_R = Reynold's number (dimensionless)

O = outflow from a reservoir, cfs (m^3/s)

p = water pressure, pounds/in^2 (N/m^2)

= wetted perimeter, ft (m)

P = precipitation, in (m)

= height of crest, ft (m), used with sharp crested weirs

P_2 = precipitation for 2-year, 24-hour storm, inches, used in NRCS Method

q_p = peak runoff, cfs, used in NRCS Method (Note: cfs is abbreviation for ft^3/s)

q_t = unit discharge at time *t*, csm/in, used in NRCS Method (Note: csm is abbreviation for cfs/mi^2)

q_u = unit peak discharge, csm/in, used in NRCS Method (Note: csm is abbreviation for cfs/mi^2)

Q = quantity or rate of flow of water, cfs (m^3/s) (Note: cfs is abbreviation for ft^3/s)

= runoff, inches, used in NRCS Method

Q_p = peak runoff, cfs (m^3/s), used in Rational Method (Note: cfs is abbreviation for ft^3/s)

R = hydraulic radius, ft (m)

ρ = density, slugs/ft^3 (kg/m^3) (ρ is the Greek letter *rho*)

s = slope of the energy grade line of a channel, ft/ft (m/m)

= slope of the ground for overland flow and shallow concentrated flow, ft/ft (m/m)

s_o = slope of the bottom of a channel, ft/ft (m/m)

s_w = slope of the water surface in a channel, ft/ft (m/m)

S = potential maximum retention after runoff begins, inches, used in NRCS Method

ΔS = change in reservoir storage during time Δt, ft^3 (m^3)

T = top width of a channel, ft (m)

τ = shear stress, lb/ft^2 (N/m^2) (τ is the Greek letter *tau*)

t_c = time of concentration, min

T_t = overland travel time, hours, used in NRCS Method

T_p = time to peak of a hydrograph, hours

TW = tailwater depth, ft (m)

TW' = vertical distance from invert of culvert (at outlet) to hydraulic grade line, ft (m)

Δt = incremental time period, min, for reservoir routing

θ = angle, degrees, made by a v-notch weir (θ is the Greek letter *theta*)

U = potential energy, ft-pounds (N-m)

v = average velocity of a cross section of water, ft/s (m/s)

V = volume, ft^3 (m^3)

W = weight, pounds (N)

     = apron width, ft (m)

z = vertical depth below a free water surface, ft (m)

UNIT CONVERSIONS

ENGLISH-METRIC CONVERSIONS

The following table states the equivalence between selected quantities expressed in both the English system and the metric system (SI). The following example illustrates how to use the table.

Example

To convert 25 cfs to m³/s, first locate the equivalence relation between cfs and m³/s

1 cfs = 0.02832 m³/s.

Then multiply 25 cfs by a fraction consisting of the two equal numbers above with cfs in the denominator:

$$25\,\text{cfs} \times \frac{0.02832\,\text{m}^3\!/\text{s}}{1\,\text{cfs}} = 0.71\,\text{m}^3\!/\text{s} \quad \text{(Answer)}$$

Length

1 inch = 0.02540 meter
1 foot = 0.3048 meter
1 mile = 1609 meters

Area

1 square inch = $6.452 \times 10^{-4}\,\text{m}^2$
1 square foot = $0.0929\,\text{m}^2$
1 acre = $4046.9\,\text{m}^2$
1 acre = 0.40469 hectare

Volume

1 cubic inch $= 1.64 \times 10^{-5}$ m^3
1 cubic foot $= 0.0283$ m^3

Velocity

1 foot/second $= 0.3048$ m/s

Force

1 pound $= 4.448$ N

Pressure

1 pound/square inch $= 6895$ N/m^2 (pascal)
1 pound/square foot $= 4.788$ N/m^2 (pascal)

Discharge

1 ft^3/s (cfs) $= 0.02832$ m^3/s
1 ft^3/s (cfs) $= 28.32$ l/s

MISCELLANEOUS UNIT CONVERSIONS

Area

1 acre $\quad= 43,560$ ft^2
1 s.m. $\quad= 640$ acres
1 hectare $= 10,000$ m^2

Volume

1 ft$^3 = 7.48$ gallons

Discharge

1 cfs $= 449$ GPM

GLOSSARY

The following terms are defined as they are used in this text.

Absolute Viscosity—A measure of the influence of the motion of one layer of a fluid upon another layer a short distance away.

Abstraction—*See* Initial Losses.

Adhesion—A property of water that allows it to cling to another body.

Apron—Concrete or riprap lining of the ground at the inlet or outlet of a storm sewer or culvert.

Attenuation—A reduction of rate of flow accomplished by a detention basin, which temporarily stores stormwater and then releases it slowly. Can also refer to the alteration in a hydrograph that occurs as water flows downstream.

Backwater Curve—A variation in the water surface profile of a channel or stream caused by an obstruction, such as a bridge crossing.

Base Flow—The constant low-level flow in streams due to subsurface feed.

Basin Divide—*See* Divide.

Berm—Earth embankment constructed on the downhill side of a detention basin to help contain the stored water.

Bernoulli Equation—Equation formulating the conservation of energy in hydraulics.

Broad-crested Weir—A commonly employed weir for dams and detention basins. The multistage weir, a variation of the broad-crested weir, is used to regulate discharge very precisely.

Buoyancy—The uplifting force exerted by water on a submerged solid object.

Capillarity—Property of liquids causing the liquid to rise up or depress down a thin tube.

Catch Basin—Stormwater inlet structure with sediment trap at bottom.

Catchment Area—Synonym for *drainage basin* or *watershed*.

Center of Pressure—Point on a submerged surface at which the resultant pressure force acts.

Cipoletti Weir—A trapezoidal variation of the sharp-crested weir devised to compensate for loss of flow quantity due to contractions at the vertical edges of a rectangular weir.

Civil Engineer—An engineer specializing in the design and construction of structures and public works.

Cleansing Velocity—The minimum velocity of water flow through a pipe to avoid deposits of silt and debris.

CMP—Corrugated metal pipe, used for storm sewers and culverts composed of aluminum or steel.

Cohesion—A property of water that allows it to resist a slight tensile stress.

Combination Drain—A storm sewer made of perforated pipe backfilled with gravel to intercept groundwater in addition to conveying stormwater.

Combined Sewer—An obsolete system once used to convey both sewage waste and stormwater through the same pipes. Combined sewers have been nearly eliminated in favor of separate storm and sanitary sewers.

Confluence—The intersection of two branches of a stream.

Contraction—A loss of energy that takes place as water flows past the vertical sides of a weir.

Control Section—Channel cross section used to start computation of a water surface profile.

CPP—Corrugated plastic pipe, used for storm sewers and culverts composed of high-density polyethylene.

Critical Depth—Depth of flow in an open channel for which specific energy is at minimum value.

Critical Slope—A slope that causes normal depth to coincide with critical depth.

Critical Velocity—The velocity of water at critical depth.

Crown—The top of the inside of a pipe or culvert.

Culvert—Conduit to convey a stream or runoff through an embankment.

Current Meter—Device used to measure the velocity of flowing water.

Density—A measure of mass per unit of volume.

Design Storm—The largest storm expected to occur in a given period of time specified in the design parameters for a hydraulic project.

Detention Basin—A facility designed to store stormwater temporarily during a rainfall event and then release the water at a slow rate.

Discharge—Flow of stormwater either overland or in a conduit; measured as a rate of flow in cfs (m³/s).

Discharge Coefficient—A dimensionless constant that accounts for a number of various hydraulic factors. Used in computing the rate of discharge over a rectangular weir.

Discharge Rating—A table important in detention basin design, which displays discharge through the outlet structure as a function of water level in the impoundment.

Divide—The line on a map that outlines the watershed. All rainfall landing outside the divide does not flow to the point of analysis. Also called *basin divide* or *watershed divide*.

Drainage Basin—Area of land over which rainfall flows by gravity to a single point called the point of analysis or point of concentration.

Emergency Spillway—A safety feature to prevent detention basins from overflowing, consisting of an additional outlet set higher than the other outlets. Water will enter only if the impoundment level rises higher than anticipated in the original design.

Energy Dissipater—A specially designed obstruction (block or blocks) placed at an outlet to create head loss in very high-velocity situations.

Energy Grade Line—Line graphed along a one-dimensional hydraulic system representing total energy or total head at every point along the system.

Energy Head—Energy of water per unit mass, expressed in length measure.

Entrance Coefficient—A dimensionless proportionality constant that accounts for the reduction of flow due to entrance head loss. Used in computing orifice flow.

Entrance Loss—A small but sudden drop of the energy grade line at the point where water enters a pipe from a larger body of water caused by loss of energy as the turbulent water enters the more restrictive pipe.

Erosion Control Mat—Mesh netting placed on the ground to protect the ground surface and anchor a vegetative cover.

Evapotranspiration—When rainfall strikes the ground, some of it is absorbed by plants and some evaporates immediately. This lost rainwater is not available for runoff.

First Flush—The first flow of runoff that picks up the loose dust that has coated the ground since the last rainfall. First flush is responsible for most transport of pollutants.

Flared End Section—A precast section of pipe made in a flared shape to use at the inlet or outfall end of a storm sewer or culvert in place of a headwall.

Flood Flow—A quick surge in stream flow due to runoff from a rainfall event.

Fluid—Material, such as gas or liquid, that flows under the slightest stress.

Freeboard—The vertical distance from the maximum or design level of water to the top of the structure containing or conveying the water.

Free Surface—The surface of water in a container or conduit exposed to the atmosphere.

Friction Loss—The constant drop in energy of water as it flows along the length of a pipe caused by contact with the inside surface of the pipe.

Froude Number—Parameter used to distinguish subcritical flow from supercritical flow.

Gabion—A rectangular wire mesh basket filled with rocks and placed on the ground as a protective lining similar to riprap.

Gauge Pressure—Water pressure in excess of atmospheric pressure.

Gradient—A measure of the slope of a channel or conduit expressed in ft/ft (m/m).

Groundwater—A large pool of underground water filling the voids between soil and rock particles.

Head—*See* Energy Head.

Headwall—Short retaining wall placed at the end of a storm sewer pipe or culvert (inlet or outlet).

Headwater Depth—Upstream water depth, which provides the potential energy to drive water through a culvert. It can therefore become a measure of the capacity of a given culvert.

Hydraulic Grade Line—A line drawn along a one-dimensional hydraulic system depicting potential energy expressed as position plus pressure head at all points along the system.

Hydraulic Jump—An abrupt transition of channel flow from supercritical to subcritical flow.

Hydraulic Path—Path traveled by the drop of rainwater landing at the most remote point in the drainage basin as it flows to the point of analysis.

Hydraulic Radius—Mathematical term defined by the ratio of cross-sectional area to wetted perimeter; a measure of the hydraulic efficiency of an open channel.

Hydraulics—The study of the mechanics of water and other fluids at rest and in motion.

Hydrograph—A graph of runoff quantity or discharge versus time at the point of analysis of a drainage basin.

Hydrologic Cycle—The natural pattern of water evaporation, condensation, precipitation, and flow.

Hydrology—The study of rainfall and the subsequent movement of rainwater including runoff.

Impervious—A ground cover condition in which no rainfall infiltrates into the ground. Typically, pavement and roofs are considered impervious.

Impoundment—Volume of water stored in a detention basin.

Infiltration—The absorption of rainwater by the ground.

Infiltration Basin—A detention basin that promotes recharge of stormwater to groundwater storage.

Inflow—Rate of flow of stormwater into a detention basin.

Initial Losses—The amount of rainfall in inches that infiltrates into the ground before any runoff begins. Also called initial abstraction.

Inlet—A component of a storm sewer system, it is a precast concrete structure placed in the ground with a cast iron grate on the top. Stormwater enters through the grate and into the storm sewer system.

Intensity-Duration-Frequency (IDF) Curve—Central to the Rational Method for determining peak runoff, IDF curves are developed by various government agencies based on data from Weather Bureau records. They show the relationship between rainfall intensity and duration for various return periods at given locations in the United States.

Invert—Lowest point on the cross section of a conduit, such as a pipe, channel, or culvert.

Kinematic Viscosity—Absolute viscosity divided by density; a measurement useful in hydraulic problems affected by density.

Lag—A parameter used in runoff analysis; the time separation between the centroid of the rainfall excess graph and the peak of the hydrograph. Related empirically to time of concentration.

Laminar Flow—Smooth, nonturbulent flow of water in a conduit, usually having low velocity.

Manometer—A device, similar to a piezometer, for measuring water pressure.

Metric System—A standard of measurement used by most of the world. The United States has not yet completed a changeover to metric units, so the civil engineer is faced with the need to be conversant with both metric and English systems of measurement. Also known as the International System of Units (SI).

Modified Rational Method—Procedure for calculating a synthetic runoff hydrograph using a modification of the Rational Method.

Normal Depth—Vertical distance from the invert of a channel or conduit to the free water surface when water is flowing without the influence of backwater.

Ogee Weir—A rectangular weir used commonly as a spillway; the smooth, rounded surface of the ogee weir is designed to reduce energy loss by contraction.

Open Channel Flow—Water that flows by gravity through a conduit with its surface exposed to the atmosphere.

Orifice—An opening in a container through which stored water may flow.

Overbank—Land immediately adjacent to each side of the channel of a stream. When flow in the stream exceeds the top of bank, it spills onto the overbank area.

Overland Flow—Stormwater runoff flowing over the ground surface in the form of sheet flow. Usually occurs at the beginning of the hydraulic path.

Outfall—The point of a storm sewer system where discharge leaves the system to enter the receiving body of water.

Outflow—Rate of flow of stored water out of a detention basin.

Outlet—Downstream end of a culvert.

Parshall Flume—Device used to measure flow in a channel.

Piezometer—A simple device for measuring water pressure, both static and dynamic.

Pipe—A hollow cylinder used in storm sewer systems to convey stormwater toward a receiving stream.

Pitot Tube—A simple device for measuring discharge in a pipe.

Planimeter—A device for measuring the area contained within a line making a closed figure on a map.

Point of Analysis—Any point on the ground or along a stream at which the quantity of runoff from the upstream catchment area is to be determined.

Point of Concentration—Synonym for point of analysis.

Precipitation—Water that lands on the ground from the sky as part of the hydrologic cycle.

Pressure—Force exerted by water against a unit area caused by the weight of the water above the point.

PVC—Polyvinyl chloride pipe; usually used for roof drains and sanitary sewer mains.

Rainfall Excess—The remainder of rainfall that reaches the point of analysis after initial losses and infiltration.

Rational Method—Procedure for calculating peak runoff based on theoretical reasoning.

RCP—Reinforced concrete pipe, used for storm sewers and culverts.

Receiving Water—A body of water into which a storm sewer system discharges. Usually consists of a stream, lake, or another storm sewer.

Recharge—Engineered effort to redirect some runoff into the ground where it would seep down to the groundwater.

Retention Basin—A detention basin that holds some water under normal non-flooding conditions. Serves as a sediment basin as well as a detention basin.

Return Period—The average number of years between two rainfall events that equal or exceed a given number of inches over a given duration.

Ridge—A land formation shaped so that runoff diverges as it flows downhill. The opposite of a swale. A drainage basin divide runs along a ridge.

Riprap—Stones placed on the ground used as a protective lining at inlets and outlets of storm sewers and culverts.

Roughness Factor—A dimensionless parameter used in Manning's equation describing the roughness of the surface of a channel or pipe.

Routing—In hydraulics, a mathematical procedure for computing an outflow hydrograph when the inflow hydrograph is known.

Runoff—The quantity of surface flow or discharge resulting from rainfall.

Runoff Coefficient—A dimensionless proportionality factor used in the Rational Method to account for infiltration and evapotranspiration.

Saddle—A topographic feature marking the transition between two ridges and two swales.

Sediment Basin—A depression in the ground lower than the invert of its outlet so that stormwater passing through will deposit its silt and sediment in the resulting ponded water.

NRCS Method—Procedure for calculating peak runoff or a synthetic runoff hydrograph based on an empirical method developed by the Soil Conservation Service, now called the Natural Resources Conservation Service.

Shallow Concentrated Flow—The form taken by stormwater runoff as it flows along the ground and converges into rivulets due to irregularities in the ground surface.

Sheet Flow—The form taken by stormwater as it flows along a smooth flat surface. Flow lines remain parallel and do not converge.

Siphon—Tube or pipe used to convey flow from an impoundment to a lower elevation by first rising above the impoundment level.

Slope—The ratio of the vertical drop to the length along a channel multiplied by 100 and expressed as a percent.

Specific Energy—A mathematical formulation equal to the flow depth in an open channel plus the velocity head. It is the total energy head above the channel bed.

Specific Weight—The weight of water per unit volume. The specific weight of water is taken as 62.4 lb/ft^3 (9.8×10^3 N/m^3).

Spillway—A structure for regulating the outflow from a reservoir or detention basin. Generally consists of a weir or orifice or both.

Spring Line—A line running the length of a pipe midway up the cross section of the pipe.

Stage—A term for elevation of water level in a stream or detention basin.

Standard Step Method—A method used to compute a backwater curve or profile.

Steady Flow—The rate of flow does not significantly vary with respect to time at any point along a stream.

Stilling Basin—A depression in the ground surface at an outlet designed to trap water and absorb excessive energy of discharge.

Storm Sewer—A pipe, usually underground, used to convey stormwater runoff.

Stormwater—Water that falls to earth as precipitation and then runs along the ground impelled by gravity.

Stormwater Management—All endeavors to control the quantity and quality of runoff in areas affected by land development.

Stream Rating Curve—A graph of discharge versus water surface elevation used to analyze stream flow.

Subbasin—A portion of a drainage basin functioning as a complete drainage basin when calculating runoff. If a drainage basin is not homogeneous, it should be partitioned into two or more subbasins. Also called *subarea.*

Subcritical—When flow depth is greater than critical depth, the flow is relatively tranquil and is called subcritical.

Subsurface Flow—Water that originates as precipitation and infiltrates a short distance into the ground, then runs laterally within the ground, eventually reaching a stream.

Supercritical—Flow depths below critical depth that flow rapidly.

Superposition—A principle used to add two or more hydrographs to obtain the resulting total hydrograph.

Surface Tension—Property of water that gives rise to cohesion and adhesion.

Swale—A land formation shaped so that runoff converges as it flows downhill. The opposite of a ridge. A basin divide never runs along a swale.

Tailwater Depth—Depth of water immediately downstream of a culvert or storm sewer outfall.

Time of Concentration—The amount of time needed for runoff to flow from the most remote point in the drainage basin to the point of analysis.

Turbulent Flow—Water flowing at a great enough velocity to develop eddies and cross currents. Turbulent flow results in more friction loss.

Uniform Flow—Flow of water in a conduit with constant shape and slope.

Unit Hydrograph—A generalized hydrograph resulting from a rainfall excess of one unit (1 inch or 1 cm).

Unsteady Flow—There is a change in the rate of water flow at any point along a stream.

Venturi Meter—Device used for the direct measurement of water flow or discharge in pipes.

Viscosity—The ability of fluid molecules to flow past each other.

Water Hammer—The extreme variation in pressure within a pipe caused by an abrupt stoppage in flow.

Watershed—Synonym for *drainage basin.*

Weir—A structure, usually horizontal, placed in a stream or pond over which water flows.

Wet Basin—A detention basin constructed to have a permanent pond at its bottom. Also called a *retention basin* or *sediment basin*, it is especially effective at trapping pollutants.

Wetted Perimeter—The distance along the cross section of a channel or conduit where the surface is in contact with flowing water.

Wingwall—Retaining wall placed at each end of a culvert to stabilize the embankment slope and help direct the flow.

INDEX